Tava vā mama vā sadānusaraṇāt
namanān mananāt prasanna-cittaḥ
bhagavan vāñchitam akhilaṃ datvā
kiṃ te bhūyaḥ priyam iti hasati

Your Lord or mine, it does not matter
With a quiet mind, meditate with humility
The Lord, pleased, gives what you seek
and happily offers more.

– T. Krishnamacharya, *Krishnamacharya Granthamala* series 1, *Yoganjalisaram śloka* 13

T0322608

नाडीशोधन
Nāḍī śodhana

Yoga in the Tradition of Sri K. Pattabhi Jois:
The Intermediate Series Practice Manual

Petri Räisänen

The practitioner, that keeps faith
and practices the limbs of *yoga*,
can achieve anything in the world.
He can even redo creation.
– Sri K. Pattabhi Jois, Yoga Mala

Photos by Alexander Berg

YOGAWORDS

The *Nāḍī-śodhana* team:
Petri Räisänen – text, translations, pictures, interviews
Alexander Berg – photos
Måns Broo – Sanskrit & *Devanāgarī*, *mantra* transliteration, editing, Guruji's interview
Eddie Stern – introduction to the Nāḍī system
Wambui Njuguna-Räisänen – translation and editing (Finnish-English)
Eija Tervonen – editorial staff (Finnish)
Lindsay Clipner – adjusting on page 74

Nāḍī-śodhana
Yoga in the Tradition of Sri K. Pattabhi Jois:
The Intermediate Series Practice Manual

First published in Finnish by Otava

This English edition first published by YogaWords,
an imprint of Pinter & Martin, 2017

ISBN 978-1-906756-50-5

British Library Cataloguing-in-Publication Data
A catalogue record for this book is available from the British Library.

Photos on pages 18, 152 by 155 Heli Sorjonen
Photo on page 14 Mikko Seppinen
Photo on page 16 from Petri Räisänen's archive
All other photos by Alexander Berg

Printed in the EU by Hussar Books

Pinter & Martin Ltd
6 Effra Parade
London SW2 1PS
United Kingdom

pinterandmartin.com

This book is dedicated to all
yoga teachers and students
who recognize the internal light of *yoga*,
bowing at the feet of their gurus,
and follow the traditional path of Yoga.

Petri Räisänen

Contents

Nāsti māyāsamaḥ pāśo nāsti yogāt paraṃ balam
nāsti jñānāt paro bandhur nāhaṃkārāt paro ripuḥ

There are no fetters like those of illusion (*māyā*)
no strength like that which comes from discipline (*yoga*)
there is no friend higher than knowledge (*jñāna*)
and no greater enemy than egoism (*ahaṃkāra*)

– Gherāṇḍa Saṃhitā (1/4)

Introduction to the system of nāḍīs

From 1927 to 1954, Śrī Pattabhi Jois undertook a voluminous amount of *yoga* practice and textual study with his teacher, Krishnamacharya, and at the Maharaja's Sanskrit College of Mysore, which gave him a perspective by which he could understand the inner meanings of *yoga*. According to Śrī Pattabhi Jois and the ancients, *yoga* was never meant merely as a physical conditioning practice, but as a methodical system of internal purification; by its practice, one could remove the physical and mental impediments that obscure self-knowledge. With this understanding, Śrī Pattabhi Jois set out to achieve this purification, applying the use of *āsana* (*yoga* postures), *prāṇāyāma* (breathing techniques), concentration and other yogic methods.

The method of *yoga* that he learned and practiced, *Aṣṭāṅga yoga*, is split up into three distinct categories: the primary, intermediate and advanced levels. In his first book, Petri Räisänen discussed the topic of the primary sequence, called Yoga-cikitsā, or, *yoga* therapy. These are the *āsanas* that are helpful for maintaining the health of the physical body. The second series of *āsanas*, called *Nāḍī-śodhana*, or *nāḍī* purification, is the subject of his second book. These *āsanas* purify the network of channels in the subtle body called *nāḍīs*.

Subtle body

What is the subtle body? The yogis have long considered the fact that beings are not made of one body only, but consist of several layers. The first is the physical body, which is made up of the food we eat and the water we drink. The second is called the subtle body, made up of our *prāṇa* (breath), *nāḍīs* (subtle tubes that carry *prāṇa*), cakras, mind, intellect and sense organs. It is called subtle because, although we can sense the aspects associated with it, we cannot see them in the same way we can see our hands, feet and other parts of the body. The third body is called the causal body and is the layer of bliss and happiness that surrounds our Inner-Self.

Once a student has learned the primary *āsanas*, and can perform them with a certain degree of capability, the intermediate series of *āsana* can be commenced, usually at the discretion of one's teacher. At this juncture, the student begins to focus on strengthening the nervous system. In the beginning, certain indications may appear. For example, one may have difficulty sleeping due to the deep back-bending *āsanas* which come at the beginning of the series. These *āsanas* have an excitable quality to them and, in turn, on the nervous system. This type of symptom usually settles down after a short while, however. If not, the student must look at the approach in which he or she is taking to the practice. If one practices in an excitable way, the result will mimic that. When working with the nervous system, it is best to have a calm and balanced approach to the practice, insuring that you can breathe in a steady manner. This will, no doubt, protect you and your subtle body, which is built largely upon, and developed largely on, the imprints that it receives through our behavior.

In the West, we have developed, through scientific endeavor, much knowledge about the sympathetic and parasympathetic nervous system, and the functions that the nerves, running from the brain stem through the spinal column and reaching the entire body – skin, muscles and bones, internal organs and sense organs, perform. We also have knowledge of the circulatory system, with its veins, arteries and blood vessels. The Yogis and *Āyurvedins* have considered these same systems, and have called all of these pathways '*nāḍīs*', which is a general term that means 'tube', 'flute' or 'channel', conveying the idea of a transport system. The general condition of the tubes must be kept in good condition for health, control of the sense organs and understanding of knowledge to be established in an individual.

Three groups of nāḍīs

Śrī Pattabhi Jois categorized *nāḍīs* into three different groups. The first is *dhamani*, which are blood vessels. The second is *śira*, which are the size of a human hair split six times, and act as the transmitter of messages from the sense organs to the brain – these basically do the job of carrying the electrical messages of the nervous system. Guruji explained that in the heart we have a 'message center'; all external information comes first to the heart and is then sent to the brain. The last group is known simply as *nāḍī*, from where *prāṇa* flows in the subtle body. The *yoga* practices work on all three levels of *nāḍīs*.

Just as our body develops knots in the muscles, our *nāḍīs* develop knots too. These knots prevent the free-flow of *prāṇa*, breath or energy, and lead us to experience several types of debilitations: sickness, apathy, doubt, carelessness, laziness, hedonism, delusion, lack of progress and inconsistency (in practice.)[1] They manifest themselves in the body through the following symptoms: pain, depression, trembling (or shaking) of the limbs, and disturbed inhalation and exhalation.[2] Two of the remedies suggested by Patañjali, the author of the *Yoga Sūtras*, the primary philosophical text regarding *Aṣṭāṅga yoga*, are telling in their objective. First, adhere to one chosen method; as Guruji quite often says, 'One Guru, one method, otherwise, one's mind will never be steady.' The second suggestion is to pause for a certain period after the exhalation of breath, which indicates that one must use breath, or *prāṇa*, to begin removing the obstructions from the *nāḍī* system. First, adopt the proper intention; second, purify the *nāḍīs*. All of this should be done, further, within the context of *yoga* practice, as the container of our inner work.

A student of *yoga* should slowly begin to understand how the physical body works in order to get maximum benefit from the primary *āsanas*; at least, a basic understanding of where each internal organ is located and the general function it fulfills. For example, we should know the location of our liver, spleen, heart and lungs and understand how the diaphragm works. In regards to the intermediate *āsanas*, at the very least, the three main *nāḍīs* that exist in the subtle body should be learned too. The *kanda-sthāna* and the main *nāḍīs* which are spoken of by Guruji in this book, are purified by the practice of the intermediate *āsanas*. The *prāṇa* that flows through the *nāḍīs* will then flow freely and unimpeded. What's more, the unimpeded *prāṇa* will then able to perform the variety of jobs that it must fulfill in order for us to remain healthy and clear individuals.

---

1. *Yoga-sūtra* 1.30.
2. *Yoga-sūtra* 1.31.

Nāḍīs rise from kanda

There are said to be 72,000 *nāḍīs*, and according to the *Yoga Yagnavalkya*, a book which Guruji held in high esteem, they all stem from a place called the *kanda-sthāna*. A *kanda* is a bulbous root or knot. Our individual karmas are actually fixed to the center of the *nāḍīs*, so we are, in a sense, knotted to the root of our birth, and our job in *yoga* is to begin to untie this knot, little by little; to untie our bondage to the idea of "I" and "mine," exposing our true nature of unbounded freedom. *Kanda* further means cloud. The *nāḍī* system exists in the subtle body, which cannot be seen by the human eye. It is therefore also cloud-like in nature. A cloud has substance, but is simultaneously vaporous and permeable; so too are our karmas, which are ephemeral, or transitory, in form, but whose effects can be felt – we cannot physically hold on to our karmas, but we can feel their results, in the same way that we cannot grasp a cloud, but can feel the rain, snow or shade it provides.

To locate the *kanda*, according to the *Yoga Yagnavalkya*, the following measurements can be considered. The measurements are made using the width of one's finger, called an aṅgula (one aṅgula is 16–21mm). Each person's physical body is approximately ninety-six *aṅgulas* in length (try measuring this against a wall). Two *aṅgulas* above the rectum and behind the genitals is a place called the *deha-madhya*, the center of a person's body. Nine *aṅgulas* above that is the *kanda-sthāna*, which is four *aṅgulas* in size and is the shape of an egg. In the Indian philosophical systems there is an alchemical maxim, "As in the Cosmic embryo, so in the individual embryo" – the Universe, and the individual, are both visualized as born from an embryo, or an egg. The Universe, in Hindu cosmology, was born from the Hiranyagarbha, the Golden Embryo. In the Western alchemical tradition it is said similarly, 'as above, so below'. As humans, not only are we born from an embryo, but the 'so below' egg can be seen in the *kanda*. Our actions that have led us to this particular birth are fixed to the *kanda*.

In the center of this egg shape is a place called the *nābhi* – or, navel – and this *nābhi* has twelve spokes, like a spider web of sorts. Within this web of spokes sits the *jīva*, the individual soul, which moves about within, according to the good and bad actions it has performed. *Prāṇa* moves with the *jīva* at all times. When *prāṇa* departs from the physical body at the end of our life span, the *jīva* departs with it, moving onto the next sheath, or body, that it will inhabit.

Three main nāḍīs

Stemming from the very center of the *kanda* is the most central of all *nāḍīs*, the *suṣumnā*, which is one of the principle rays of the sun. The sun, for yogis, signifies the light of all knowledge, of illumination. Resting to the left and the right of the *suṣumnā-nāḍī* are the *īḍā* and *piṅgalā-nāḍīs*. The *ida* and *piṅgalā-nāḍīs* are those which carry the moon and the sun within an individual; the properties of cooling and heating. The moon insures that the body does not become dry, as the moon moves the tides and all things juicy and liquidy. The sun insures that all undesirable elements are purified from us, as the sun has the power to burn. These two qualities circulate day and night, with the *prāṇa* first flowing through one *nāḍī* for a fixed period of time and then through the other. *Ida* is also said to be tamas, the property of heaviness and inertia, while *piṅgalā* is rajas, or the property of activity and the *prāṇa* flowing within has the quality of sattva, or purity. All the aspects of our existence which make up the pairs of opposites – hot and cold, pleasure and pain, honor and dishonor, and which thereby bind us with a sense of separation – are flowing through the *ida* and *piṅgalā*. When these pairs of opposites are completely harmonized, then *prāṇa* ceases to circulate in the two channels, and enters into the central channel, the *suṣumnā-nāḍī*, the pathway of singularity, which leads to the non-dual experience of reality. At this point, one does not need to breathe the air of duality, that is, through the nose and into the lungs, for the *prāṇa* has been absorbed into *suṣumnā* and one breathes only within the spinal column. Guruji calls this internal-breathing, and is the height of achievement for the yogi. When a yogi is able to breathe internally, he or she may extend his or her life span indefinitely, remaining in a state of complete absorption.

All the remaining 72,000 *nāḍīs* arise from the *kanda* as well, reaching from the tip of the toes to the top of the head, to the eyes, ears, nose and mouth, genitals, anus and every internal organ. When one grasps the thumb to the big toe in *Pādāṅguṣṭhāsana*, the *hastajihva-nāḍī* is stimulated; when one engages *mūla-bandha*, the *alambuṣa-nāḍī* which ends in the rectum, is purified; when one places the elbows in the belly for *Mayūrāsana*, the *viśvodara-nāḍī*, along with the entire *kanda*, is purified. Each *āsana* purifies and stimulates a different *nāḍī*, or set of *nāḍīs*, and each has its origins in the *kanda-sthāna*. If a student can manage to grasp the location of the main *nāḍīs*, and focus the breath within them while practicing, surely their *nāḍīs* and practice will give positive results.

Five important prāṇas

The next process that must be considered is the *prāṇa* that flows through the *nāḍīs*. For it is not just the *nāḍīs* that are important to yogis, but the *prāṇa* that flows through them that we want to develop and cultivate as well.

Prāṇa, according to Guruji, is breath. It can also be called the life-force of the universe, as this whole universe, indeed, breathes. However, in the individual, it manifests as the breath. *Prāṇa* is one, but is divided into different categories depending on the jobs it needs to perform. There are five major and five minor *prāṇas*, of which the five major will be considered here. These five (*pañca*) *prāṇas* are also called the *pañca-vāyus* – *vāyu* also means breath. Just as I am a son to my parents, a husband to my wife, a student to my teacher and a father to my daughter, *prāṇa* is called by a different name for each relative job. As the controlling energy, *prāṇa* resides in the head, and dictates how all the other *prāṇas* should move. Some say that *prāṇa* also performs this job from the heart. *Prāṇa* is responsible for our respiration, for with *prāṇa* comes the idea of nourishment and the breath being our primary source of nourishment. With the influx of any nourishment, one must also expect waste. The transformation of *prāṇa* into an energy that can expel waste gives us *apāna*, which is the waste-removing energy. *Apāna* is situated in the anus and is responsible for removing all waste that moves out of the body, such as the carbon dioxide carried by the exhalation of breath, feces, urine, semen and menstruation. It is also the force responsible for childbirth.

For nourishment to be made possible, assimilation must also exist. We must be able to assimilate not only food, but ideas and information as well. *Samāna*, which resides in the abdomen - near the *agnī*, or fire, that is constantly burning and is the source of our vitality and longevity- is responsible for assimilation. It carries assimilated food to each and every part of the body, and to each and every *nāḍī*.

Uḍāna resides in the chest, throat and head; some say *uḍāna* is in all the joints. If it remains in the chest and throat, *uḍāna* becomes responsible for respiration, as dictated by the chief *Prāṇa*; by remaining in every joint, it becomes responsible for the movements of the body.

Lastly comes *vyāna*, which has its seat in the heart. It is through *vyāna-vāyu* that all the messages transported throughout the entire body are distributed. The transmission of messages to the brain falls under the jurisdiction of *vyāna*. *Vyāna* is the pulsation that indicates the level of health, in the form of *vāta, pitta* and *kapha* (the three conditions of wind, fire and phlegm), which *āyurvedic* doctors examine while reading our pulse. Our breathing and lifestyle make an imprint upon the subtle body of our heart, which is reflected by *vyāna* through the whole body and nervous system. Clearly, our breath and lifestyle should make a positive imprint from the start, so that our hearts are balanced and calm, and this message of calm is sent to our entire system. From even this cursory examination, we can see that all of the functions that are ascribed to the nervous and digestive systems are under the control of the *pañca-vāyus*.

Nāḍīs – the doorways to Self-knowledge

The five *prāṇas* and the 72,000 *nāḍīs* have been described in various texts in many different ways. What is important for us is to have a general grasp of the concepts contained in them. As living beings, we depend on nourishment. We must also expect that waste will be produced with this essential nourishment and will need to be expelled. That which is not expelled should be assimilated and carried to each and every part our body, and then stored in the body as energy so that we may perform our daily tasks. Lastly, the messages that need to be sent throughout the body for movement, reflex action, pain perception and the like, should be carried out without obstruction. If each of these jobs is performed properly, then all of our *prāṇas* can be said to be in the proper place, performing their proper jobs, and being transported in vessels that are free from blockages. At this point, it can be said with certainty that we are on the road to health and balance.

Nāḍī-śodhana, the purification of the *nāḍīs*, is an important step in linking the physical aspects of *yoga* with the deeper, more internal aspects. The *nāḍī* system is the link between the physical body and the causal body. By clearing the subtle body from blockages, and balancing the five *prāṇas*, a doorway is opened by which one may begin the journey inward towards Self-knowledge. Our sense organs will become purified, and thus turning our gaze inward becomes possible, as we turn our vision from absorption in the outer world to absorption into our inner world. When this system is put into order, then clarity will be reflected in the mind and mental confusion will begin to dissipate. Hence, we should pay careful attention in our attempt to understand the *nāḍī* system as an integral part of our journey in the practice of *yoga*.

Eddie Stern
18.6.2008
New York City

Adapted from the forthcoming collection of essays on *Aṣṭāṅga* Yoga, entitled *One-percent Theory*

Translator's note

This English edition of *Nāḍī-śodhana* has been translated as faithfully as possible from the original Finnish edition. Shortly after the first edition was published in 2008 by Otava, Petri began translating it into English. I joined in the process after moving to Helsinki, Finland in 2010. This was done primarily to learn the *vinyāsas* and details of each *āsana* of the intermediate series as I was learning and practicing it. It also seemed like a natural and captivating way to start engaging with the Finnish language. I started by translating the charts, managing short words and phrases and found the repetition of these words and phrases to be beneficial for the memory. What followed was a slow and inelegant process where, by using the strengths of our respective native languages, Petri and I would swap the Finnish to English drafts back and forth, from which we would edit and further refine the text. We had already had practice with this kind of process, when we updated the English edition of his primary series book, which was published by YogaWords in 2013.

Petri has mentioned on several occasions that, in comparison to the primary series book, this book on the intermediate series documents a deeper and more direct account of his interactions with Guruji. In Petri's own words, he has stated that the essential value of this book is that, "It is all Guruji." A testament, perhaps, to the final few moments a student had with his Guru.

It is our sincere endeavour to have created an edition that is not only informative and instructional, but inspiring as well. One which maintains the essential tone of Petri's unique and lyrical Finnish voice.

Wambui Njuguna-Räisänen

Helsinki, Finland, July, 2017

Nāḍī-śodhana – Intermediate series
According to Śrī K. Pattabhi Jois, Guru of Aṣṭāṅga yoga

The God Shiva gave humankind 72,000 *yoga* poses, the same amount as there are *nāḍīs* or energy channels in the body. Of these, only a few poses – those that were considered the most important – were recorded in old scriptures (śāstra) such as the *Upaniṣads*. Over the course of his life, my guru T. Krishnamacharya learned approximately 3,000 poses, how they are performed and what their impacts are. The *Yoga Korunta*, the 'handbook' of *Aṣṭāṅga yoga* written by Ṛṣi Vamana at around the start of the Christian era, features almost 300 poses, sequenced in three different series, all of which affect the body in a different way. The first of them is *Yoga-cikitsā* or *yoga* therapy, which is designed to increase flexibility and strength and eliminate impurities that are the cause of illnesses. The intermediate series is *Nāḍī-śodhana*, which purifies and relaxes the physiological and energetic nervous system. The advanced series, *Sthira-bhāga* (*sthira* = steady, firm, complete; *bhāga* = graceful, prosperous), stands for strength and beauty and is divided into the A, B, C and D series, all of which intensify the impacts of *Yoga-cikitsā* and *Nāḍī-śodhana*, thus making both the body and mind strong, healthy, pliable and receptive. These *Aṣṭāṅga yoga* poses, their impacts and the *vinyāsa* krama (*krama* = method), as well as the philosophical implications and practicalities of *yoga*, I learned from T. Krishnamacharya during the years 1927–1953.

The *āsana* sequence in *Nāḍī-śodhana* (*nāḍī* = energy channel, *śodhana* = cleansing), or the intermediate series, purify the energy channels and the nervous system. Some of the poses are anyhow considered as a *Yoga-cikitsā* poses, as they has more therapy benefits than purification benefits (like *Pāśāsana* and *Krauñcāsana*). All the poses can be performed safely only after the body has been appropriately prepared through the primary series, or *Yoga-cikitsā*, which makes the body supple, strong and clean. According to the traditional method, mastery of each pose requires at least one thousand repetitions, which translates into four to five years of regular daily practice, including the days off (Saturdays, moondays, public holidays and ladies holidays).

Practice makes the body pliable and strong. Strength cannot be achieved without pliability and control of the bandhas. A body which is outwardly strong but lacks pliability is easily injured and fatigued.

The correct breathing technique, sound or *ujjayī* breathing, and application of the *vinyāsa* method in performing the poses warms up the blood and makes it rich in nutrients and oxygen. When warm, blood circulates easily throughout the body, thereby making the muscles flexible while healing illnesses and eliminating tensions. Poor circulation increases tension and illnesses and prevents the body from becoming pliable and strong.

The body has impurities (*duḥkha*), which cause blockages and illnesses. These impurities must be removed. The seven dhatus (plasma (*rasa*), blood (*rakta*), flesh or muscle tissue (*mansa*), fat (*meda*), bones (*asthi*), bone marrow (*majja*), and the sexual fluids (*śukra*: vīrya, male fluid or semen and *śoṇita*, female fluid or ova) of the body have to be purified in order to achieve the goals of *yoga*.

Yoga practice achieves purification on both the physical body, *sthula shatira* or *annamaya kosha* (made from the food we eat and drink) and subtle body, *sukshma sharira*, *linga sharira* or *pranamaya kosha* (related to the breath, mind and *prāṇa*), energy centres (*cakras*), mind or *manonmaya kosha* with five main senses and intelligence or *vijnamaya kosha*-layers.

All the poses in *Nāḍī-śodhana* has almost similar benefits. The poses are as many as the species in the world; *"Asanāni ca tavanti yāvanto jīvarāśayah"* (Dhyānabindu Upaniṣad 42). The benefits from the one position will effect for the all other positions. All the individual positions are connected to each other. When you learn how to perform one position, all the other positions will become easier. They all purify the body and mind and support each other in the purification process. Anyhow, some positions has still specific benefits (like in *Mayurāsana*).

The primary series begins the process of making the body pliable and purifying the nerves, and this process is taken deeper in the intermediate series. The *nāḍīs*, which are purified through the practice of *yoga āsanas* and a yogic (*sattvic*) lifestyle, breathing practices (*prāṇāyāma*), correct mind focus (*pratyāhāra*), concentration (*dhāraṇā*), meditation (*dhyāna*) and other practices, fall into three categories: 1. *Dhamini* (flute; it has a hole similar to that of a flute), is called also *Nara*, which means rope. *Dhamini* is the largest in size of all the *nāḍīs*. 2. *Nāḍī*, which is transporting the *prāṇa*, energy. 3. *Sira* (the size of a split hair, a very sensitive nerve).

When performed correctly, *yoga āsanas* purify and strengthen the *nāḍīs*, allowing for an unrestricted flow of *prāṇa* within the *nāḍīs*, which resides in a central place called *Kanda*, located on the pelvic floor. In contrast, incorrect performance of *yoga āsanas* can harm the sensitive *Sira nāḍī* system. One example of this includes *Śīrṣāsana* (headstand), where too much pressure can be placed on the crown of the head if the pose is held for several minutes without using the arms to lift the head off the floor. Excessive pressure on the crown of the head may prevent blood circulation in the area and block the *Sira nāḍīs*. If the student comes out of the pose too quickly, the release of pressure may be too rapid and result in mental problems. That is why it is important for students to learn poses from a qualified teacher.

The practice of *Aṣṭāṅga yoga* begins with the primary series, which traditionally is practiced six days a week at a maximum. Saturday (or Sunday) is a rest day and no practice is taken on the days of the full and new moon, as well as on national holidays and days following long travels. In addition, women should withdraw from practice during the first three days of menstruation, the first trimester of pregnancy and three months after labour. New poses are added to the series one by one as, and when, the student is ready. This means that the student must be able to perform the preceding pose with a calm breath and concentration.

When the student has progressed to *Setu-bandhāsana*, the last pose of the primary series, and mastered all the preceding poses, he or she can be introduced, under the guidance of a competent teacher, to the poses from the intermediate series, starting with the first pose, *Pasāsana*. Once the student has advanced half way through the series and has reached *Eka-*

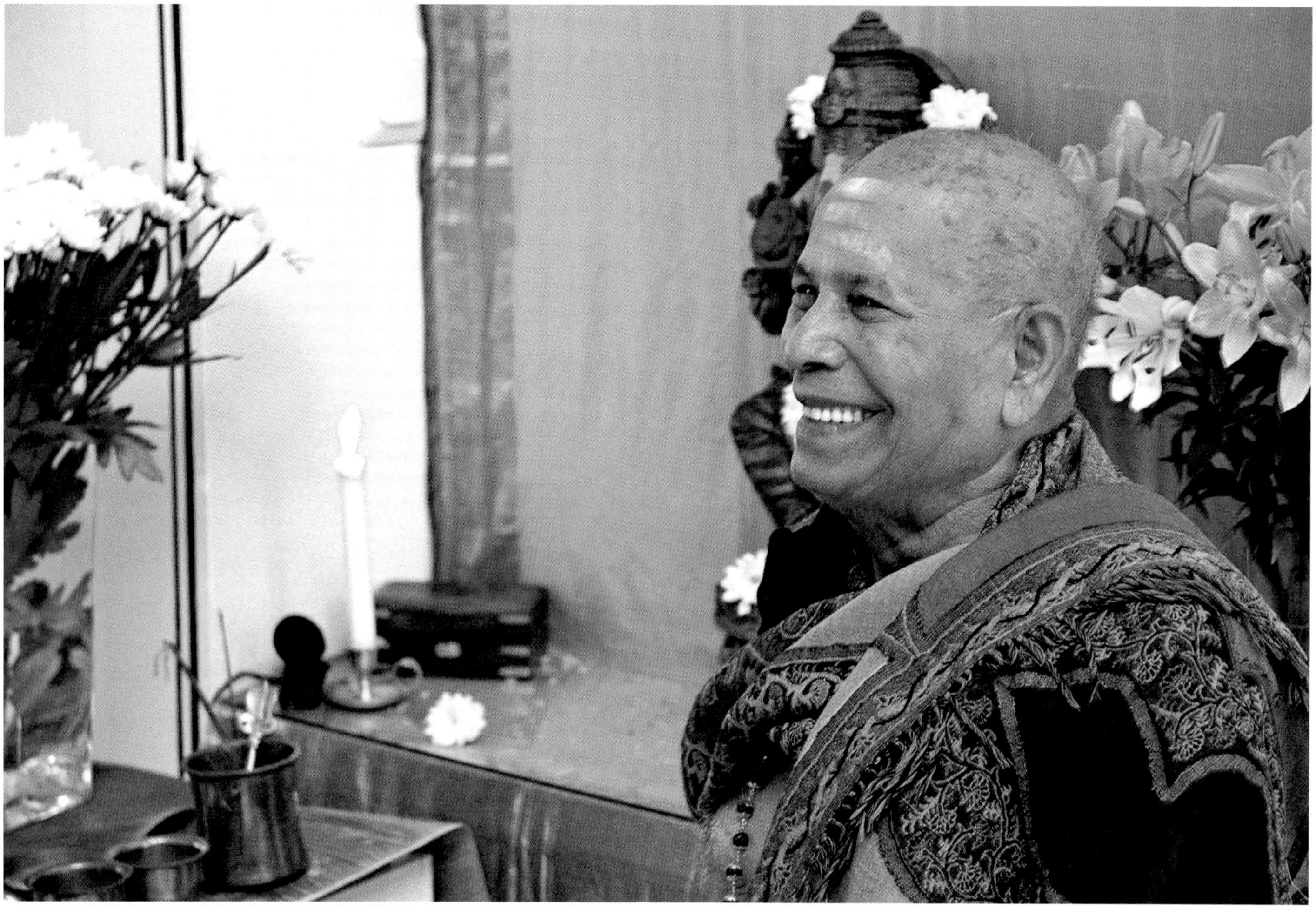

pāda-śīrṣāsana, he or she can 'split' the primary series. This means that from Sunday to Thursday, the student practices only the *Nāḍī-śodhana* sequence until *Eka-pāda-śīrṣāsana*, and on Friday, the last day before the rest day, he or she practices the full primary series. When the student has progressed systematically to the last pose of the intermediate series and mastered all the preceding poses, he or she can start to practice poses from the Advanced series or *Sthira-bhāga*, starting with the first pose, *Viśvāmitrāsana*.

The intermediate series requires that the student is ready for different poses much sooner than in the primary series, because there are fewer preceding poses that prepare the student for the next pose (i.e., poses from *Kapotāsana* to *Eka-pāda-śīrṣāsana*, halfway through the intermediate series). This makes the body and mind increasingly sensitive, stronger and more adept at handling physical and psychological changes, thus reducing the mind's desire to become attached to things.

You should always endeavor to practice under the guidance of a competent teacher. It is not advisable to learn poses from books, friends or teachers who lack the necessary understanding and experience of the traditional practice method of *Aṣṭāṅga yoga*. Only regular and patient practice delivers mental detachment from obstacles and impediments and brings about clarity that is otherwise beyond reach.

When the mind is quiet, the *āsana* is correct.

Śrī K. Pattabhi Jois
February 2007, Mysore, India

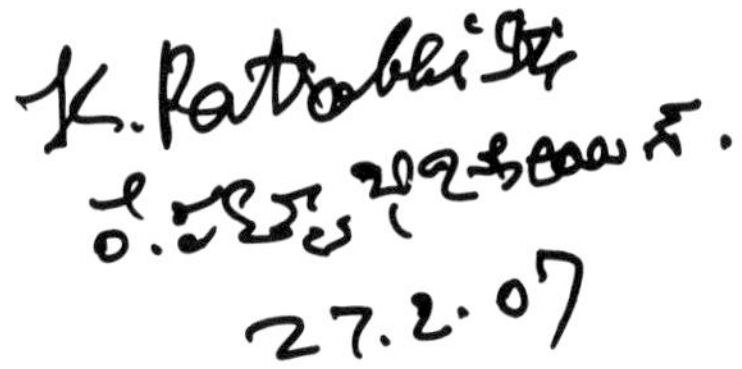

* There is a section about the moon days and its effects in Petri's first book: *Ashtanga: Yoga in the tradition of Śrī K. Pattabhi Jois*.

Foreword

Nāḍī-śodhana is a continuation of my first book *Aṣṭāṅga Yoga: Yoga in the Tradition of Śrī K. Pattabhi Jois*. This second book documents the practice of the intermediate series, known as *Nāḍī-śodhana*, as it is practiced and taught in Mysore, India by my Guru, Śrī K. Pattabhi Jois, R. Sharath Jois (Pattabhi's grandson) and Saraswathi Jois (Pattabhi's daughter and Sharath's mother). Nothing more, nothing less.

During my stay in Mysore in 2006 and 2007, I asked my 90-year-old guru permission to interview him for this book. In turn, he asked to see and review my first book, and wanted to know what my purpose was in writing a second. I explained my intentions and, as he considered my first book to be truthful and in line with the traditional method, he agreed to offer his words and thoughts to my second book. His decision was no doubt influenced by the fact that I have practiced *Aṣṭāṅga yoga* since 1989, and have been his devoted student since 1997, when I first traveled to Mysore to practice at his "old" shala in Lakshmipuram. Since then, I have spent time with him in India every year, save for one winter (1998/99), when my oldest child, Julian, was a baby. I have also participated in a number of his workshops in the West and was one of the principal coordinators of his family's visits to Helsinki in 2001 and 2006. It was in 2001, in Boulder, Colorado, when I realized Śrī Pattabhi Jois was my guru.

To conduct our interview, Guruji and I met in his small office in Mysore for eight days in both years (2006 and 2007) and discussed the *Nāḍī-śodhana* practice. We were occasionally joined by Sharath Jois, who deepened my understanding of our guru's wisdom by clarifying some translations and highlighting details about the postures. We went through the *vinyāsa* techniques for the intermediate series and discussed relevant philosophical issues. In order to preserve the authenticity of the information, I taped most of our discussions and transcribed them immediately after the interviews, while they were still fresh in my mind. This was necessary, not only because a face-to-face discussion involves a lot of facial expressions and hand gestures, but because I had also performed some poses on the Guruji's office floor, in between two tables and three chairs. I did this to illustrate and clarify exact details of the poses under Guruji's guidance, such as the angle of the feet or the correct placement of the hands in certain lifts.

Our meetings were very fascinating. Guruji was in a very open mood and wanted to make sure I truly understood everything he said. These meetings became more like private teachings, rather than an interview. He spoke deeply about yogic philosophy and in detail about the intermediate series *āsana* techniques and the benefits of these *āsanas*. He also gave translations of *āsana* names that I had never come across before.

The idea for this book originated from the need of thousands of *Aṣṭaṅga* practitioners, including myself, for a clear and comprehensive documentation of the intermediate series. Although a number of *Aṣṭāṅga* books are now available, none of them cover all the practical techniques, and physical and mental impacts of the intermediate series. This book comes as an important tool for students and teachers alike, who wish to consolidate their understanding of the intermediate series. It is written to honor and preserve the traditional method of *Aṣṭāṅga yoga*.

Over the years, the second (intermediate) series' *āsanas*, like in the primary series, have gone through small changes, which will surely hit the eye of the *aṣṭāṅgis* who started their practice with Guruji in the 70s and 80s and with Sharath in the 2010s. These few reforms have occurred in a few *vinyāsas*, *āsanas*, *dṛṣṭis* and number of breaths, and are the result of Guruji's research from over 70 years of teaching experience. They are designed to improve the benefits of the practice and support the student's progress. *Aṣṭāṅga yoga* is still evolving over time and with recurrent practice, which follows the guru's teaching; as it always has throughout history of *yoga*, and as it will continue to do so in the future. How I see it, *Aṣṭāṅga yoga* in its current stage has returned back to more essential roots. In contrast to the 70s and 80s (and earlier), 'extra' positions which started appearing in the series, for a number of reasons, have been cut out. What remains now is a more direct sequencing of *āsana*, without the fancy and oftentimes simply unnecessary 'ego-swelling' techniques, which can, not only be harmful to the practitioner's body and mind, but counterintuitive and detrimental to the spirit of the practice. I was thus relieved to hear from Guruji and Eddie Stern, who also discussed this topic with our guru, that the sequences of the *āsanas* are now complete, after years of refinement. They are now a graceful, benevolent expression of *Aṣṭāṅga yoga*.

In order to broaden our collective understanding of the history and lineage of *Aṣṭāṅga yoga*, I was pleased to be able to include in this book, interviews with Śrī Pattabhi Jois, Sharath Jois and Saraswathi Jois. What's more, I was able to document Śrī Pattabhi Jois's commentaries on the opening and closing mantras which we recite during in every practice.

In addition, I asked my friend Måns Broo, Professor of Comparative Religion and Indology, author and commentator of Patanjali's *Yoga-sūtras* (in Finnish) and Sanskrit language scholar, to collaborate on the Sanskrit language chapter. This chapter demonstrates the pronunciation of *āsana* names, how to chant the mantras and also increases one's basic understanding of the Sanskrit language. Guruji's interview, conducted in Helsinki in 2006 and published in the Finnish magazine *Ananda* (4/2006), was also primarily Måns' work, of which I completed with a few extra questions in Mysore the following year. Måns has also worked with the spellings and translations for the benefits of the *āsanas* and other Sanskrit terms.

Just before I delivered the manuscript to my Finnish publisher (Otava) in 2007, I had a discussion with Eddie Stern, my friend, one of my teachers and a faithful follower of Śrī Pattabhi Jois, at his *yoga shala* in New York. Eddie has contributed significantly to the book, with an introduction on the body's energy channels (*nāḍīs*) and the movement of *prāna* and its effects on the body, mind and energy flow, based on his discussions with Śrī Pattabhi Jois. This introduction highlights the most important *nāḍīs*, demonstrates how *nāḍīs* are cleansed through the *āsana* practice and explains how to fill these purified *nāḍīs* with prāna. This is one of the most important benefits of the *yoga* practice which, surprisingly, has rarely been discussed.

I have inserted between the chapters, collections of *mantras*, *ślokas* and *sūtras*, which have had a strong influence on me during my *yoga* path.

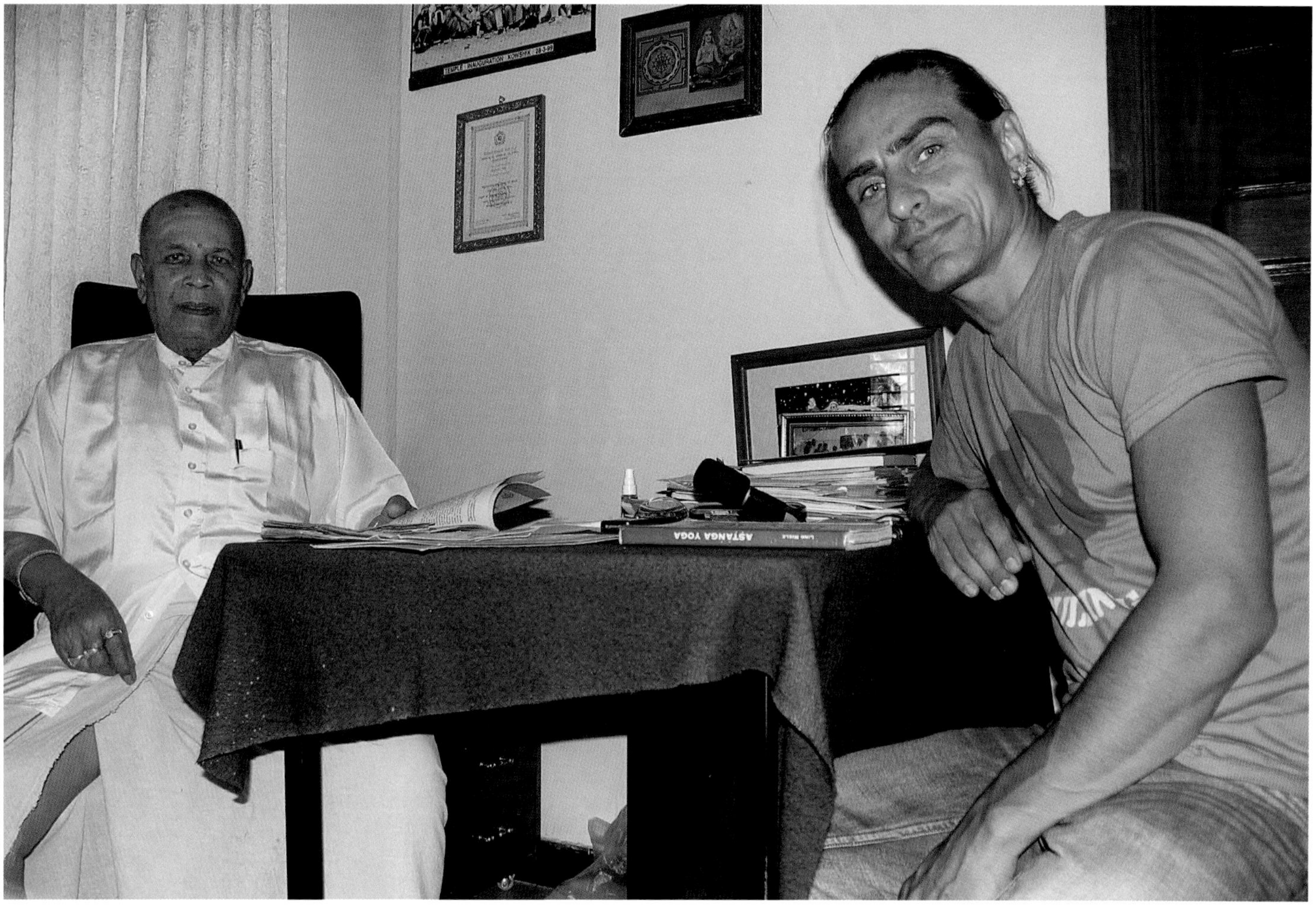

They have upheld my faith and determination for the practice for over two decades, and continue to do so. *Svādhyāya* – the study of self through practice, observation and yogic texts – is truly an essential part of the process.

This book uses the traditional *vinyāsa* counting method in the Sanskrit language (e.g., *ekam, dve, trīṇi* – one, two, three) as well as the Sanskrit names of postures, with an added English translation (e.g., *Utthita-trikoṇāsana*, triangle pose). Also mentioned in Sanskrit are *daśa dṛṣṭi* (ten gazing points) and *bandhas* (*mūla-bandha* – root lock and *uddīyana-bandha* – lower abdominal lock). It is recommended that the student study the Sanskrit names of the postures in order to facilitate communication with the teacher, as well as to internalize the idea and feeling of the *yoga* practice in more detail.

I remain deeply and sincerely grateful to Guruji for giving me the information needed to compile a book such as this. *Aṣṭāṅga yoga* was his passion, his work and his tradition, which he taught with determination and devotion for over 70 years. His own disciplined work ethic, which followed his guru's (T. Krichnamacharya) teachings, resulted in him taking *Aṣṭāṅga yoga* from a small *yoga shala* in Lakshmipuram, Mysore, and bringing it to a world-wide awareness of this method of physical, mental and spiritual development for all human beings. This book is a token of my respect and gratitude for the man whose efforts have resulted in the benefit for so many.

Guruji, in your memory, may the light of *Aṣṭāṅga yoga* continue to shine brightly and lead us, unhesitatingly, to discover the unending joy of knowing our true nature.

I am grateful to R. Sharath Jois, Saraswathi Jois, Eddie Stern, Lino Miele, Derek Ireland, Tove Palmgren, Måns Broo and my sister, Karola Räisänen, for all their help and teachings. I would also like to pay tribute to my father, Matti Räisänen (1939–2000), and to my mother, Ritva Räisänen (1942–2014), who raised me with love and imparted the seed of freedom of thought, encouraging me to choose my own way.

I extend my appreciation to my first son Julian's mother, Kati Rosendahl, for her patience and understanding over the years. This is also for my dear son, Julian Räisänen, who has been involved, sometimes bored and at other times enthralled, but patiently following his father's practice along the mystic path of *yoga*.

And finally, a deep, heartfelt thank you goes to Wambui Njuguna-Räisänen, my wife, colleague and mother to our delightful boys, Sesam and Sumu, for translating and editing this book with me. It has been one of our most fulfilling projects together, along our yogic path and in the life we share together.

Petri Räisänen
Helsinki, July 2017

Interview with Śrī Pattabhi Jois

Sir, your students call you Guruji, but what really is the meaning of guru?

Guru means "supreme". The student should see the guru as God. This is stated in the scriptures: *gurur brahmā gurur viṣṇuḥ gurur devo maheśvaraḥ/guruḥ sākṣāt paraṁ brahma tasmai śrī-gurave namaḥ* – "Guru is Brahmā, guru is Viṣṇu, guru is Maheśvara Śiva, guru is directly the highest divinity! Obeisance to this holy guru."

It is also said: *Hariḥ ruṣṭe gurus trātā guruḥ ruṣṭe na kaścana*, "If God becomes angry, the guru can save you, but if the guru becomes angry, no one can."

So if the guru curses someone, nobody can help.

So your students should beware of making you angry!

[*Laughter*] The guru doesn't really curse anyone; that is very rare. But there are many stories about that in the scriptures. It is said that one guru had many students. One of them decided to become an ascetic and went away to live in the forest. On the way he met another student, who took care of a huge herd of cows, from which he would kill one daily, chop it up and eat it. The first student was terrified, "How can you kill holy cows? What sin could be worse?" He asked his fellow student to never kill a cow again and went back to his guru to tell him what he had seen. To his astonishment the guru wasn't at all pleased with him but rather cursed him: "May you become a *cāṇḍāla*, an outcast, until your black hair turns white and your white cloth(es) turns black!"

To get rid of the curse, the student travelled to all the holy places of India, but nobody could help him. Years later, he sat on the steps of a temple of the goddess, *Kālī*. He happened to overhear someone speaking about wanting to give *bali*, a sacrificial offering to the goddess, but lacked the means to do so. Thinking that his life was useless anyway since he couldn't get rid of his guru's curse, the student decided to offer himself as a human sacrifice! He was smeared with ghee and turmeric, they offered *aarti* (ritual waving of lamps) to him and he was led into the temple to be sacrificed. He awaited his death in a small room, but because of the darkness, the priest couldn't find his sacrificial knife. While the priest was thus groping around the room, the student happened to find the knife, lost his nerve, quickly killed the priest and escaped. When he was finally safe, he noticed that his hair had turned white and his clothes black! The guru's curse was gone.

The student then returned to the guru. "I tried to protect the cows and you cursed me. Now I killed a Brahmin, and the curse was lifted. What is the point of all of this?" The guru replied, "That other student killed cows to keep himself and his family alive. He was so poor that he had no other option. The *Kālī*-priest, again, was no real Brahmin – in the name of *Kālī*, he slit the throat of so many people and took their money. By killing him, you did a good deed."

So fortunately the guru doesn't curse anyone. He tells people the truth. The guru is like a father, the disciple like a child, but the guru won't ask you to find a job and get married. He asks you, "Who are you? If that's your hand; that, your foot; that, your body, then who are you, yourself?" That is what the guru tells you, and for that reason, he is called supreme.

You have studied *Aṣṭāṅga-vinyāsa-yoga* under Śrī T. Krishnamacharya. Did he also teach you the scriptures?

No, I studied them at the Sanskrit College of Mysore. I studied there for 13 years and went through so many *yoga* books: *Bhagavad Gīta, Yoga Sūtra,Gheraṇda Saṁhitā, Śiva Saṁhitā, Kaśhyapa Saṁhitā, Agastya Saṁhitā* and so on. From Krishnamacharya I only learned the five or six-thousand year old *Yoga Korunta* of Vāmana Ṛṣi. This book had been written on palm leaves and was kept in the University of Calcutta, where my guru visited three times to study it. He wrote down notes, and I studied those. I never saw the book itself, and it was later destroyed. In that book, Vāmana Ṛṣi says: *Vinā vinyāsa-yogena āsanādin na kārayet*. This means, "Do not do *āsanas* without the *vinyāsa* system." If you do, your breath will not work properly, and you will become *alpa-āyus*, short-lived. It is said that God has given the human being a hundred years of life, but if our mind is disturbed, our senses will become distracted and our duration of life decreases. The mind is controlled through the breath, that is *prāna*, and this is done through *vinyāsa*, proper breathing. In the *Bhagavad Gīta*, it is said (5.27): *Prāṇāpanau samau kṛtvā*, "Make your in-breathing and out-breathing equal." If you follow the *vinyāsa*-system, there will be no danger in the practice. This is what I have taught for 65–70 years, but not everyone follows this, and they get all kinds of problems.

In the *Śvetāśvatara Upaniṣad* (2.8) it is said: *Trir-unnātam sthāpya samaṁ śarīram tristhānam avalokayet*, "When the body is threefold straight, one should consider three things". First, posture, then sight or *dṛṣṭi*, and finally breath or *vinyāsa*. Without *vinyāsa*, breathing cannot be controlled and diseases will come. That is why this method is so important.

In the *Yoga Sūtra* (1.2) *yoga* is defined as *citta-vṛtti-nirodhaḥ*, or the stopping of the functions of the mind, but the mind can be controlled only by controlling the breath, since (mind) follows (breath), and the senses are controlled by the mind. The *Kaṭha Upaniṣad* says (2.1.1): *Parañci khāni vyatṛnat svayaṁ-bhūs tasmāt parān paśyati nāntarātman*, "The creator drilled holes in the outside of the eyes, and therefore one can only see outside, not in towards the soul." But *kaścid dhīraḥ pratyag-ātmanam aikṣad āvṛtta-cakṣur amṛtatvam icchan*," Some *dhīras* or *yogis* have been able to turn their senses inward and see inside," towards the self, towards God. But that cannot be done just like that, only after life-long practice. Practice, practice, practice, and some day you will achieve it.

Could you tell us something about other verses from the Yoga Korunta?

This book has been destroyed, but I have committed a number of verses to memory. To recite them would take a long time, however – many days – and we do not have time for it now.

I have heard that Krishnamacharya was a very strict teacher. Could you tell us something of your own experiences?

He was very strict! He hurt us all. When I began, there were hundreds of students, but only three of us stuck it through to the end! For me, all the *āsanas* were difficult in the beginning, and I struggled especially with *Baddha-konāsana*, until one day my guru stood on top of me when I did it. What pain – I could not sleep the next night at all, but after this, it wasn't a difficult *āsana* anymore.

The guru should in fact be strict. If he is not strict, he cannot give *brahma-vidyā*, knowledge about spirit.

How do the different paths of *yoga* of the Bhagavad-gītā (karma-*yoga*, *jñāna-yoga*, *bhakti-yoga*) relate to *Aṣṭāṅga yoga*?

They are all included within it. In the *Gītā*, Arjuna is afraid of fighting because he cannot control his mind. Kṛṣṇa tells him, "You are a *kṣatriya*, a nobleman, so your *dharma* or duty is to fight." First he encourages Arjuna by saying that he has taught this same science to other kṣatriyas, and then he starts teaching him *yoga*.

Arjuna, however, voices an argument, "What if I do not achieve perfection in *yoga*? Will my life then not be a complete waste, neither materially nor spiritually successful?" Kṛṣṇa answers by saying (BG 6.41–42): *Sucinām śrīmatāṁ gehe yoga-bhraṣṭo 'bhijāyate/ atha vā yogināṁ eva kule bhavati dhīmatām* - "No, because an unsuccessful *yogi* is reborn into a pure and prosperous family, or into the family of *yogis*." From this he can then go on – in *yoga*, nothing is ever lost.

In the eighteen chapters of the *Gītā*, the system of *Aṣṭāṅga yoga* is perfectly taught. So also in all other ancient texts on *yoga*, such as the Saṁhitas, which deal exclusively with *Aṣṭāṅga yoga*. That which we learn here – *yama,niyama*, *āsana*, *prāṇāyāma* – these four are the outer side of *Aṣṭāṅga yoga*. Ādi Śaṅkarācarya has explained its inner side, *pratyāhāra*, *dhāraṇa*, *dhyāna* and *samādhi* in his book *Yoga Tārāvalī*. There are 72,000 *nāḍīs* or nerves in the body, and when one, through *recaka* and *pūraka* breathing, has purified them all and controls the three locks of the body (the *bandhas*), the *prāṇa* or life-air moves only through the *suṣumnā-nāḍī*. When that stage has been achieved, the *yogi* may stop the aging process. If he is, for example 25 years old when he achieves breathing through the *suṣumnā-nāḍī* and stays in that state for ten years, his body remains 25 years old even after that! This is how all the 68 great *mūla-ṛṣis* or original seers such as Vashiṣṭa, Jamadagni and Kaśyapa have been able to live for thousands of years. Viśvāmitra performed penance for 5,000 years, another sage for 7,000 years. According to the *Rāmāyana*, Rāma ruled over Ayodhyā for 14,000 years! In this way, *Aṣṭāṅga yoga* is not a new system; it is the most ancient.

Now we live in the *Kali-yuga*, the last and worst of the ages of the world, and the old systems of *yoga* have been forgotten. In the *Gītā* it says (3.14): *Tasmāt tvam indriyāny ādau niyamya bharatarṣabha/ pāpmānaṁ prajahi hy enaṁ jñāna-vijñāna-nāśanam* - "Oh Arjuna, first control your senses, and thus slay this sinfulness, the destroyer of knowledge and realisation." In the beginning, one must practice *yoga* to get control over the senses.

All of these subjects are dealt with in the *Bhagavad-gītā*. It is a great book, but it must be read carefully and repeatedly.

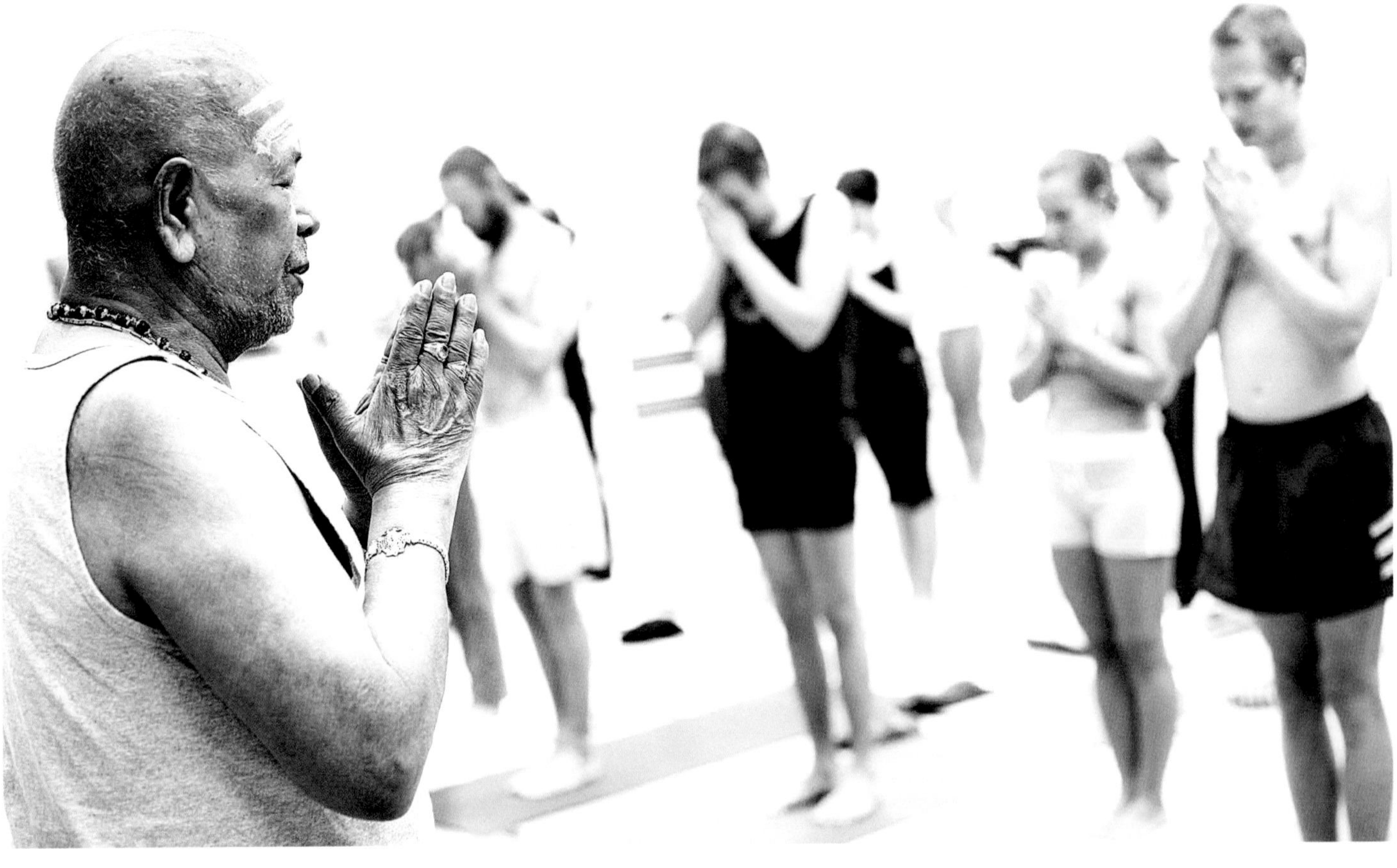

How would you define brahma-vidyā?

There are many different kinds of knowledge (*vidyā*) species, but only one through which you understand the true nature of yourself. *Brahma-vidyā* is the knowledge of the spirit, about God, how you are basically a God. This is what guru teaches, and what you should follow.

Does this mean that *brahma-vidyā* comes only through the practice, or does it require some special instruction?

No, no, no, through practice. Practice, practice and the guru will teach you. How long? *Dīrgha-kāle nairantaryeṇa* - "For a long time and uninterruptedly." Do your practice this whole life, and in the next life you will be born into a good family. In that life, again practice your whole life, and then again. In this way, you will collect good saṁskāras, mental impressions, and slowly *brahma-vidyā* will awaken in you.

How many lifetimes of *Aṣṭāṅga yoga* practice does it then take to achieve *mokṣa*, final liberation?

Mokṣa is not achieved easily. The *Gītā* says (6.44): *pūrvābhyāsena tenaiva hrīyate hy avaśo 'pi saḥ* – "The interest towards *yoga* is born from the practice of earlier lifetimes." It is no coincidence that some are more interested than others. "*Asānāni ca tāvanti yāvantyo jīva-rāśayaḥ.*" There are 22,000 different stages of life that have to be passed through, one after the other. You may have passed through many of them already, but it cannot be done in one lifetime. Śaṅkarāchārya collected good *saṁskāras* life after life and finally achieved *mokṣa*. Some *yogis* such as Brahmānanda Saraswatī have achieved *mokṣa* in one lifetime, but this is very rare. Now it is *Kali-yuga*, and very few practice *yoga* faithfully. But if you practice, practice, practice, in some lifetime you will achieve *mokṣa*.

After a long practice, you will come to the stage where there are no more bad thoughts. In the Yoga Yajñavalkya it is said: *Tritīya-kāla-storvihe svayaṁ saṁbharate prabhā/ tritīyāṅge sthito yogī vikāram mānaso tataḥ* – "At the third time, that is at sunset, the sun draws back its power into itself." Similarly, when the yogi has completely mastered the three *aṅgas* of *yama*, *niyama* and *āsana*, he draws back the functions of the mind into himself. Now the situation is different: you may sit in one place, but your mind is working in a completely different place. Sit straight and do not bend your spine. Do your practice, and gradually you will get control over your mind.

Swami Vivekananda used to say that if you can control your mind even for a second, you can control the whole world! Once he was supposed to give a lecture at six o'clock, but he did not arrive until seven. Everybody was angry and scolded him: "You Indians! You have no sense of time." Vivekananda said, "But it is only six o'clock", and asked them to look at their watches. Everyone's watch showed six! At this occasion, he mentioned the sentence I just quoted. Controlling the mind is very important. *Yoga* is *citta-vṛtti-nirodhaḥ*, the stopping of the functions of the mind. It is difficult, but possible through practice.

One has to practice for a long time, for one's whole life. Not only *āsanas*, but *prāṇāyāma* and *pratyāhāra* as well. Finally, wherever you look, you will see God. Whatever you hear, you will hear God. Now we think that we are surrounded by the world, so how could we see God, but it is possible. One must practice constantly.

One should think of God also during *āsana*-practice, all the time. At first we may see God in only one form, but later we will see all as God. It is possible. If we have good *saṁskāras*, it may be achieved even in one life.

Can anyone attain *brahma-vidyā*, or is it just for those who are born as brahmins?

No, it is for everyone. Control your senses and think about God daily. Have you heard about *bhramarī-kīṭa-nyāya*, the exemplary story of a wasp and larva? Once a wasp was chasing a larva. The larva crawled into a small hole to protect himself and thought continually about the wasp out there. "It's coming, it's coming and it's going to eat me!" The larva was afraid and thought about the wasp until it developed into a wasp itself. In the same way, you're really not a man until, if the guidance of a guru, you constantly remember God, you too will one day become God. This is possible for all people.

You have said that the air, *vāyu*, is God. Are we thus breathing God?

God is everywhere, in humans, but also elsewhere. You cannot understand it now, but sometime you will come to realize it. All comes from God. *ṁtmana ākāśaḥ saṁbhūtaḥ. ṁkāśād vāyuḥ, vāyor agniḥ, agner āpaḥ, adbhyaḥ pṛthiviḥ.* (Taittirīya Upaniṣad 2.1.1)- "Space originates from God. The air is born from space, fire from air, water from fire and earth from water." All these originally come from God. It is about understanding. Now, if you look at a wall you will only see the wall, but if you think about God, you can also see God in the wall. You are a thinking human being. Think strongly and you will become God.

What does the concept in the *Yoga Sūtras*, *Īśvara-praṇidhāna*, mean?

Īśvara-praṇidhāna in the *Yoga Sūtras* means surrendering to God, that you surrender completely, giving over your whole self, your body, your mind and all to him. Whatever you do, think that you do it for God, and give over all the fruits of your actions to him as well. Whatever happens to you, try to think that it comes from God.

Who is this God? Krishnamacharya, according my understanding, worshipped *Viṣṇu*.

Indeed, he was a *Vaiṣṇava* (worshipper of the God *Viṣṇu*), but only by birth. He was really an *Advaitin* (follower of Advaita Vedānta philosophy), that is, he saw all the gods as one. *Viṣṇu, Śiva* - all is one.

You've been practicing *yoga* throughout your life. Have you got to this level?

I'm thinking about God all the time, not about bad things. That is why I have so many students in my *yoga shala*. I teach the same method as the ancient sages, I do not hurt anyone, and I do not speak bad of anyone.

This is your second time teaching on a European tour (2006). Have your students made progress since the last time?

They do better *āsanas*, and they think more – about the world! [*Laughter*]. But really, there is a big difference. The students are sincere with *yoga* and have a very good attitude.

How to use this book

Nāḍī-śodhana is a continuation of my first book, *Ashtanga Yoga: Yoga in the tradition of Śrī K. Pattabhi Jois*. Therefore, the principles of the practice of *āsana*, *bandhas* (muscular and energetic locks), *dṛṣṭi* (gazing points), and *ujjayī* or sound breathing, along with the translation of *mantra*, the importance and purpose of the finishing *āsanas*, including the final relaxation pose, and the practical philosophy behind the practice have all been defined in detail in the first book. For this reason, I have not included these aspects in detail in this book, although they are naturally an essential part of the intermediate series practice.

Nāḍī-śodhana is intended to give a comprehensive picture of the intermediate series *āsana* practice of *Aṣṭāṅga yoga*, according to the tradition of Śrī K. Pattabhi Jois. This book features the positions in the intermediate series, but it also reflects the multidimensionality of the *Aṣṭāṅga yoga* philosophy and how it relates to everyday life.The practice of the intermediate series is aimed for teachers and students who have been practicing *Aṣṭāṅga yoga* for some years, have completed the primary series in the traditional manner and have begun the intermediate series.

On the other hand, it is fine, and even recommended, to take a peek at the intermediate series poses and discover the tradition of *Aṣṭāṅga yoga*, as it has been documented in this book, even if your own practice is still at the primary series level, or if you haven't yet started the yogic path.

The book provides a detailed and accurate account of the linking together of the poses in the two traditional ways:

1. The original "full-*vinyāsa*" technique
2. The practical "half-*vinyāsa*" practice

The original full-*vinyāsa* method describes the postures from the beginning to the end, meaning starting and ending each pose in samasthitiḥ. Whereas, in the practical half-*vinyāsa*, the *āsanas* are linked to each other in an abbreviated version of the full-*vinyāsa*. Nowadays, this half-*vinyāsa* technique is how most practitioners work with the various series. The full-*vinyāsa* technique is particularly important for teachers and for those who wish to become thoroughly familiar with the *vinyāsa* system, but it is also useful information for all those who are interested.

In the old guru-student tradition, the teachers tested their students to ensure whether the student was ready to advance further in the series. The student had to be able to do the postures unwaveringly, while keeping the breathing calm and steady, as well as know by heart the number of *vinyāsas* in each position. This pedagogy is still alive and well in India today.

The *āsana* charts, at the side of the *āsana* pages, list and describe each *vinyāsa*, from *samasthitiḥ* to *samasthitiḥ*, which follows the traditional full-*vinyāsa* count. The orange colored *vinyāsas* shows the practical "half *vinyāsa*" method. The first *vinyāsa* and pose is *ekam* (*ekam* = one), the second is *dve* (*dve* = two), etc. *Prāṇa* means breath, *āsana* what to do, *dṛṣṭi* where to look and the bandhas tell which muscle locks to engage during the pose. (⊙ is the sign for *mūla-bandha* or anal contraction and ⓥ is the sign for *uddīyana-bandha* or lower abdominal contraction).

The charts can also be used as a quick reference to check the details (the *vinyāsa*, breaths, gazing points, muscle locks, etc.) of a particular *āsana*. Please be aware that this "full-*vinyāsa*" technique is not recommended as a daily practice, but it can be beneficial sometimes for energizing the practice and to release the body after the most challenging poses found in the series.

The main text in the *āsana* pages describes the techniques for the regular (half-*vinyāsa*) intermediate series practice. The poses, breathing, gazing points and muscle locks, as well as the *vinyāsa* counting system have been presented according to how Śrī K. Pattabhi Jois was teaching the intermediate series in Mysore, India during 2006-2007. All postures are shown from start to finish, and include getting into the pose and how to transition into the next posture.

The final state or sthiti of each pose is presented with a clear picture. If the *sthiti* of the pose has both a right and left side, the picture has been taken from the first side (with the exception of *Gomukhāsana*), which shows the shape and alignment of the posture, as well as the details.

All *vinyāsas*, including the transition from pose to pose, are numbered and described in the small pictures at the top of the page. The angle of the picture was chosen carefully to show the details and techniques of each pose. As a result, some of the poses are shot from a different angle as they normally would be done in the practice. The right direction of the posture can be easily found by reading the *āsana* description.

In some postures, there is more than one 'approved' way of jumping into or out of the pose. These techniques are explained separately in the "jump techniques" (pp 28–29), as well as in each position's own *vinyāsa*.

Some *dṛṣṭis*, or gazing points, have changed since Śrī Pattabhi Jois wrote his book Yoga Mala (1958–60). Most of the brūmadhya (between the eyebrows) *dṛṣṭis* have been moved to nasāgra (tip of the nose). In fact, the only *brūmadhya-dṛṣṭi* which still remains in this series is in *Yoga-nidrāsana* (pp 91–92). Changes and special details are mentioned in the notes on the side of the page. In addition to the practical techniques of each posture, the physical, mental and energetic benefits are listed, as well as other important aspects of the practice.

The benefits of the positions come from both practical and theoretical research of *yoga* tradition which is thousands of years old. It is quite safe to assume that even though the ancient *ṛṣis* (sages) and seers who observed, experimented and compiled this knowledge didn't have the parallel equivalent for modern medicine, this hardly means that the ancient research has been less valuable. *Yoga* is a tradition which has been growing in the West over the last hundred years, more or less, and only recently has modern science and allopathic medicine started to take *yoga* more seriously and incorporate aspects of it into treatments and preventative care.

In the case of severe illness, it is always better to discuss with your doctor how to combine the treatment of disease with *yoga* therapy. In the intermediate series, there is no mention of modified positions if the student is not ready to make the original pose. This is because the student should not continue forward in the series if the previous positions are not yet under control. Anyhow, *yoga* is an individual sight and it is recommended to discuss with your main teacher about your progress in the practice. The body should be prepared peacefully for the intermediate series by practicing the primary series postures thoroughly for a sufficient amount of time.

The general rule is that all the poses of the primary series should be done correctly and students should be able to drop-back into the bridge (pp 124–125) and stand up without help. Remember that for every general rule, there is an exception; as well, in *yoga*.

If injuries or muscle soreness occur during or separately from the practice; if you have been ill, or if you are not, for one reason or another, able to do the practice, you should first recover your body completely by doing the primary series sequence until you are ready to get back to the intermediate series.

If you are not sure how to practice after an illness or injury or if are still in the recovery phase, it is advisable to discuss the details of the *yoga* therapy with an experienced *yoga* teacher. The intermediate series requires much more dedication for the practice than the primary series. Its effects also extend deeper into the body, nervous system and psyche.

Remember to always keep track of the body's condition and the mind's possibilities and limits. The safest and most efficient way to proceed forward with the practice is to seek the guidance of a qualified teacher. Enjoy the process!

Yoga liberates us from the devil
known as disease.

– Sri K. Pattabhi Jois, *Yoga Mala*

Sanskrit – The sacred language of India

Sanskrit, India's ancient sacred language, is the universal language of the Yoga tradition. In its most ancient form, it is embodied in the many thousand year old Vedic literature. Its name, *saniskṛta*, meaning "perfectly embodied," refers to the fact that in the first centuries of the common era, Sanskrit became the universal language of learning and culture all over South and South-East Asia, functioning in a way similar to Latin in mediaeval Europe. The linguist Panini's system of grammar (ca 400 BC) gave Sanskrit its classical form, which is still followed, even as new words are continuously added. Unlike Latin, Sanskrit is not a 'dead' language, as it is still used in Hindu, Jain, and in Mahāyāna Buddhist rituals. It is also being taught, read and written all over South Asia. There are even some initiatives to revive its status as a spoken language in many parts of India. In the 2011 population census of India, 14135 people reported Sanskrit as their mother tongue. Sanskrit is an Indo-European language, so it is distantly related to most European languages, such as English, German or French.

The sound of mantras

Practitioners of *yoga* do not necessarily need to know Sanskrit, but it is useful to know something about the pronunciation. There are plenty of mantras, that is, syllables, words and verses which are thought to contain mystical powers in the Yoga tradition. What's more, Sanskrit is considered to be the language of the gods, and out of all known and classified languages, it is credited as the one closest to the original cosmic vibration. In this way, it is thought that through Sanskrit, we can access the driving forces of the universe in an easier and more effective way than though other languages. Even if the student does not fully understand the meaning of a *mantra*, benefits can still occur from chanting or repeating them. However, the right effect can only be achieved if the *mantra* is pronounced properly.

The difficulty in Sanskrit pronunciation and translation does not mean that the sadhaka (practitioner) shouldn't make the effort to find out the meanings of mantras. Mantras work best when they are pronounced correctly, and when their meanings are meditated on in the mind. When understood well and pronounced correctly, Sanskrit is an extremely beautiful language, full of harmony and inner power.

Mantras link the yogi and yogini to the living tradition, in which countless *yoga* practitioners since ancient time, have chanted the same mantras as they have been passed down through a paraṃparā or disciplic succession. Through chanting mantras, even modern practitioners can create a connection to ancient yogis and yoginis and obtain support and strength for their yogic path.

If the Sanskrit words are mispronounced, the meaning of words may change. For example, the words Rāma and Ramā refer to two different people: the first one is one of Lord Vishnu's descents (avatāras), and the second to the Viṣṇu's spouse, Lakṣmī.

The Devanāgarī script

Over the centuries, Sanskrit has been written in several different scripts. *Devanāgarī* – the writing of the cities of the gods – which was developed in the 12th century, is currently the most common script in use. In this book, the mantras and names of *āsanas* are written in this script. Since the *Devanāgarī* alphabet has more letters than are found in the Latin alphabet, diacritical marks need to be added to the letters so that we can distinguish all the sounds and letters from each other. Among the diacritical marks, the most important ones are the lines above vowels, e.g., ā, which show that these are long vowels, something that must be indicated in pronunciation.

Devanāgarī is written from left to right, as we are commonly used to. However, it differs from the Latin alphabet, in that it is generally written in syllables rather than individual phonemes. If a vowel does not begin a word, it will be linked to the preceding consonant by a vowel mark. If the consonant does not have such a separate vowel mark, the consonant is by default followed by a short "a". Thus kāla (time) is written as काल, while kula (school) is कुल.

Below we have listed both the independent forms of the vowels (used especially when a vowel begins a word) as well as the vowel marks (in parentheses). The place for the consonant is in the latter case marked with a circle (◌). When two or more consonants follow each other, they are written together, either side by side (अम्बा , a + m + bā, ambā, the mother) or below each other (अक्क a+k+kā, akkā, an old woman). The case is further complicated by the fact that there are also a number of special forms of conjunct consonants!

Letters and pronunciation

The *Devanāgarī* alphabet begins with the vowels, followed by the consonants, in the order of how and where they are pronounced. After that comes the four half vocals, the three sibilants, and ends with the last letter, "h".

Vowels

अ a - short a (as in u in cut)
आ ā (◌ा for example, बा , bā) - long a (as in father)
इ (ि◌) i - short i (as in bit)
ई (◌ी) ī - long i (as in beet)
उ (◌ु) u - short u (as in put)
ऊ (◌ू) ū- long u (as in brute)
ऋ (◌ृ) ṛ - also a vowel, a resonant r-sound, pronounced also "ri" in North India; "ru" in South India
ॠ (◌ॄ)ṝ - the long version of the previous vowel
ऌ (◌ॢ) ḷ - vocalic l-sound (as in table)
ए (◌े) e - long e (as in bay)
ऐ (◌ै) ai - (as in sight)
ओ (◌ो) o - long o (as in Rome)
औ (◌ौ) au - (as in sound)
◌ः ḥ - visarga, the previous vowel is repeated (e.g., aha)
◌ं - anusvāra, nasal m (as in French bon)

Consonants
The consonants are organized into five categories according to where they are pronounced in the mouth (see figure).

1. Velar
क k – as in cat
ख kh – as above, but with a clear-h aspiration
(the expulsion of air will result with an additional h-like sound)
ग g – as in gazelle
घ gha – as above, but aspirated
ङ ṅ – as in sung

2. Palatal
च c – as in chill
छ ch – like the previous one, but aspirated
ज j – as in joy
झ jh – as above, but aspiration
ञ ñ – as in Kenya

3. Retroflex
ट ṭ – as in tub, but sharper
ठ ṭh – as above, but aspirated
ड ḍ – as in dame, but sharper
ढ ḍh – as above, but aspirated
ण ṇ – sound with aspiration, as in renown

4. Dental
त t – as in tinderbox
थ tha – as above, but aspirated
द d – as in lady
ध dha – as the previous one, but aspirated
न n – as in Nile

5. Labial
प p – as in petrified
फ ph – as above, but aspirated
ब b – as in Balthasar
भ bh – as above, but aspirated
म m – as in March

Semi-vowels
य y – as in young
र r – as in right – this is a strong sound
ल l – as in limited
व v – as in very

Sibilantit
श ś – palatal, sibilant s, as in ship
ष ṣ - pronounced today as the previous one; originally retroflex
स s – as in sauna
ह h – as in Heidi

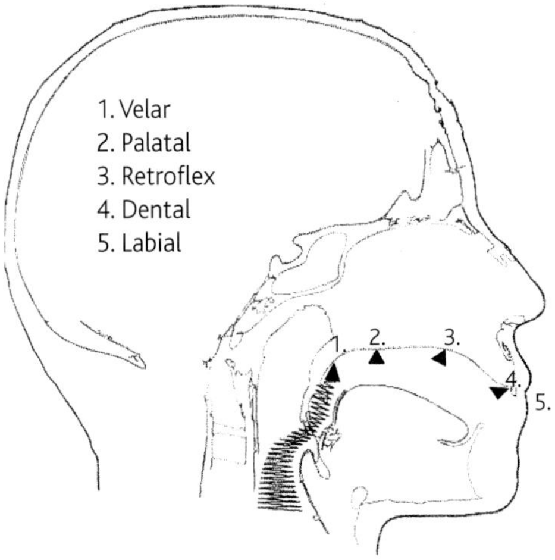

Illustration: Vyaas Houston

General pronunciation guide

When pronouncing Sanskrit, it is necessary to take into account the difference between short and long vowels. Note that the vowels "e" and "o" are always long. Commonly, there are no breaks between the words in Sanskrit verses and all the words are pronounced in a row. There is also a clear distinction between aspirated and nonaspirated consonants i.e., between "k" and "kh". For most English speakers, the vowels are easy, but retroflex words are often tricky and require a lot of practice.

About Sanskrit grammar

Sanskrit is an Indo-European language, and therefore the grammar has a number of similarities with languages such as Ancient Greek and Latin. Sanskrit uses place cases instead of prepositions, of which are only eight. As a point of comparison, Finnish, which belongs to the Finno-Ugric language group has fifteen cases. For example, the nominative for the word *yoga* is yogaḥ, the genitive yogasya and accusative yogam.

One special feature in Sanskrit is sandhi, which literally means connection. In all languages, this feature of assimilation, in which the beginning and the end of the words affect each other when pronounced, occurs. An English example of this could be the "linking r" which occurs in many dialects (Law-r-and order). In English, the only sandhi which occurs in the written language is the difference between "a" and "an", but since Sanskrit grammar is based on the spoken language, sandhi occurs there regularly in writing as well. Sometimes the sounds meeting each other assimilate, such as when the words matsya and *āsana* make up the word matsyāsana. At other times, a vowel may change into a semivowel, as in the case of marīci and *āsana* forming marīcyāsana, or into a developed form of itself, as when ā and i combine into e (mahā and indra form mahendra). Consonants may also change: sat, cit and ānanda becomes sac-cid-ānanda; yogaḥ and citta-vṛtti-nirodhaḥ form yogaś citta-vṛtti-nirodhaḥ (Yoga-Sūtra 1.2). Note that sandhi does not change the meaning of the words, only the pronunciation and spelling.

Sanskrit uses many compound words, which is why words can sometimes seem extremely long. Take the previously mentioned citta-vṛtti-nirodhaḥ, which can be divided as follows; cittasya vṛtter nirodhaḥ, i.e., stopping the fluctuations of the consciousness. The different parts of the compound words are combined together in *Devanāgarī* writing, but in transcription they are separated for readability.

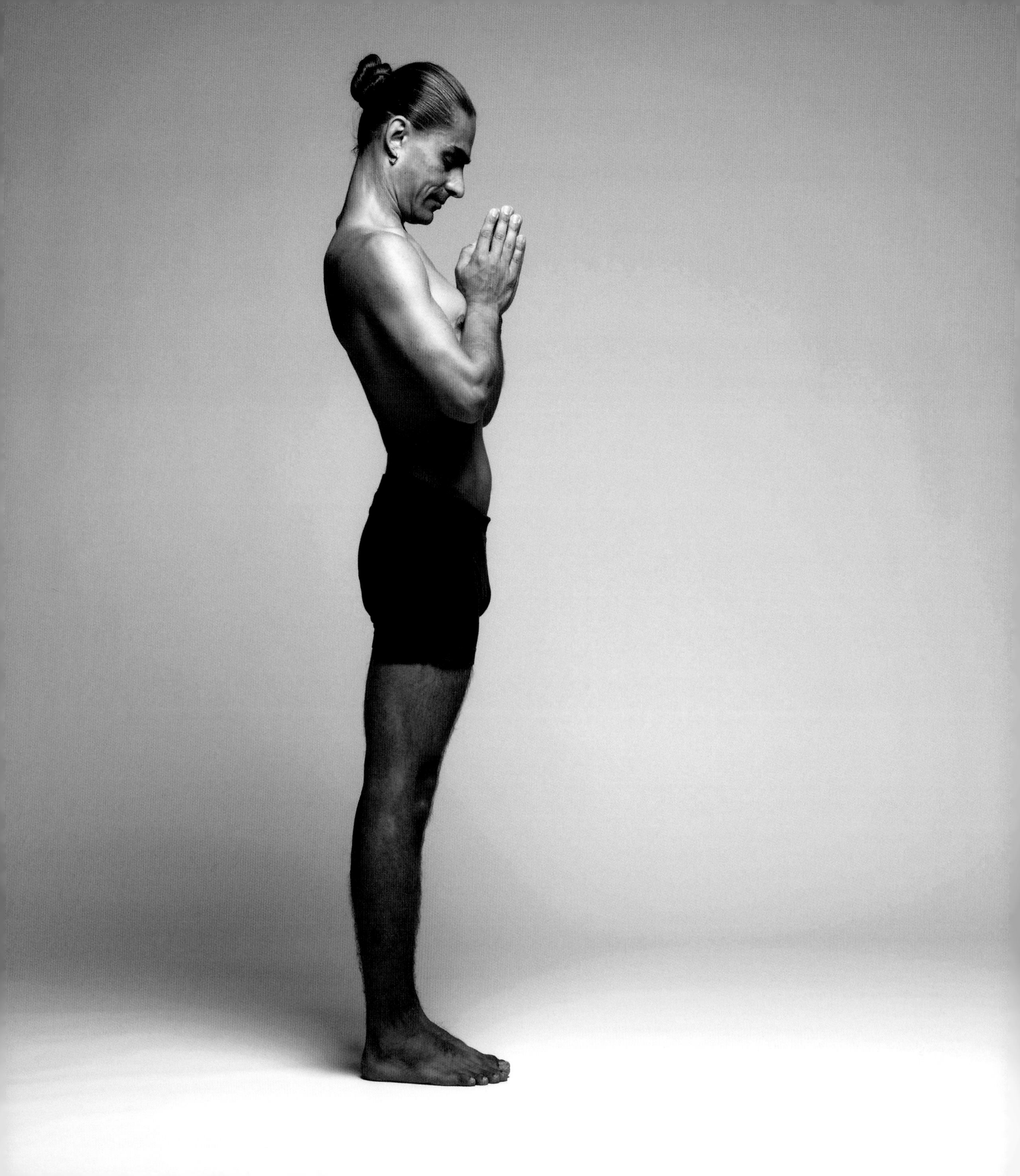

Opening invocation

ॐ

वन्दे गुरूणां चरणारविन्दे
सन्दर्शितस्वात्मसुखावबोधे।
निःश्रेयसे जाङ्गलिकायमाने
संसारहालाहलमोहशान्त्यै॥

आबाहुपुरुषाकारं शङ्खचक्रासिधारिणम्।
सहस्रशिरसं श्वेतं प्रणमामि पतञ्जलिम्॥

ॐ

Oṃ
vande gurūṇāṁ caraṇāravinde
sandarśita-svātmā-sukhāvabodhe
niḥśreyase jāṅgalikāyamāne
saṁsāra-hālāhala-mohaśāntyai

ābāhu-puruṣākāraṁ
śaṅkhacakrāsi-dhāriṇam
sahasra-śirasaṁ śvetaṁ
praṇamāmi patañjalim
OM

Translation
I bow to the lotus feet of the gurus,
that awaken the happiness of one's self revealed;
that are the ultimate good;
that take the form of a medicine man
for curing the delusion of the poison of birth and death.

Who takes the form of a man
up to his shoulders,
bearing conch, disc and sword
thousand-headed, white
I salute Patañjali!

The meaning of the first verse
Oṃ – the sound of Brahman, God
vande – I bow; *gurūṇām* – to the gurus; *caraṇa* – feet; *aravinde* – (of) lotus; *sandarśita* – revealed; *svātmā* – own Self; *sukha* – happiness; *avabodhe* – (who) enlightens, awakens; *niḥśreyase* – (who are) highest good; *jāṅgali* – jungle medicine man; *kāyamāne* – (those who) take (that) form; *saṁsāra* – the cycle of life and death; *hālāhala* – poison; *moha* – delusion; *śāntyai* – to remove.

Śrī Pattabhi Jois's commentary
Who is a guru? Guru is Brahmā, Viṣṇu and Mahesvara (Śiva) - He is the highest God. The guru should teach the student, and the student should be loyal to the guru's knowledge. Do not do that, what the guru does not teach. The guru reveals to you what is svātmā, what is your true self, where you came from, why have you come, and who, after all, you are.

You are looking for God, but you don't know that God is within you. Listen to the guru's message, "You are not human, you are God." The scriptures say, "Ahaṁ brahmāsmi", "I am God!" This is what a real guru teaches; others do not teach the same (method). When you follow the *yoga* method, and practice, practice and practice, your real self will be revealed.

Before you, a countless number of fathers and mothers have come and gone, one after another.

"Punar api jananaṁ punar api maraṇam that", "We are born and we die again and again and again."

You are circling around with 22,000 other living species again and again. Why? Because you do not know your own self. In this life, you were born from one mother; in next life you will be born from another. There are numerous species on the planet. Between human lives, you will be born as a cow or a dog and many others, but common to all is that you stay ignorant of your true self.

Once you realize that you are also God, you will no longer be reborn. Species die. Your body will not stay here long, it dies, but you will not be born again. You will reach "niḥśreya" which is the highest good, the highest goal. This can be achieved by following the method which the guru is teaching. The guru is jāṅgali, jungle doctor, who will give you the medicine against samsara's snake poison. As a guru teaches you the philosophy that you are God, this guru is important; therefore, in this *mantra* we worship the feet of our gurus.

The meaning of the second verse
ābāhu – up to the shoulders; *puruṣa* – man, person; *ākāram* – (who) has taken, adopted, incarnated; *śaṅkha* – conch; *cakra* – disc; *asi* – sword; *sahasra* – thousand; *śirasam* – headed; *śvetam* – white; *praṇamāmi* – I salute; *patañjalim* – sage *Patañjali.*

Śrī Pattabhi Jois's commentary
When the heavenly Adiśeṣa-serpent took the form of Patañjali (sage, yogi) on earth, he was a man up to the shoulders. His head, however, remained in the terrifying thousand-headed form of Adiśeṣa. Patañjali taught the same philosophy as all the other gurus. He carried the conch (śaṅkha) to scare enemies with the sound, the discus weapon (cakra) to fight against them and the sword (asi) to cut the heads off these enemies of the mind. The thousand -headed Adiśeṣa is completely white in color, and is the object to whom we bow.

Closing invocation – Mangala or Śānti mantra

ॐ स्वस्ति प्रजाभ्यः परिपालयन्तां

न्यायेन मार्गेण महीं महीशाः।

गोब्राह्मणेभ्यः शुभमस्तु नित्यं

लोकाः समस्ताः सुखिनो भवन्तु॥

ॐ शान्तिः शान्तिः शान्तिः॥

Oṃ
svasti prajābhyaḥ paripālayantaṁ
nyāyena mārgeṇa mahīṁ mahīśāḥ
go-brāhmaṇebhyaḥ śubham astu nityaṁ
lokāḥ samastāḥ sukhino bhavantu

Oṃ santih, santih, santih

Translation

Fortune to the people,
and to the rulers of the earth,
who protect the countries
by following the path of righteousness!

May there always be prosperity
for the cows
and the Brahmins
May all the worlds be happy!

The meaning of the words

Oṃ – the sound of Brahman, God; *mangala* – auspicious; *śāntiḥ* – peace; *svasti* – fortune, success; *prajābhyaḥ* – folk, nation, people; *paripālayantam* – protected, preserved; *nyāyena* – righteousness, lawfulness, by virtue; *mārgeṇa* – follow the path; *mahīm* – country, the earth; *mahī-īśāḥ* – rulers of the earth; *go-brāhmaṇebhyaḥ* – for cows and brahmins (priests); *śubham* – goodness; *astu* – may it become, be; *nityam* – always; *lokāḥ* – words; *samastāḥ* – all, every; *sukhinaḥ* – happy; *bhavantu* – may it be.

Śrī Pattabhi Jois's commentary

In this *mantra*, it is hoped that the kings and rulers would follow the path of truth and walk the path of righteousness. If you defend the truth, you are moving in the right direction at all times. Do not choose the wrong path. Protect the Brahmans (priests, scholars and virtuous people), and cows (representing peace, wealth, innocence and Mother Earth). Don't ever kill them. Let all people have a chance for happiness in every world!

Dṛṣṭi – gazing points

The gaze and mental focus are directed and held towards certain points in the poses, using what is known as *dṛṣṭi*. These gazing points are important tools for the body and mind in the *Aṣṭāṅga yoga* method. *Dṛṣṭi* is not only used to align the body to the right position, but it also guides prāna throughout the body, and so opens the pathways for energy to flow through the *nāḍīs*. When the body is in motion, the different *dṛṣṭis* are not normally used; rather, the eyes follow the movement, to how and where the body is placed in the main part of the pose. Once the movement has slowed down and the state, sthiti, of the position has been established, the gaze is then focused to a specific point. There are also certain *dṛṣṭis* during the *vinyāsas*, i.e., between the states of the poses. The primary *āsana* sequence has nine *dṛṣṭis* (nava-*dṛṣṭi*). The intermediate sequence includes a tenth *dṛṣṭi*, *Adho-mukha-dṛṣṭi* in *Ṭiṭṭibhāsana* C, which means to gaze down at the floor.

1. *Nāsāgra-dṛṣṭi* – the tip of the nose
Example positions: *Samasthitiḥ*, *Bakāsana* A & B and *Ṭiṭṭibhāsana* A.

Nāsāgra-dṛṣṭi is the most common gazing point during the *āsana* practice. If you are not sure of the correct *dṛṣṭi* in a certain position, nāsāgra is a good "all-purpose" *dṛṣṭi* to refer back to and focus on.

2. *Aṅguṣṭha-madhya-dṛṣṭi* – the thumbs or Aṅguṣṭhāgra-*dṛṣṭi* - the tip of the thumbs (synonymous)
Example position: The first *vinyāsa* in *Sūryanamaskāra* A.
When gazing at the thumbs, we also, for all purposes, gaze upwards. Due to this, some of the positions may have two *dṛṣṭis* mentioned, thumbs or upwards.

3. *Bhrūmadhya-dṛṣṭi* – in between the eyebrows
Example position: Yoga-nidrāsana.

4. *Nābhi-cakra-dṛṣṭi* – the navel center
Example position: *Adho-mukha-svanāsana* (the 6th *vinyāsa* in *Sūryanamaskāra* A)
Note: During *Adho-mukha-svanāsana*, *uddīyana-bandha* is held in, making it practically difficult to see the navel. For this reason, it is commonly mentioned to gaze towards the navel, while your mental focus stays at the navel.

5. *Hastāgra-dṛṣṭi* – the fingertips or the "end of the hand"
Example position: *Utthita-trikonāsana* A and B.

6. *Pādayor agra dṛṣṭi* – the toes or Pādāṅguṣṭha-*dṛṣṭi* – the big toe
Example position: Krauncāsana.

7. and 8. *Pārśva-dṛṣṭi* – right and left sides
Example positions: *Ardha-matsyendāsana* and *Bharadvājāsana*.

9. *Urdhva-dṛṣṭi* or *antara-dṛṣṭi* – upwards
Example positions: *Vātāyanāsana* and *Parighāsana*.

10. *Adho-mukha-dṛṣṭi* – down, the floor
Example position: *Tittibhāsana* B (when walking forwards and backwards).

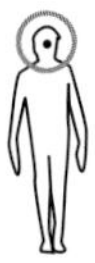

Nāsāgra-dṛṣṭi
the tip of the nose

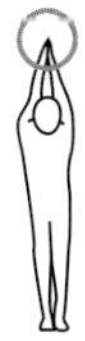

Aṅguṣṭha-madhya-dṛṣṭi
the thumbs or
aṅguṣṭhāgra-dṛṣṭi
the tip of the thumbs

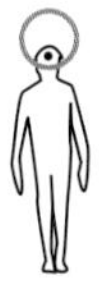

Bhrūmadhya-dṛṣṭi
between the eyebrows

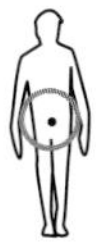

Nābhi-cakra-dṛṣṭi
the navel center

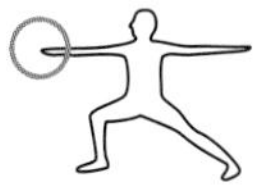

Hastāgra-dṛṣṭi
the fingertips
or the "end of the hand"

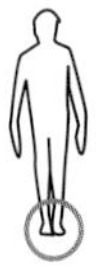

Pādayor agra dṛṣṭi
the toes or
pādāṅguṣṭha-dṛṣṭi
the big toe

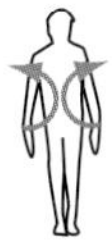

Pārśva-dṛṣṭi
the right and left sides

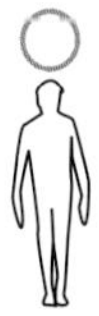

Urdhva-dṛṣṭi or
antara-dṛṣṭi
upwards

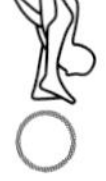

Adho-mukha-dṛṣṭi
down, the floor

Jumping techniques between vinyāsas

Between some of the intermediate series positions, there are several different ways to jump back (into *Catvāri*) through the arms. The usual jump will be done with crossed legs (photos 1 & 4), unless the position doesn't have a specific jump-back technique. If the specific techniques are too challenging or you are currently in the process of developing these jump-back techniques, the crossed legs jump is always recommended.

The forward-jump through usually has the legs crossed (photo 2) or uses the straight legs technique (photo 3).

Traditionally, there has been a smooth jump, rather than stepping, into the standing poses in the first *vinyāsa* and jumping back to *Samasthitiḥ* in the last *vinyāsa*. While landing after the jump, there is a slight tremor or vibration in the body, which has a positive effect on the muscles and nerves.

Listed below are the *āsanas*, which have several ways to transition both into and out of. Other *āsanas* can follow the basic crossed-legs jump.

Asana	Hyppytekniikka
Basic jump (1, 2 or 3)	crossed legs forward or backward jump; forward jump with straight legs
Bharadvājāsana (4, 5 or 6) भरद्वाजासन	half lotus; lotus; crossed-legs jump
Ardha-matsyendrāsana (4 or 7) अर्धमत्स्येन्द्रासन	crossed-legs jump; jump straight from the pose
Gomukhāsana (4 or 7) गोमुखासन	crossed-legs jump; jump straight from the pose
Supta-ūrdhva-pāda-vajrāsana (4, 5 or 6) सुप्तोर्ध्वपादवज्रासन	half lotus; lotus; crossed-legs jump

1 Jump back

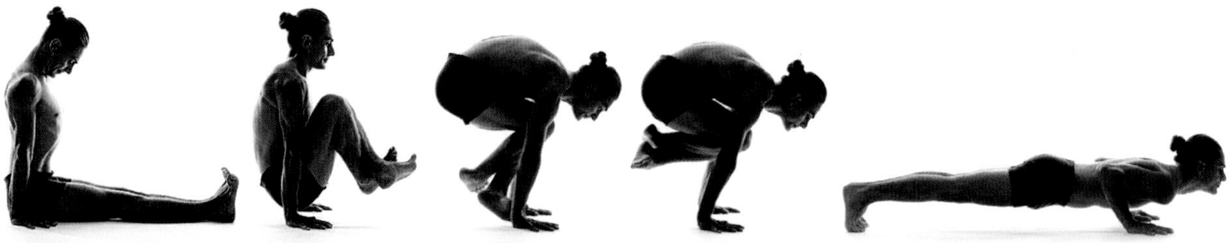

2 Jump forward

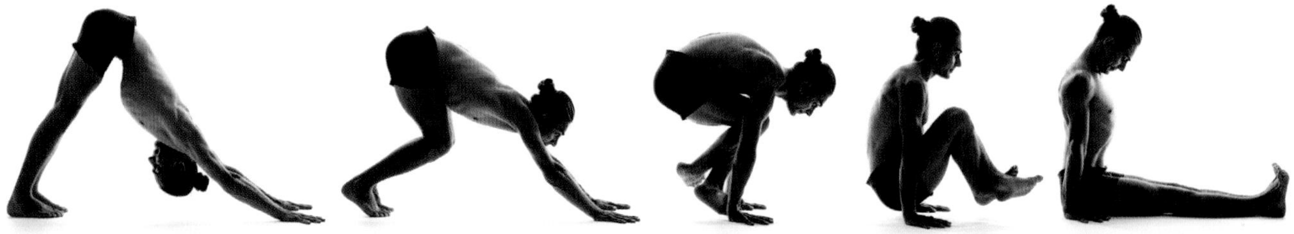

3 Jump forward

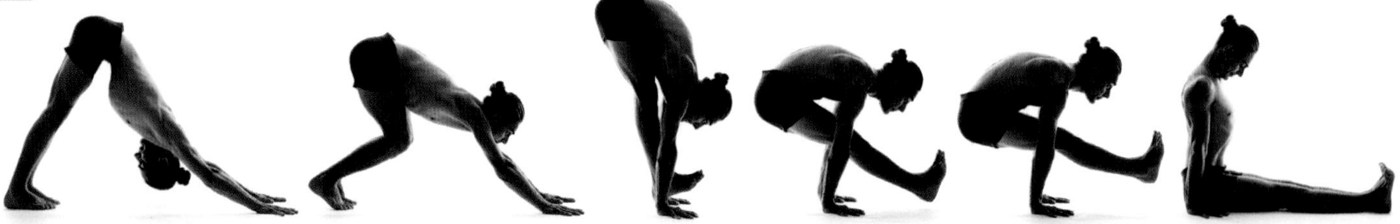

4 Jump back

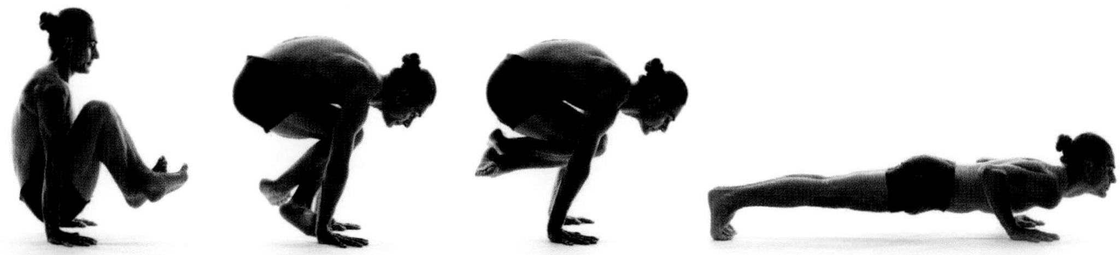

5 Jump back

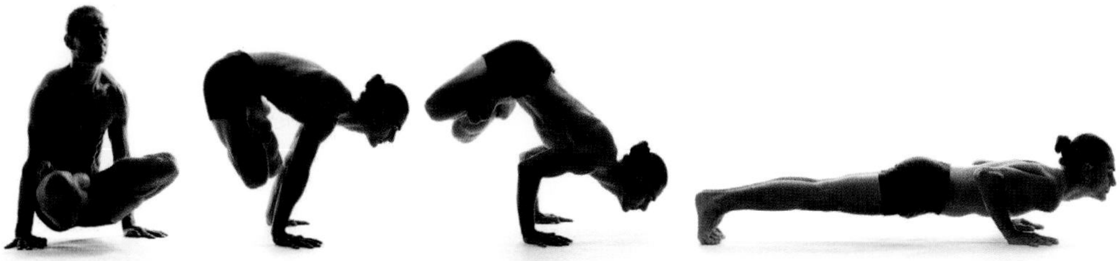

6 Jump back

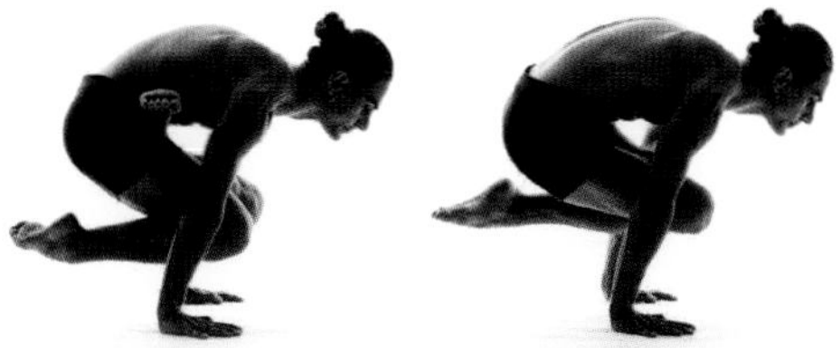

7 Jump back

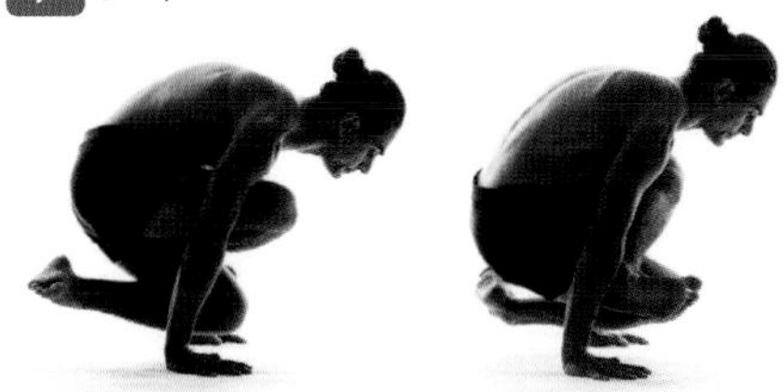

Na veṣa-dhāraṇaṃ siddheḥ kāraṇaṃ na ca tat-kathā
kriyaiva kāraṇaṃ siddheḥ satyam etan na saṃśayaḥ

Wearing the garb of a renunciant is not the cause of perfection,
neither is speaking about it.
Perfection comes from practice.
This is the truth, no doubt about it.

– *Haṭha Yoga Pradīpikā* 1/66

सूर्यनमस्कारः

Sūrya-namaskāra A

Sun salutation A | 9 *vinyāsas*

Sūrya – sun, the Sun God; *namaskāra* – salutation

Note 1: Repeat *Sūrya-namaskāra* A 3–5 times.
Note 2: On *vinyāsas* 3, 5, and 7, you can either gaze to the tip of the nose (*nasāgra*) or between the eyebrows (*bhrūmadhya*).
Note 3: It is traditional to chant the opening invocation (*mantra*) before doing the first sun salutation, and honor the guru or teacher and the ancient tradition of *Aṣṭāṅga yoga*. The chant also helps to shift the mind inward and bring about a favorable state and presence for the practice (*Pratayāhāra*).

Samasthitiḥ

Stand straight with the feet together, arms by the sides, and gaze at the tip of the nose.

1 Ekam

Inhale, lift the arms up overhead, either from the front, on a diagonal or from the sides of the body. Follow the hands with the gaze, and lean the head back. Let the inhalation broaden the chest and the back, and bring the palms and fingers together overhead. Stretch the shoulders and straighten the elbows, lifting the hands up to the ceiling at the same time that you hold the feet firmly on the floor. Straighten the back and lengthen the entire body. Direct the gaze up at the tip of the thumbs.

2 Dve

Uttānāsana (*uttāna* – strong, deep stretch)
Exhale, bend forward from the hips with straight legs and lower the arms towards the floor. Actively draw in *uddīyana-bandha*, sinking the torso onto the thighs. Place the fingertips in line with the toes, and press the palms onto the floor with the fingers spread wide. Relax the back of the neck, press the head into the knees or between the shins. Gaze at the tip of the nose.

3 Trīṇi

Inhale, open the chest, draw the shoulders back and down and fully elongate the spine. Straighten the arms and keep pressing the palms firmly onto the floor, which is the grounding action, working in opposition to the upward-moving actions of the head, chest and spine. Lift the head and gaze between the eyebrows.

4 Catvāri

Chaturāṅga-dandāsana (*chatur* - four; *aṅga* - limb; *daṇḍa* - stick)
Exhale, keep the palms pressed into the floor, hold *mūla* and *uddīyana bandha*, and lift the feet from the floor with the strength of the arms. Float (or jump) the legs back and land the feet hip-width apart (about 1/2 to one foot-length's width). The weight rests only on the hands and the balls of the feet and the legs are straight. Keep the whole body in a straight line, with the help of *mūla* and *uddīyana bandhas*, and bend the arms to 90 degrees, keeping the elbows in towards the sides of the body. Move the chin forward and gaze at the tip of the nose.

5 Pañcha

Ūrdhva-mukha-śvanāsana (ūrdhva – upward; *mukha* – facing; *śvana* – dog)
Inhale, move the body forward through the arms, slowly straighten the arms and roll over the toes until the tops of the feet are on the floor. Keep the feet straight and engage the thighs so that the kneecaps lift. Keep the knees and hips raised off the floor the entire time you move through this *vinyāsa*. Stretch the arms, open the chest and bend the back into an arch. Draw the shoulders back and lift the head. At the end of the movement, let the head fall backwards and gaze between the eyebrows.

6 Ṣaṭ

Adho-mukha-śvanāsana (*adho* – downward; *mukha* – facing; *śvana* – dog)
Exhale, lift the hips up, roll over the toes again so that you are on the soles of the feet, and press the heels into the floor. While you roll over the toes, keep your arms, back, legs, and feet fully extended and the knees and hips off the floor. With the arms shoulder-width apart, press the palms and fingers onto the floor, fingers wide, with the index finger pointing forward. Broaden the shoulders and lengthen the spine. Draw uddīyana bandha deeply inwards to facilitate the lengthening and stretching of the entire body. Using *mūla-bandha*, lift the hips up and find your center of gravity. This lightens the body and makes it easier to press the hands and heels into the floor. Be sure to place the feet evenly, hip-width apart, with the toes in line with each other. Draw the chin in towards the chest, round the back slightly and gaze at the navel, or towards the navel (oftentimes it is difficult to see the actual navel when uddīyana bandha is drawn in). Hold this position for a count of five deep breaths.

7 Sapta

Inhale, lift the head up and look for a moment in between the hands. Softly jump forward and, with straight or bent knees, land the feet between the hands, supporting yourself with the strength of the arms. After landing, stretch the arms and legs, keep pressing the hands onto the floor, and open the chest. Draw the shoulders back, straighten out the back, lift the head and look up between the eyebrows.

8 Aṣṭau

Uttānāsana
Exhale, bend forward from the hips with straight legs. Relax the back of the neck, press the tip of the nose into the knees, or in between the shins. Direct the gaze to the tip of the nose.

9 Nava

Inhale, lift the head and come up to standing. At the same time, raise the arms from the front, on a diagonal, or from sides of the body up overhead and press the palms together. Tilt the head back, keeping control in the neck, and gaze up at the tip of the thumbs.

Samasthiti

Exhale, gently lower the arms down straight to the sides, straighten the head, and gaze at the tip of the nose.

Benefits:

In the sun salutation sequence, we establish the physical and mental techniques (*vinyāsa*, sound breathing, *dṛṣṭi* and bandhas) which continue throughout the whole practice.

The sun salutations are a simple and safe series of poses that heat up the body and create a sweat which starts the purification process. This heat keeps the body warm, making it safe to move through the *āsanas*. The breathing initiated in the sun salutations creates a meditative and soothing rhythm for the mind which, in turn, provides space for the sacred dimension of the practice to unfold.

Through practicing the sun salutations and doing *āsanas* correctly, we can heal the body from physical (*deshika*), mental (*manasika*), and spiritual (*adhyāmika*) illnesses and lead a happy life.

The sun salutations in *yoga* are traditionally not only done to cleanse the body and mind, but also to pray to the sun god, "the health minister of the world," for health, prosperity and longevity.

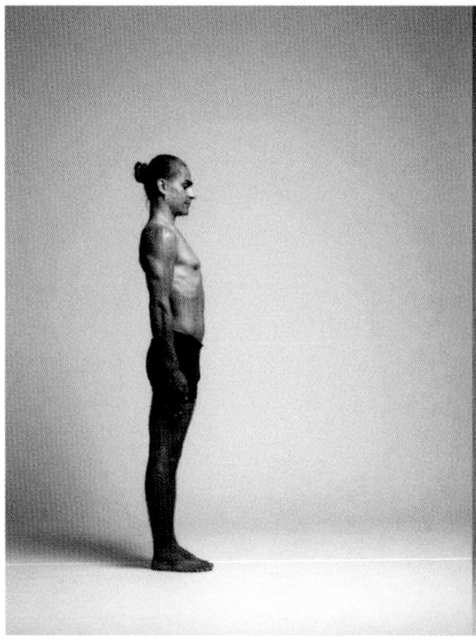
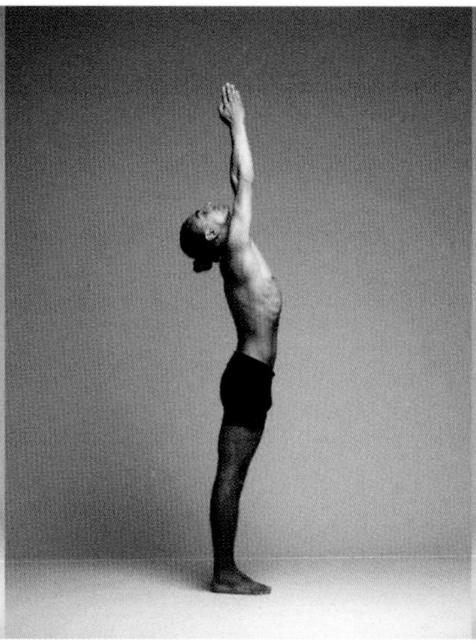
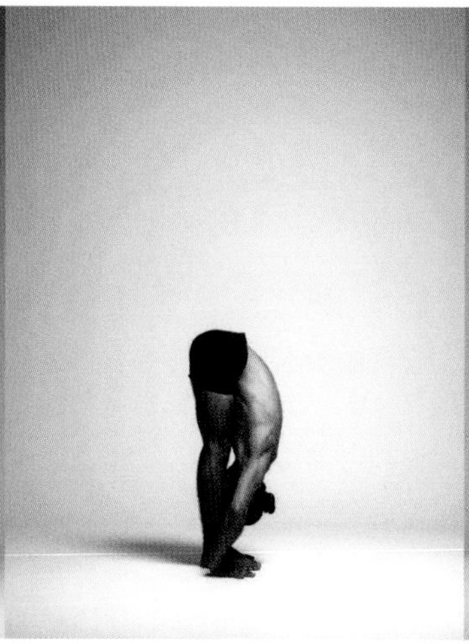
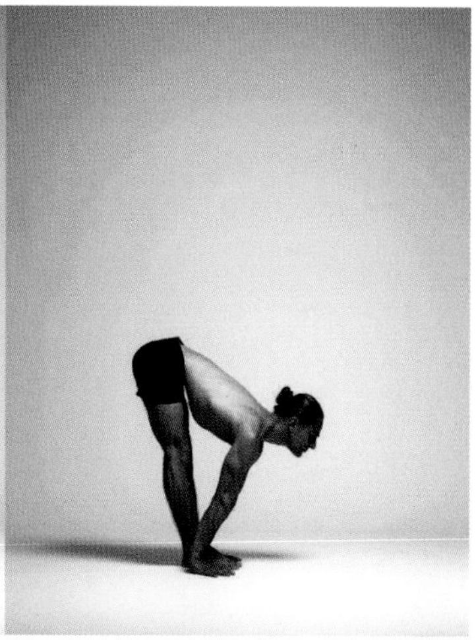
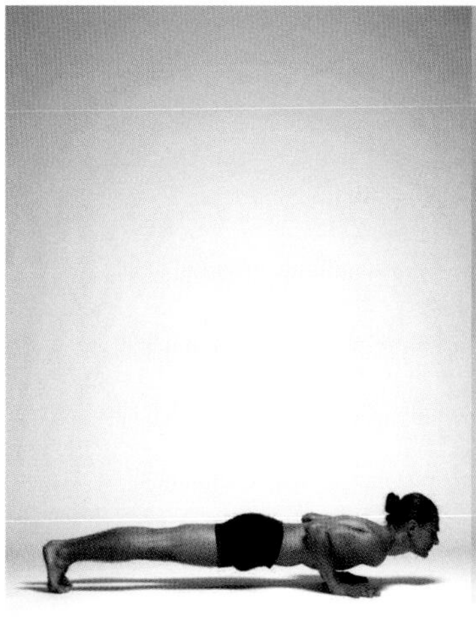
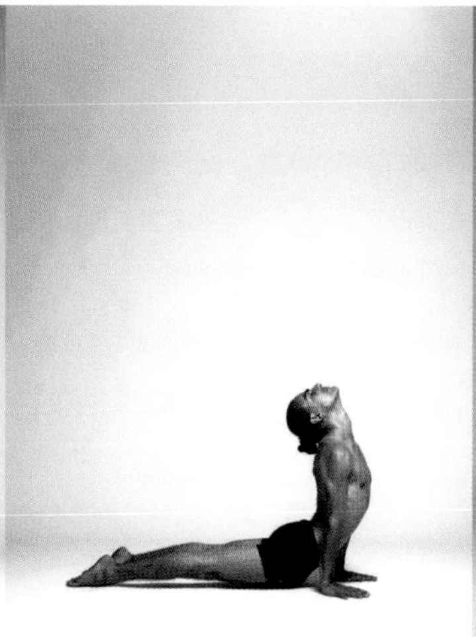
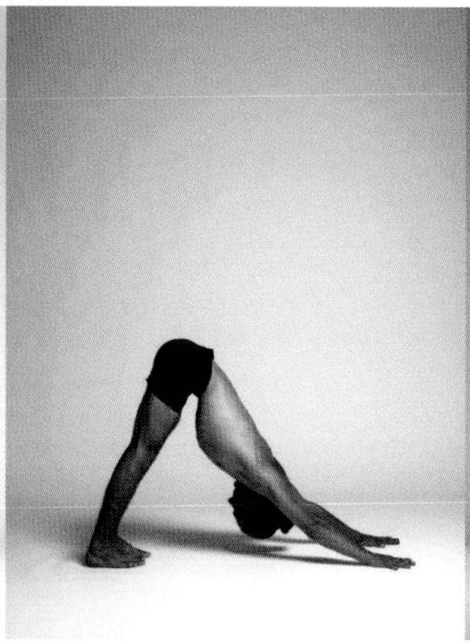
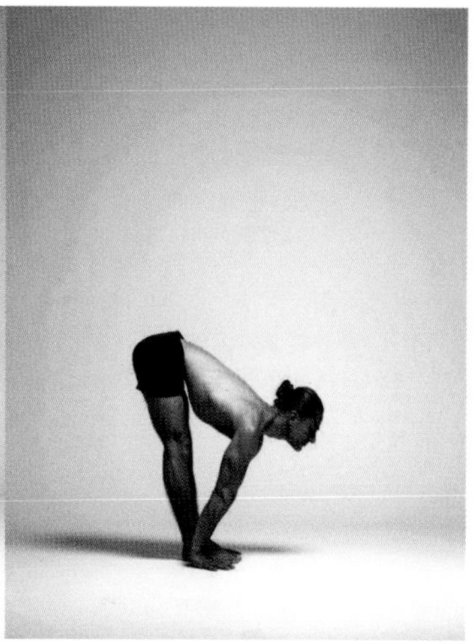
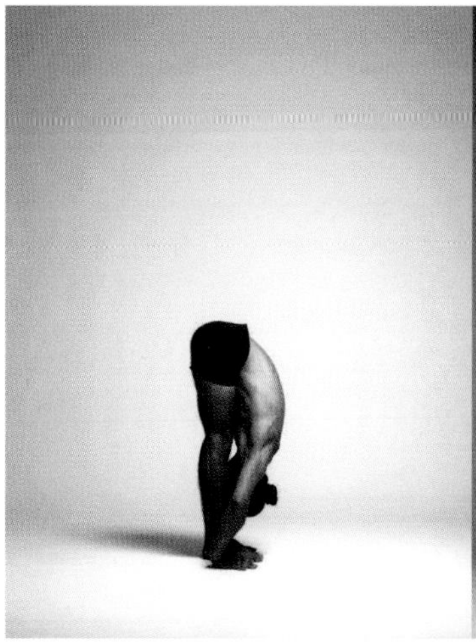
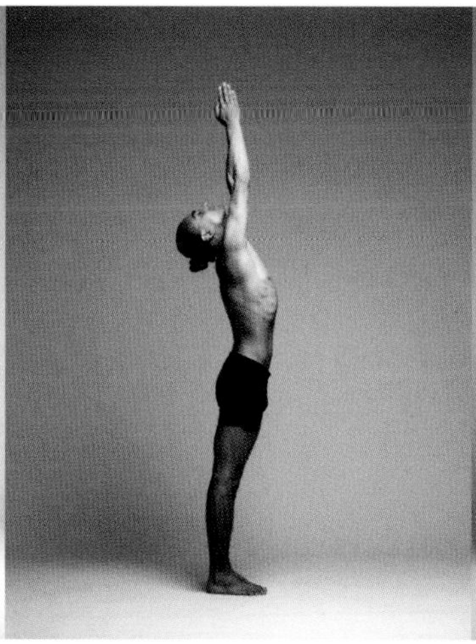
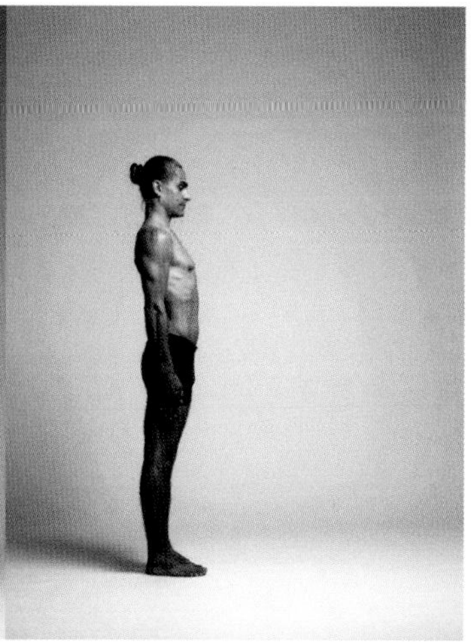

सूर्यनमस्कारः

Sūrya-namaskāra B

Sun salutation B | 17 *vinyāsas*

Note 1: Repeat *Sūrya-namaskāra* B 3–5 times.

Note 2: On *vinyāsas* 3, 5, 9, 13 and 15, you can either gaze to the tip of the nose (*nasāgra*) or between the eyebrows (*bhrūmadhya*).

Samasthitih
Stand straight with the feet together, arms by the sides, and gaze at the tip of the nose.

1 Ekam
Utkaṭāsana (*utkaṭa* – powerful, strong, fierce, uneven)

Inhale, bend the knees and lower the hips as much as possible while keeping the heels on the floor. The feet and knees are pressed together and the back is straight. Lift the hands overhead with straight arms, following the movement of the hands with the head and tilting the head back when the arms are directly overhead. Let the inhalation expand your chest and back, and press the palms and fingers together. Direct the gaze to the tip of the thumbs.

2 Dve
Uttānāsana
Exhale, straighten the legs, release the head and bend forward from the hips, while lowering the arms to the floor. Draw in *uddīyana-bandha*. Place the fingertips in line with the toes, and press the palms onto the floor with the fingers spread apart. Relax the back of the neck and press the tip of the nose onto the knees, or in between the shins. Gaze at the tip of the nose.

Vinyāsas 3–6 are the same as in *Sūrya-namaskāra A.*

7 Sapta
Vīrabhadrāsana (*vīra* – warrior; *bhadra* – good, blessed; Goddess of the hunt)

Inhale, rotate the left heel 85-90 degrees in, so the sole of the foot touches the floor, and the left heel faces the right foot. Lean forward onto the arms and extend the shoulders. Create enough space in order to take a long step forward, and direct the gaze for a moment in between the hands. Lift your right knee towards the sternum, take a long step with the right leg and place the right foot in between the hands; the palms and the left foot stay grounded. Once your right foot is on the floor, bend the right knee just over 90 degrees, and reach the arms up overhead, pressing the palms together. Widen the chest and back with the breath as you lengthen the shoulders and straighten the elbows. The hips, sternum, and chest should face forward, in the same direction as the right knee. Engage the left thigh so that the kneecap lifts up and the whole leg stretches out, and press both feet firmly onto the floor. By drawing in *mūla-bandha*, one creates a strong pelvic floor which can support the body. *Uddīyana bandha* lengthens the spine and sternum. Lean the head back and gaze up.

8 Aṣṭau
Chaturaṅga-daṇḍāsana (*chatur* – four; *aṅga* – limb; *daṇḍa* – stick)
Exhale and lower the hands onto the floor, placing them on either side of the right foot. Take the right foot back to meet the left, placing them hip-width apart. Adjust the left foot so that you are on the balls of both feet. Keep the body straight with both *mūla* and *uddīyana bandha* engaged. Bend the elbows to 90 degrees. Move the chin forward and direct the gaze to the tip of the nose.

Vinyāsas 9 and 10 are the same as the 5th and 6th *vinyāsas* in *Sūrya-namaskāra* A.
Vinyāsas 11 and 12 are the same as the 7th and 8th *vinyāsas* in *Sūrya-namaskāra* B, but the step is taken with the left foot.
Vinyāsas 13–16 are the same as the 5th-8th *vinyāsas* in *Sūrya-namaskāra* A.
Vinyāsa 14 is held for five deep breaths.

17 Saptadaśa
Utkaṭāsana
Inhale, bend the knees, lower the hips as much as possible and press the heels into the floor while squeezing the feet and knees together and elongating the back. Raise the hands, following the movement of the hands with the head, and tilt the head back with a control. Let the inhalation expand the chest and back, and press the hands together overhead, with the palms and fingers together. Gaze at the tip of the thumbs.

Samasthitih
Exhale, straighten the legs, gently bring the head back up; lower the arms alongside the body and gaze at the tip of the nose.

Benefits:
The effects of the *Sūrya-namaskāra* A and *Sūrya-namaskāra* B are similar, although *Sūrya-namaskāra* B opens more the hips, back and arms.

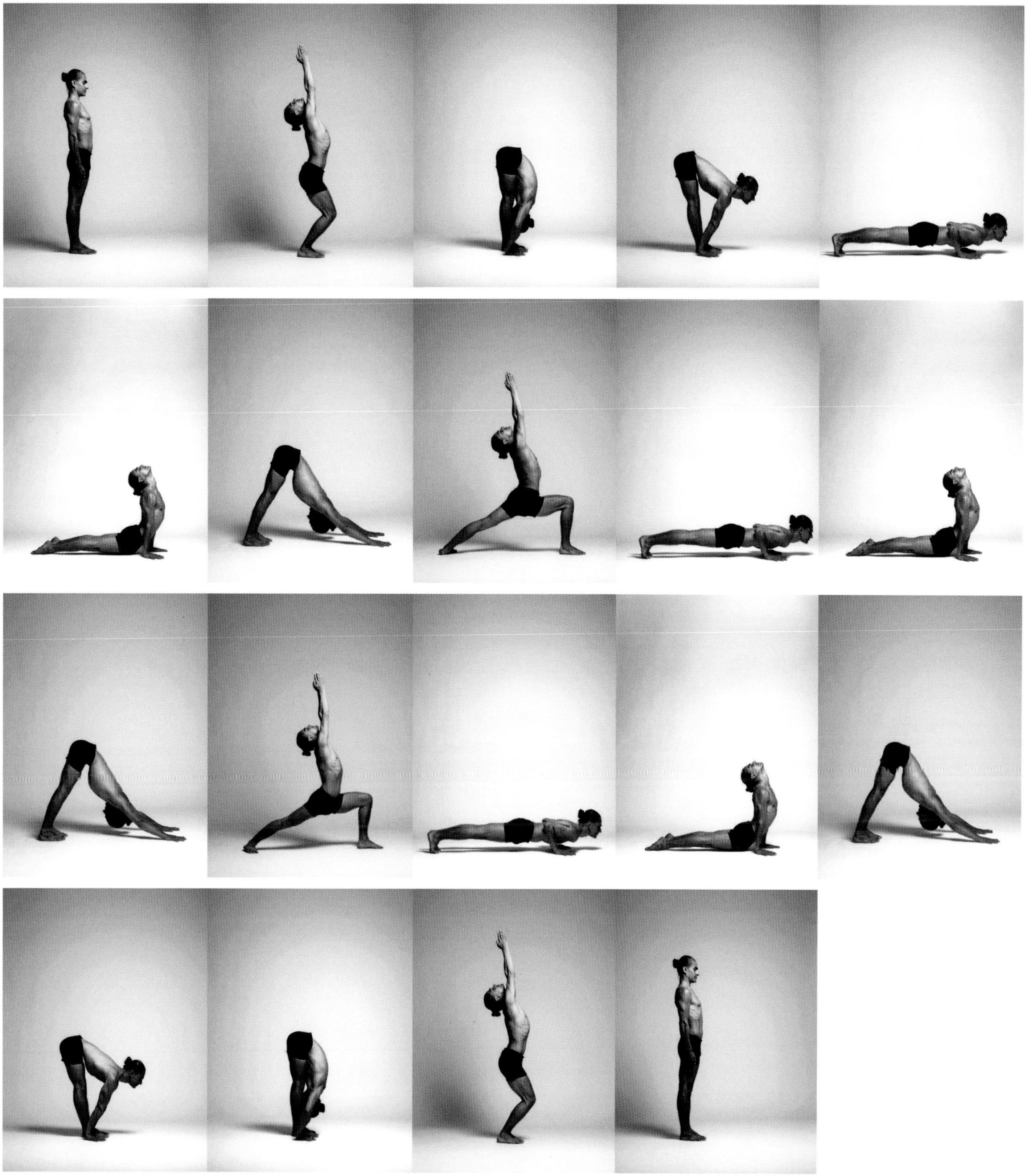

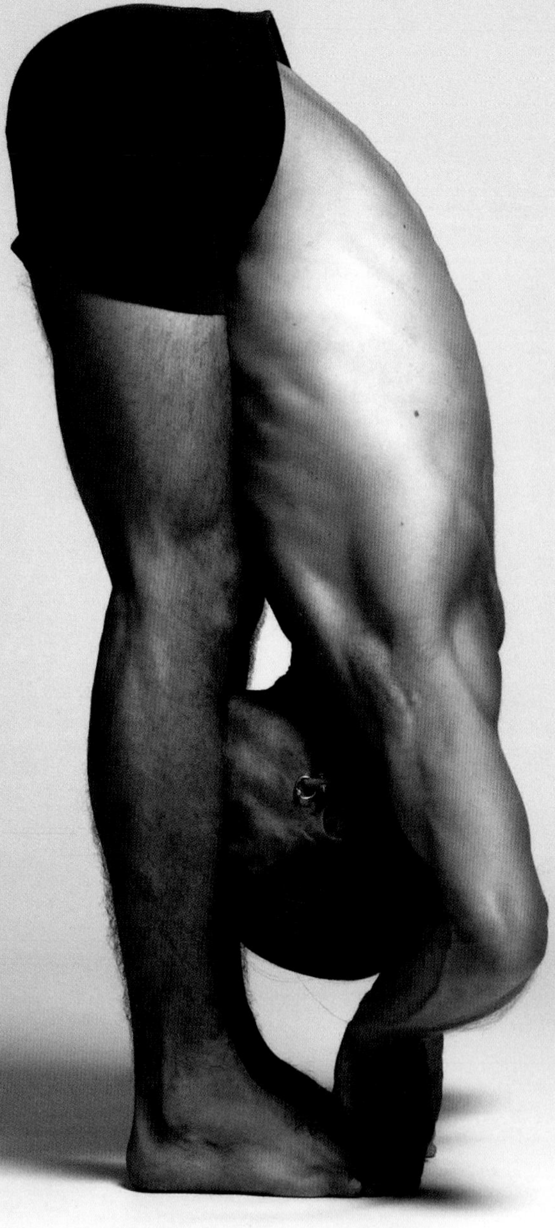

पादाङ्गुष्ठासन

Pādāṅguṣṭhāsana

Big toe pose | 3 *vinyāsas*

Samasthitih 1. *vinyāsa* 2. *vinyāsa* 3. *vinyāsa*

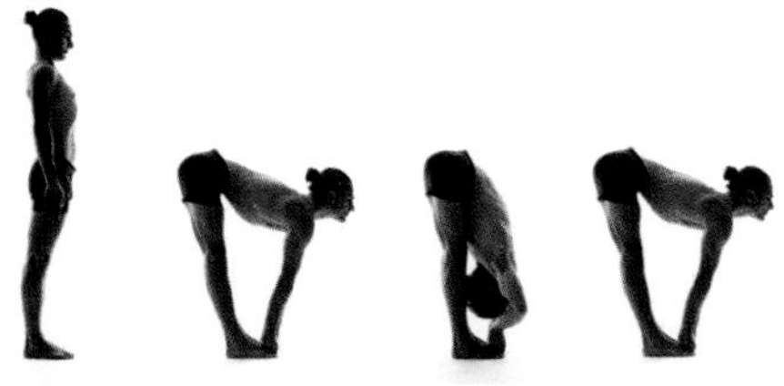

Pādāṅguṣṭhāsana

Pāda – foot; *aṅguṣṭha* – big toe; *āsana* – seat, posture

Note: There are two breaths in the third *vinyāsa*.

Samasthitiḥ
Stand straight with the feet together, arms by the sides and gaze at the tip of the nose.

1 Ekam
Inhale, jump the feet slightly apart, about half the length of your own foot. Bend forward and take hold of your big toes. Open the chest and sternum, stretch out the entire back and lift the head. Straighten the arms and lightly pull on the big toes, in opposition to the upward-moving stretch. Look at the tip of the nose.

2 Dve
Exhale, lower the head, fold forward from the hips with straight legs, and strongly engage *uddīyana-bandha* to straighten the back and to create space to fold in towards the thighs. Pull slightly on the toes, pitch the weight slightly forward into the balls of the feet, keeping both the heels and toes on the floor. Relax the back of the neck and press the tip of the nose in towards the knees, or between the shins, and gaze at the tip of the nose. This is the state of the *āsana*. Stay here for five deep breaths.

3 Trīṇi
Inhale, return to the same position as in the first *vinyāsa*. Lift the chest, lengthen the spine and raise the head. Straighten the arms and pull on the big toes. Exhale, hold the pose and gaze at the tip of the nose.

After the third *vinyāsa*, go directly to the first *vinyāsa* of *Pāda-hastāsana*.

Benefits
The benefits of this pose are similar to the next one. Refer to the list of benefits found in the following position, *Pādā-hastāsana*.

Vinyāsa	Prāṇa	Āsana	Dṛṣṭi	Bandha
Samasthitih		Stand straight		
1 Ekam	in	Jump 1/2 feet apart, take hold of the big toes, lift the head		
2 Dve	out	Bend forward		
This is the state of the *āsana*, hold for 5 deep breaths				
3 Triṇi	in & out	lift head, hold the position		
Samasthitih	in & out	come up, jump feet together		

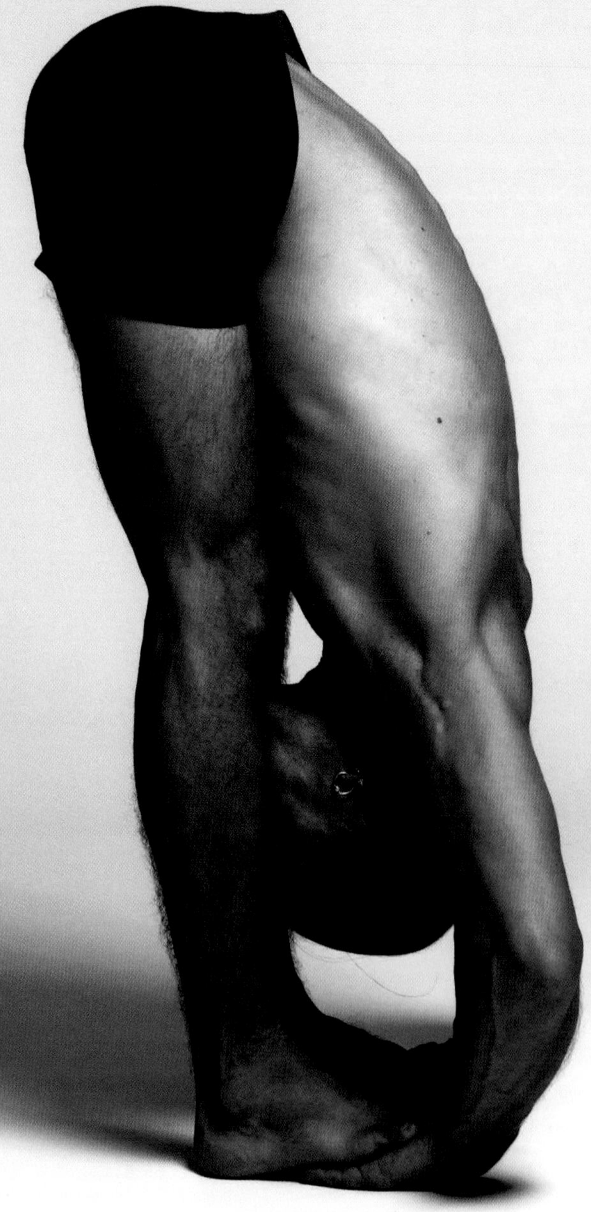

पादहस्तासन

Pāda-hastāsana

Hand to foot pose | 3 *vinyāsas*

1. *vinyāsa* 2. *vinyāsa* 3. *vinyāsa* Samasthiti

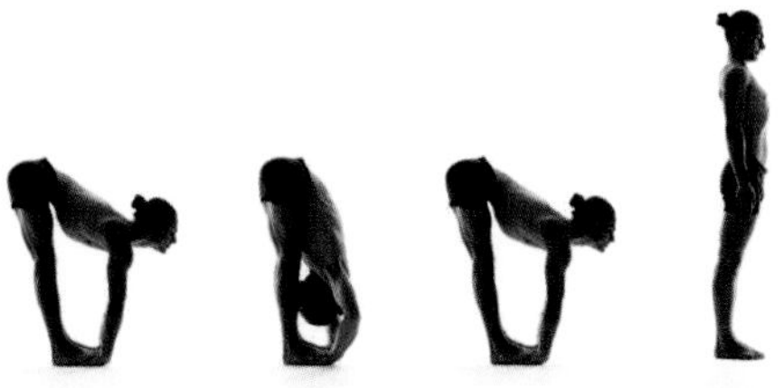

Pāda-hastāsana

Pāda – foot; *hasta* – hand

Note: There are two breaths in the third *vinyāsa*.

Pāda-hastāsana comes directly after the third *vinyāsa* in *Pādāṅguṣṭhāsana*.

1 Ekam
Inhale, place the palms under the soles of the feet with the toes touching the crease of the wrist. Open the chest, lengthen the spine, lift the head and gaze at the tip of the nose.

2 Dve
Exhale, lower the head and bend forward from the hips with straight legs. Relax the back of the neck and bring the head towards the knees or between the shins. Press the feet onto the hands while pulling up with the hands. Pitch the weight slightly forward onto the balls of the feet while keeping the heels grounded. Relax the hamstrings and the lower back, and keep the knees straight. This is the state of the *āsana*. Stay here for five deep breaths, directing the gaze to the tip of the nose.

3 Trīṇi
Inhale, open the chest, lengthen the spine and lift the head up. Straighten the arms and press down lightly on the soles of the feet, in opposition to the upward-moving stretch of the upper body. Hold this position for a full exhalation. Gaze at the tip of the nose.

Samasthitih
Inhale, come up to standing with a straight spine, the arms relaxed against the sides of the body. Exhale, jump the feet together and gaze at the tip of the nose.

Benefits:
The effects of the *Pādāṅguṣṭhāsana* and *Pāda-hastāsana* are similar, although *Pāda-hastāsana* is a bit deeper position. Both of these positions:

- strengthen the stomach, hips and leg muscles
- stimulate and purify the liver and spleen
- cleanse the urine and increase the quantity of digestive fluid
- heal the rectum and anus
- reduce gas
- dissolve excess fat from the stomach and hips.

Full vinyāsa technique

Vinyāsa	Prāṇa	Āsana	Dṛṣṭi	Bandha
Samasthitih		Stand straight		
1 Ekam	in	Jump 1/2 feet apart, hands under the feet, lift the head		
2 Dve	out	Bend forward		
This is the state of the *āsana*, hold for 5 deep breaths				
3 Trīṇi	in & out	Lift head, hold the position		
Samasthitih	in & out	Come up, jump feet together		

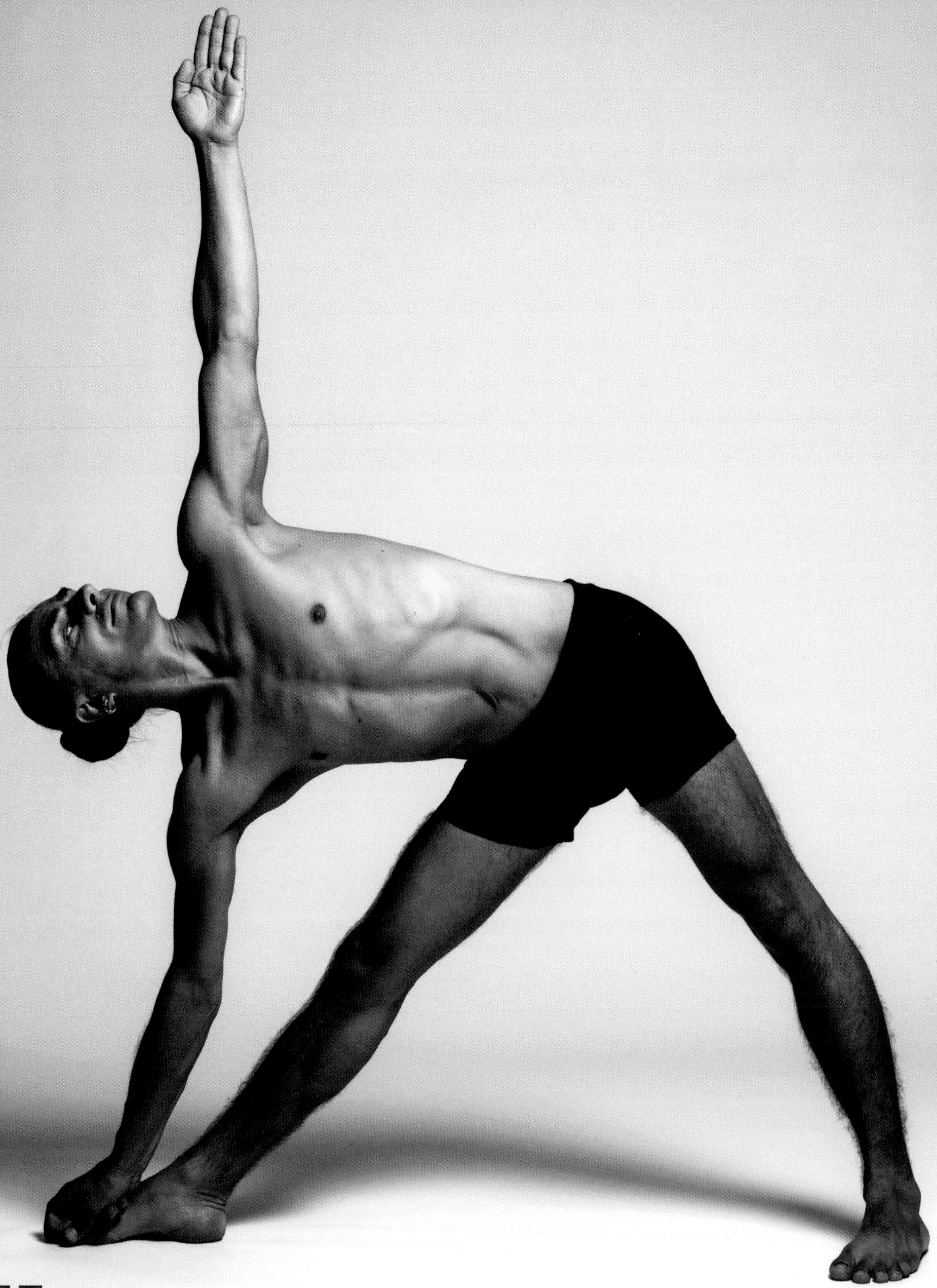

उत्थितत्रिकोणासन क

Utthita-trikoṇāsana A

Extended triangle pose A | 5 *vinyāsas*

Samasthiti 1. *vinyāsa* 2. *vinyāsa* 3. *vinyāsa* 4. *vinyāsa* 5. *vinyāsa*

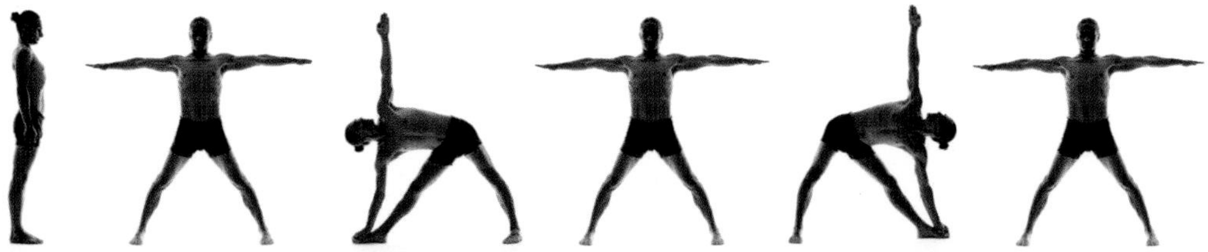

Utthita-trikoṇāsana A

Utthita – extended, intense; *tri* – three; *kona* – angle

Samasthitih
Stand straight with the feet together, arms by the sides, and gaze at the tip of the nose.

1 Ekam
Inhale, jump out to the right and separate the legs about three feet from each other (use your own foot to determine the proper length, rather than using any official measurement). While jumping, extend the arms out to the sides, palms down. Both feet will be facing forward upon landing. Broaden the shoulders by extending through the arms, open the chest and straighten the spine. Gaze at the tip of the nose.

2 Dve
The state of the āsana on the right side
Exhale, and turn the right foot 90 degrees out, so that the toes point towards the back of the mat. The right heel should remain on the floor and the left foot will point directly to the side of the mat in an 85-90 degree angle. Both feet should be firmly grounded.

Note: Unlike many other forms of *yoga* where the left foot is turned about 45 degrees inward, the left foot remains 85-90 degrees out to the side in *Aṣṭāṅga yoga*. This position creates the side and hip-opening effects of the *āsana*.

Reach the right arm out and over the right leg, and take hold of the right big toe with the first two fingers and thumb. Extend your left arm straight up to the ceiling, in line with the sternum, keeping the elbows straight and fingers together. Engage *mūla-bandha* and *uddīyana-bandha* to ground yourself in the pose. Lift the left hip up slightly, rotate the chest out towards the side, and turn the head to gaze up at the left hand. The neck should be straight, in a relaxed yet controlled position. Place the right side of the body over the right thigh, so that the body is in line with the legs. Straighten the legs and engage the thigh muscles. This is the state of the *āsana* on the right side. Stay here for five deep breaths. Gaze at the left hand.

3 Trīṇi
Inhale, and come up with straight arms and a firm body using the support of the bandhas. Turn the right foot forward (to face the side of the mat), and stand in the same position as in the first *vinyāsa*. Direct the gaze to the tip of the nose.

The 4th and 5th *vinyāsas* are the same as the 2nd and 3rd, but are done on the left side.

The 4th *vinyāsa* is the state of the left side position. Breathe deeply five times.

After the 5th *vinyāsa*, move directly into the 2nd *vinyāsa* in *Utthita-trikoṇāsana* B.

Benefits
The benefits of this pose are similar to the next one. Refer to the list of benefits found in the following position, *Utthita-trikoṇāsana* B.

Vinyāsa	Prāṇa	Āsana	Dṛṣṭi	Bandha
Samasthitih		Stand straight		
1 Ekam	in	Jump 3 feet apart to the right		
2 Dve	out	Turn right foot out, take hold of the right big toe		
This is the state of the *āsana* for the right side, hold for 5 deep breaths				
3 Trīṇi	in	Come up, straighten the right foot		
4 Catvāri	out	Turn left foot out, take hold of left big toe		
This is the state of the *āsana* for the left side, hold for 5 deep breaths				
5 Pañca	in	Come up, straighten the left foot		
Samasthitih	out	Jump to the front of the mat		

उत्थितत्रिकोणासन ख

Utthita-trikoṇāsana B

Extended triangle pose B | 5 *vinyāsas*

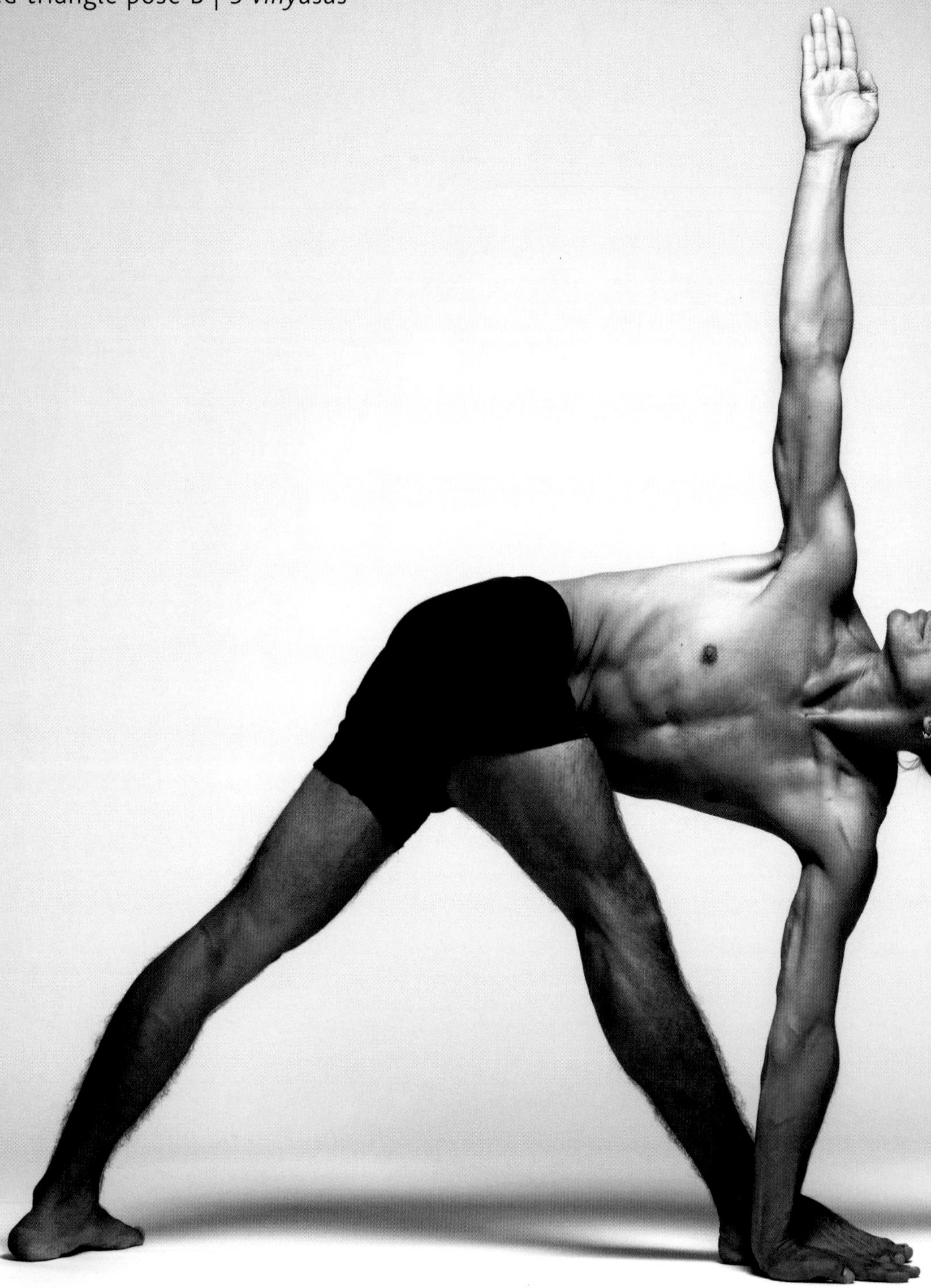

continuing | 2. *vinyāsa* | 3. *vinyāsa* | 4. *vinyāsa* | 5. *vinyāsa* | Samasthiti

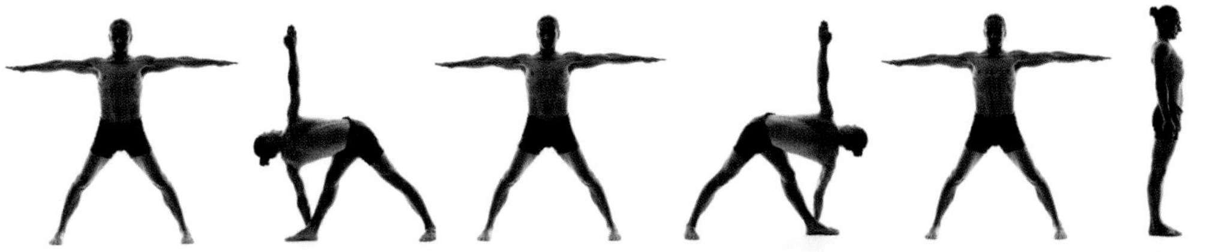

Utthita-trikoṇāsana B

Utthita-trikoṇāsana B comes directly after the fifth *vinyāsa* in *Utthita-trikoṇāsana* A.

2 Dve

The state of the āsana on the right side

Exhale, turn the right foot 90 degrees out towards the right, facing the back of the mat. With the arms out to the side, lift up from the left hip to relieve pressure from the left knee and turn the hips and the chest towards the right leg. Place the left arm onto the floor beside the outer edge of the right foot and stretch the right arm directly up to the ceiling. Place the left palm on the ground, with the fingers spread wide, the middle finger pointing forward, and the fingertips in line with the right toes. Keep the right hand aligned with the sternum, and press the fingers together. Open the chest out to the side and rotate the head to gaze towards the right hand, keeping the neck relaxed and straight. The left side is directly above the right thigh and in line with the legs, as you twist deeply in the spine. Keep the hips evenly lifted. Press the left hand and right foot firmly onto the floor, and stretch the right shoulder and arm up to the ceiling. Straighten the legs and engage the thigh muscles. This is the state of the *āsana* on the right side. Stay here for five deep breaths, gazing at the right hand.

3 Trīṇi

Inhale and come up, turning the right foot forward and stand as in the first *vinyāsa*. Come up with a straight body, fully engaging through the bandhas. Direct the gaze to the tip of the nose.

The 4th and 5th *vinyāsas* are the same as the 2nd and 3rd, but are done on the left side.

The 4th *vinyāsa* is the state of the left side position. Breathe deeply five times.

Samasthitih

Exhale and jump to the front of the mat, with the feet together, lowering the arms to the sides of the body. Gaze at the tip of the nose.

Benefits:

Utthita-trikoṇāsana A and *Utthita-trikoṇāsana* B have similar benefits. Both poses:

- strengthen the feet, hip, and back muscles
- dissolve excess fat from the hips and waist
- improve digestion and increase production of digestive fluid
- relieve difficulties in breathing and expand the trachea and chest
- circulate the breath more freely in the throat and chest
- correct the alignment of the spine (such as scoliosis)
- relaxe the nervous system (in the rotation in *Trikonāsana* B).

Vinyāsa	Prāṇa	Āsana	Dṛṣṭi	Bandha
Samasthitih		Stand straight		
1 Ekam	In	Jump 3 feet apart to the right		
2 Dve	out	Turn right foot out, left palm on the outer side of the right foot		
This is the state of the *āsana* for the right side, hold for 5 deep breaths				
3 Trīṇi	In	Come up, straighten the right foot		
4 Catvāri	out	Turn left foot out, right palm on the outer side of the left foot		
This is the state of the *āsana* for the left side, hold for 5 deep breaths				
5 Pañca	In	Come up, straighten the left foot		
Samasthitih	out	Jump to the front of the mat		

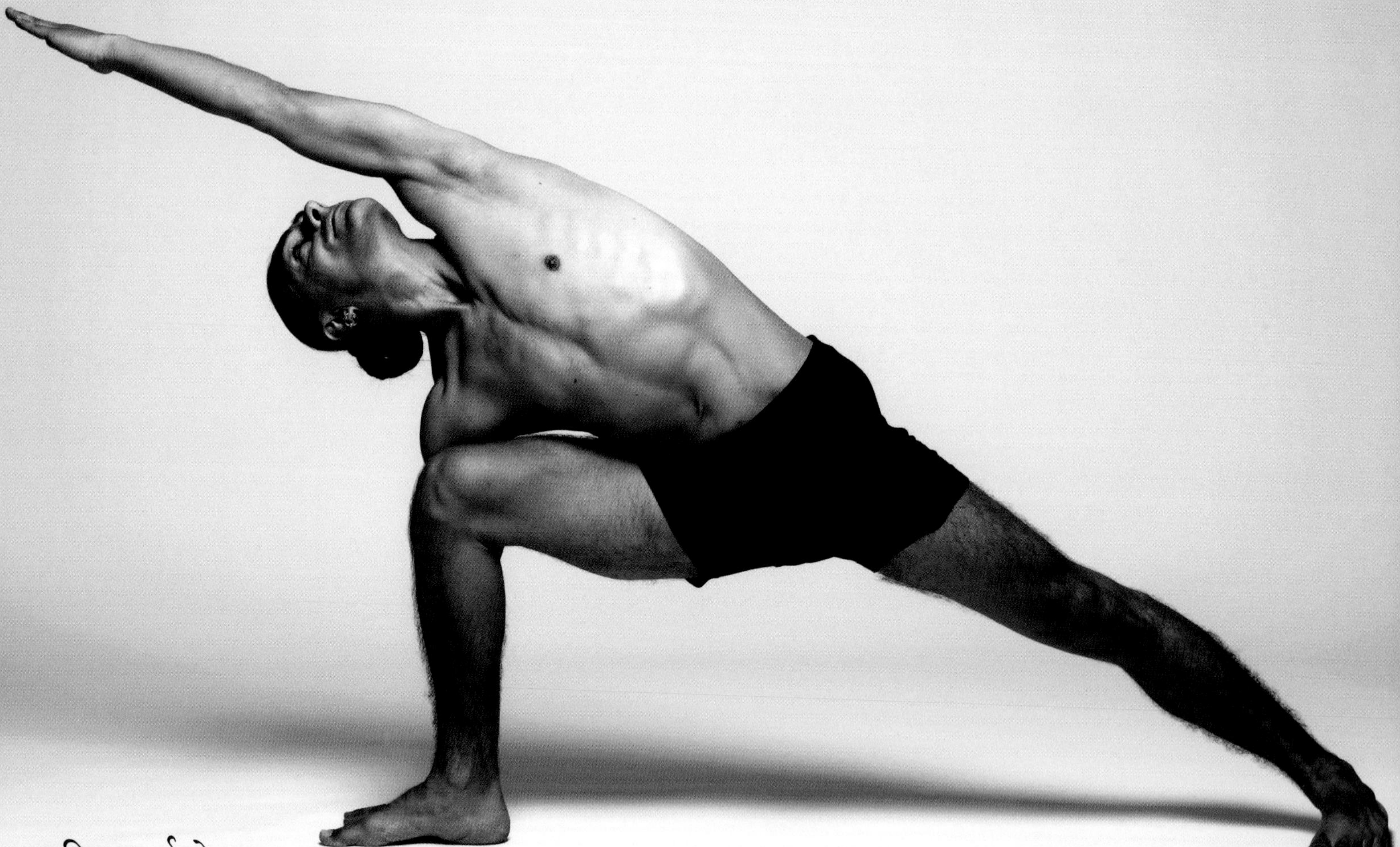

उत्थितपार्श्वकोणासन क

Utthita-pārśvakoṇāsana A

Extended side angle pose A | 5 *vinyāsas*

Samasthitih 1. *vinyāsa* 2. *vinyāsa* 3. *vinyāsa* 4. *vinyāsa* 5. *vinyāsa*

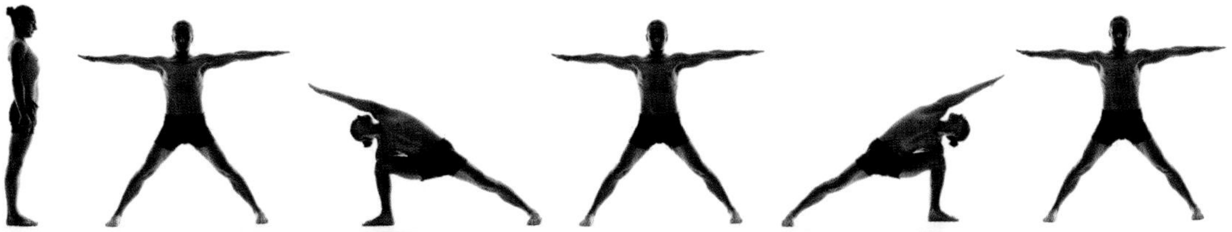

Utthita-pārśvakoṇāsana A

Utthita – extended, intense; *parśva* – side; *koṇa* – angle

Samasthitih

Stand straight with the feet together, arms by the sides, and gaze at the tip of the nose.

1 Ekam

Inhale, jump to the right and land five feet apart with the toes forward. While jumping, reach the arms out to the side and the palms facing down. Stretch the shoulders by elongating the arms away from one another. Gaze at the tip of the nose.

2 Dve
The state of the āsana on the right side

Exhale, turn the right foot 90 degrees out to the right, towards the back of the mat, keeping the heels down and in line with each other. The left foot stays pointing forward to the side of the mat in an 85-90 degree angle.

Note: Unlike many other forms of *yoga* where the left foot is turned about 45 degrees inward, the left foot remains 85–90 degrees out to the side in *Aṣṭāṅga yoga*. This position creates the side and hip-opening effects of the *āsana*.

Bend the right knee just over 90 degrees and, following the right hand with the gaze, place the palm on the floor, on outer side of the right foot. The fingertips are spread wide, in line with the toes, with the middle finger pointing forward. Extend the left arm straight up over the ear, forming a long line with the left side of the torso and left leg. Open the chest, turn the head up towards the underside of the arm, and relax the back of the neck. Keep the fingers together and gaze at the fingertips of the left hand, with the palm facing down. Press the left foot onto the floor, creating a strong base from which the left side can stretch. Straighten the left leg and stretch the left hip, shoulder and upper body by extending the left arm forward. Relax through the shoulders and engage *mūla-bandha* to stabilize the hips, and *uddīyana-bandha* to lengthen the body. This is the state of the *āsana* on the right side. Stay here for five deep breaths. Gaze at the fingertips of the left hand.

3 Trīṇi

Inhale and with the strength of the legs and bandhas, come up with straight arms and a stable body. Shift the right foot forward and come to stand as in the first *vinyāsa*. Gaze at the tip of the nose.

The 4th and 5th *vinyāsas* are the same as the 2nd and 3rd, but are done on the left side.

The 4th *vinyāsa* is the state of the left side position. Breathe deeply five times.

After the 5th *vinyāsa*, move directly into the 2nd *vinyāsa* in *Utthita-pārśvakoṇāsana B*.

Benefits:

The benefits of this pose are similar to the next one. Refer to the list of benefits found in the following position, *Utthita-pārśvakoṇāsana B*.

Vinyāsa	Prāṇa	Āsana	Dṛṣṭi	Bandha
Samasthitih		Stand straight		
1 Ekam	In	jump 5 feet apart to the right		
2 Dve	out	Turn right foot out, bend the right knee, right hand to floor, left arm over ear		
This is the state of the āsana for the right side, hold for 5 deep breaths				
3 Trīṇi	In	Come up, straighten the right foot		
4 Catvāri	out	Turn left foot out, bend the left knee, left hand to the floor, right arm over ear		
This is the state of the āsana for the left side, hold for 5 deep breaths				
5 Pañca	In	Come up, straighten the left foot		
Samasthitih	out	Jump to the front of the mat		

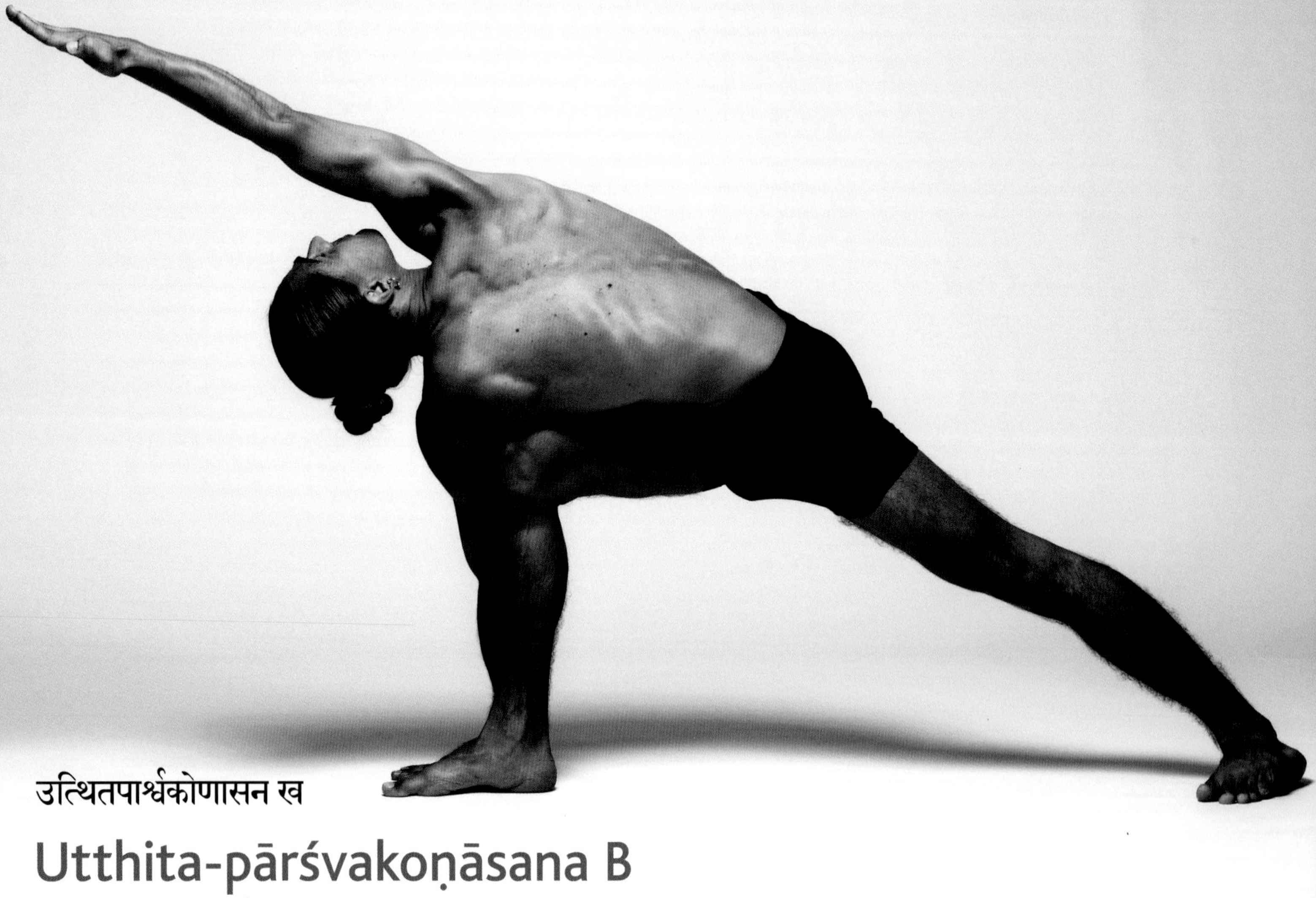

उत्थितपार्श्वकोणासन ख

Utthita-pārśvakoṇāsana B

Extended side angle pose B | 5 *vinyāsas*

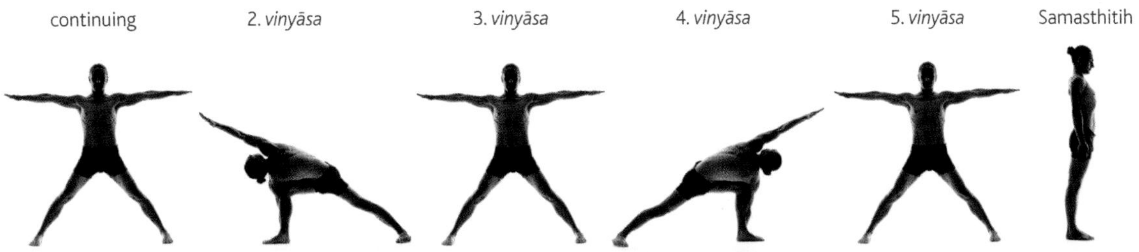
continuing
2. vinyāsa
3. vinyāsa
4. vinyāsa
5. vinyāsa
Samasthitih

Utthita-pārśvakoṇāsana B

Utthita-pārśvakoṇāsana B follows the 5th *vinyāsa* in *Utthita-pārśvakoṇāsana* A.

2 Dve
The state of the āsana on the right side
Exhale, turn the right foot 90 degrees out to the side, keeping the heels grounded and in line with each other, as in *Utthita-pārśvakoṇāsana* A. Bend the right knee just over 90 degrees and twist the chest and hips over the right leg. Lift up from the left hip to relieve any pressure in the left knee. Bend down as you twist the spine and chest towards the right. Place the left upper arm over the right thigh, slightly above the knee. Hold it in place, so it doesn't slide over the knee, and place the left palm onto the floor. The fingers should be spread wide, with the middle finger pointing forward and the fingertips aligned with the toes. Follow the left hand with your gaze. Straighten the right arm up and over the ear, in line with the left leg and upper body. Turn the chest and head upwards, relax the back of the neck and gaze at the right fingertips, with the palm facing down and fingers together. Press the left foot into the floor, engage the thighs, and straighten the leg. Keep the hips stable by engaging *mūla-bandha* and release the entire spine into the twist. Engage *uddīyana-bandha* to lengthen and open the body up. This is the state of the *āsana* on the right side. Stay here for five deep breaths. Gaze at the right fingertips.

3 Trīṇi
Inhale, come up with straight arms and a stable body using the support of the legs and both bandhas. Shift the right foot forward, and come to stand as in the first *vinyāsa*. Direct the gaze to the tip of the nose.

The 4th and 5th *vinyāsas* are the same as the 2nd and 3rd, but are done on the left side.

The 4th *vinyāsa* is the state of the left-side position. Breathe deeply five times.

Samasthiti
While exhaling, jump forward to the front of the mat, feet together, arms to the side, and the gaze at the tip of the nose.

Benefits:
Utthita pārśvakoṇāsana A and Utthita-pārśvakoṇāsana B have similar benefits. Both poses:
- strengthen the back, hips and legs
- open the ankles and knees
- dissolve excess fat from the hips and waist
- stimulate the digestive organs
- relieve lower back pain
- alleviate breathing issues (mainly from the rotation in Parshvakonāsana B)
- correct the alignment of the spine
- release the nerves around the spine.

Vinyāsa	Prāṇa	Āsana	Dṛṣṭi	Bandha
Samasthitih		Stand straight		
1 Ekam	In	Jump 5 feet apart to the right		
2 Dve	out	Turn right foot out, bend the right knee, left hand to floor, right arm over ear		
This is the state of the āsana for the right side, hold for 5 deep breaths				
3 Trīṇi	In	Come up, straighten the right foot		
4 Catvāri	out	Turn left foot out, bend the left knee, right hand to the floor, left arm over ear		
This is the state of the āsana for the left side, hold for 5 deep breaths				
5 Pañca	In	Come up, straighten the left foot		
Samasthitih	out	Jump to the front of the mat		

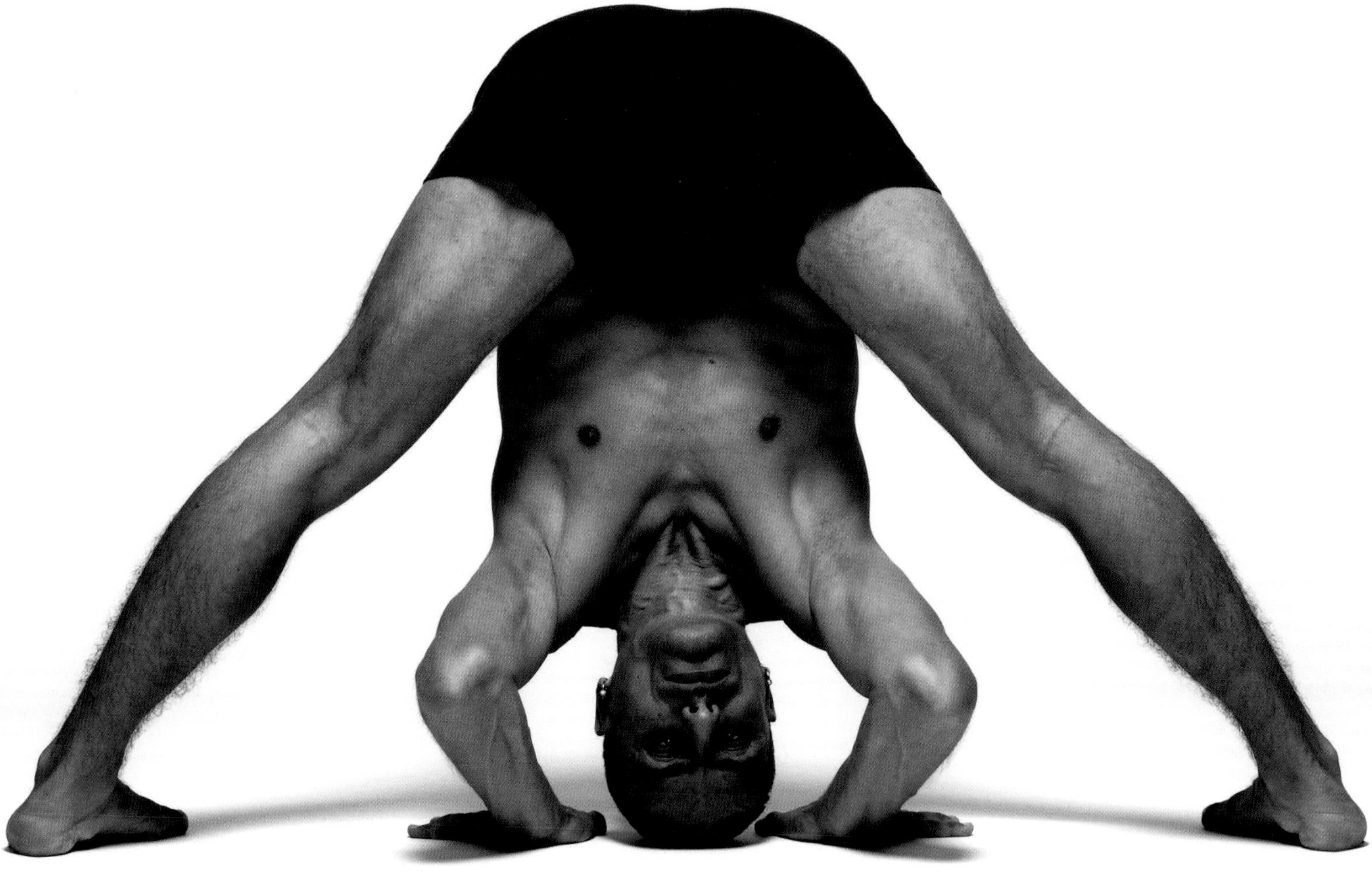

प्रसारितपादोत्तानासन क

Prasārita-padottānāsana A

Wide-foot forward bend pose A | 5 *vinyāsas*

Samasthitih 1. *vinyāsa* 2. *vinyāsa* 3. *vinyāsa* 4. *vinyāsa* 5. *vinyāsa*

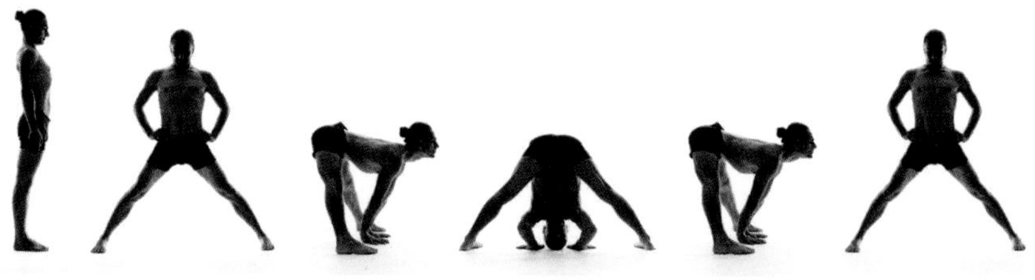

Prasārita-pādottānāsana A

Prasārita – wide, opened, outstretched; *pāda* – foot; *ut* – deep, strong, intense; *tāna* – stretch, extend, lengthen

Note: There are two breaths in the 2nd and 4th *vinyāsas*.

Samasthiti
Stand straight with the feet together, arms by the sides, and gaze at the tip of the nose.

1 Ekam
Inhale, jump five feet out to the right, with the toes pointing straight forward. While jumping, bring both hands to your waist, with the fingertips pointing in towards *uddīyana-bandha* (i.e. lower abdomen) and lift the chest. Gaze at the tip of the nose.

2 Dve
Exhale, bend forward from the hips. Place the hands shoulder-width apart on the floor, fingertips in line with the toes. Gaze at the space between the hands and check their placement. Spread the fingers wide, with the middle finger pointing forward, and press the palms into the floor.

Inhale slowly, pressing the palms down, straighten the arms and lift the head. Lengthen the spine and expand the chest. Apply *mūla-bandha* to support the hips, as the feet remain grounded into the mat. Draw in *uddīyana-bandha* to open the chest and straighten the back. Gaze at the tip of the nose.

3 Trīṇi
Exhale, lower the head, strongly engaging *uddīyana-bandha* and bending forward down between the legs. Release *mūla-bandha* slightly to relax through the hips. Press the hands into the floor to ease the forward bend and lower the crown of the head to the floor with a straight and relaxed neck. This is the state of the *āsana*. Take five deep breaths here, gazing at the tip of the nose.

4 Catvāri
Inhale, keep pressing the palms into the floor and straighten the arms. Open the chest, lengthen the spine, and lift the head up, as in the second *vinyāsa*. Gaze at the tip of the nose.

Hold this position for an exhalation as well.

5 Pañca
Inhale, place the hands on the hips. Come to stand up, while simultaneously keeping uddīyana and *mūla-bandha* engaged to support the movement. Exhale, to complete this *vinyāsa*. Gaze at the tip of the nose.

From here, move directly into the next *āsana*. On the next inhalation, stretch the arms out to the sides. Count this as the first *vinyāsa* in *Prasārita-pādottānāsana* B.

Benefits:
Refer to the list of benefits found at the end of the description for *Prasārita-pādottānāsana* D.

Vinyāsa	Prāṇa	Āsana	Dṛṣṭi	Bandha
Samasthitih		Stand straight		
1 Ekam	in	Jump 5 feet apart to the right, hands on the hips		
2 Dve	out & in	Hands to floor, stretch out, head up		
3 Trīṇi	out	Bend forward		
This is the state of the āsana, hold for 5 deep breaths.				
4 Catvāri	in & out	Stretch out, head up, hold pose		
5 Pañca	In (& out)	Hands to hips, come up hold the pose		
Samasthitih	out	jump to the front of the mat		

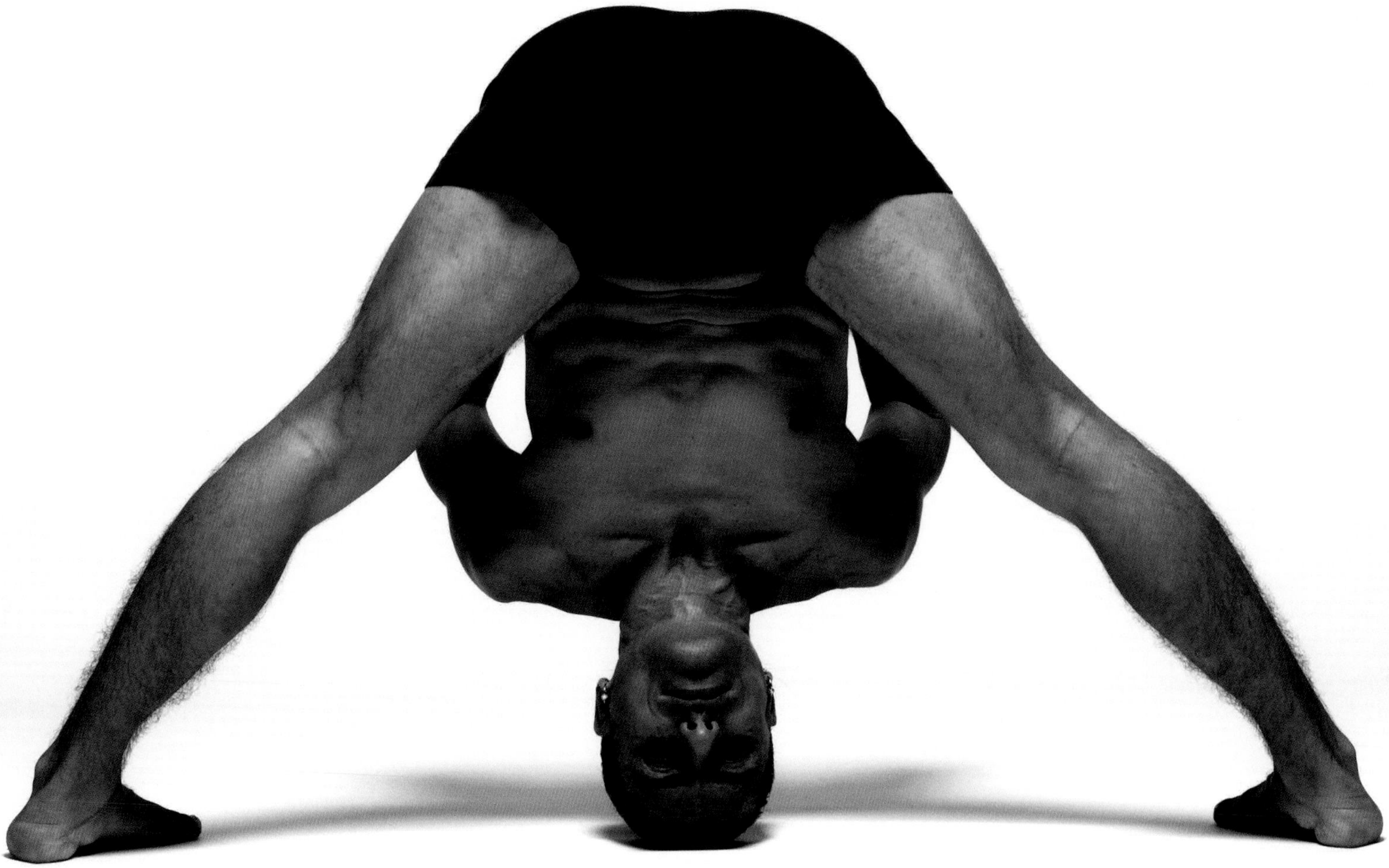

प्रसारितपादोत्तानासन ख

Prasārita-pādottānāsana B

Wide-foot forward bend pose B | 5 *vinyāsas*

1. *vinyāsa* 2. *vinyāsa* 3. *vinyāsa* 4. *vinyāsa*

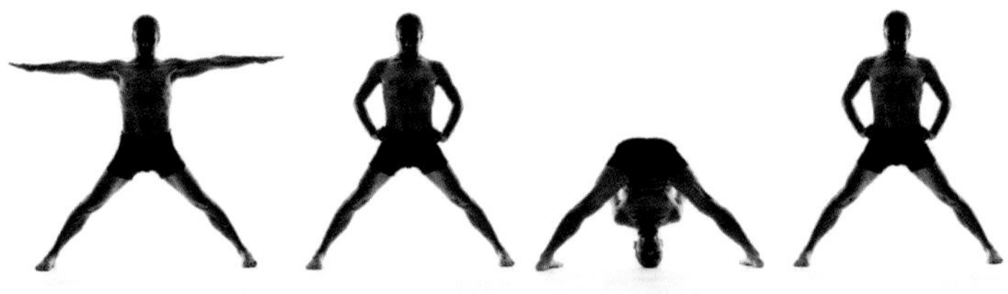

Prasārita-pādottānāsana B

Note: Two breaths in the 2nd and 4th *vinyāsas*.

Prasārita-pādottānāsana B follows directly after the 5th vinyāsa in Prasārita-pādottānāsana A

1 Ekam
Inhale, extend the arms out to the side, palms facing down and shoulders relaxed. Gaze at the tip of the nose.

2 Dve
Exhale, place the hands on the hips, while keeping the chest open.

Inhale and draw in *uddīyana-bandha* as you widen the chest, while engaging *mūla-bandha* to support the hips. Gaze at the tip of the nose.

3 Trīṇi
Exhale, strongly engage *uddīyana-bandha* and bend forward between the legs. Lower the crown of the head to the floor in between the feet, relaxing and lengthening the back of your neck. Release *mūla-bandha* slightly to relax through the hips. Straighten the legs, press the feet into the ground and engage the thighs. This is the state of the *āsana*. Take five deep breaths here and gaze at the tip of the nose.

4 Catvāri
Inhale and keep hold of your hips as you come up to stand. Fully engage uddīyana and *mūla-bandha* to support the lower back.

Stay in this posture as you exhale completely. Gaze at the tip of the nose.

From the 4th *vinyāsa*, go directly to the next *āsana*, *Prasārita-pādottānāsana* C. Stretch the arms out to the sides while inhaling, counting this as the 1st *vinyāsa* in *Prasārita-pādottānāsana* C.

Benefits:
Refer to the list of benefits found at the end of the description for *Prasārita-pādottānāsana* D.

Vinyāsa	Prāṇa	Āsana	Dṛṣṭi	Bandha
Samasthitih		Stand straight		
1 Ekam	in	Jump 5 feet apart to the right, hands out to the sides		
2 Dve	out & in	Hands on the hips, open the chest		
3 Trīṇi	out	Bend forward, keeping the hands on the hips		
This is the state of the āsana, hold for 5 deep breaths				
4 Catvāri	in & out	Come up, hold the pose		
5 Pañca	in	Hands out to the sides		
Samasthitih	out	Jump to the front of the mat		

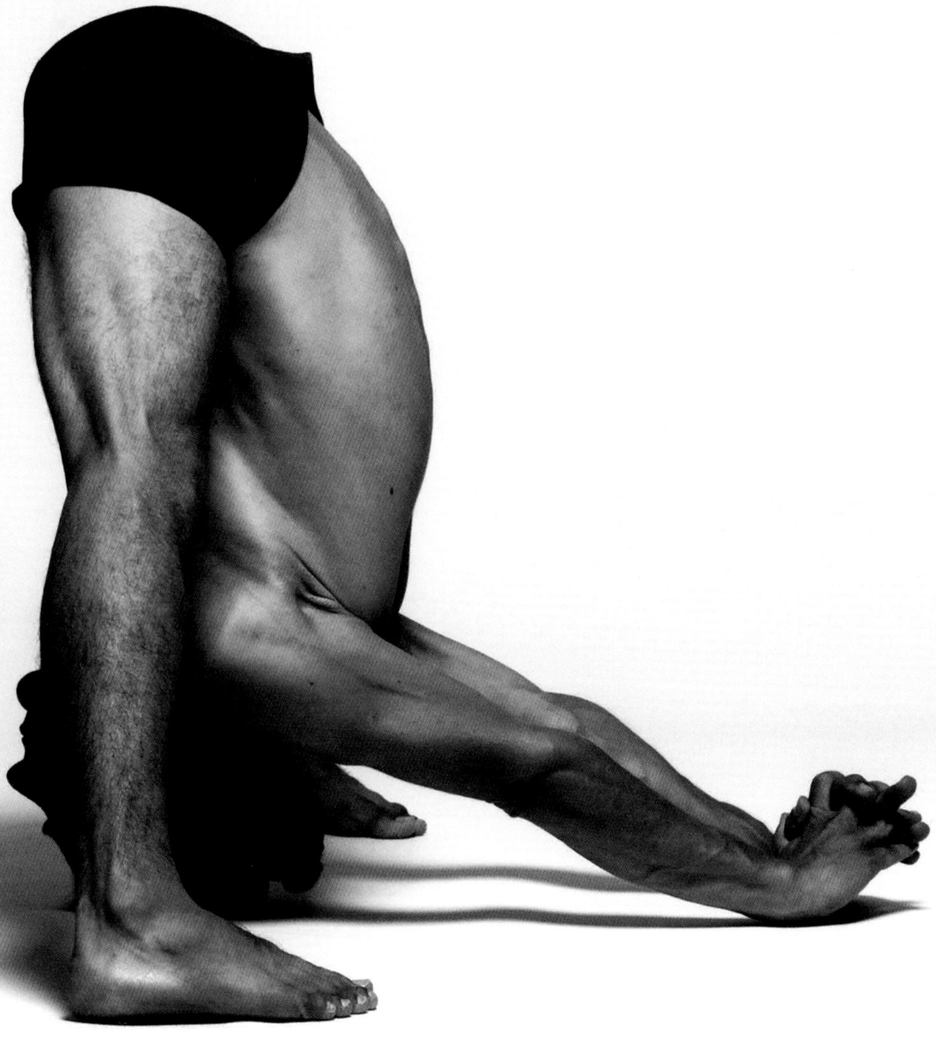

प्रसारितपादोत्तानासन ग

Prasārita-pādottānāsana C

Wide-foot forward bend pose C | 5 *vinyāsas*

1. *vinyāsa* 2. *vinyāsa* 3. *vinyāsa* 4. *vinyāsa*

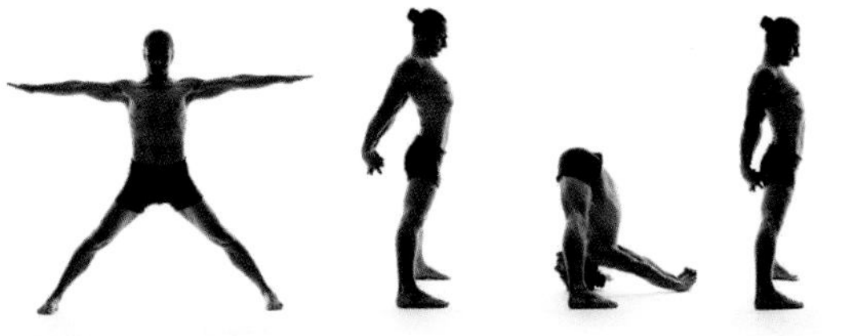

Prasārita-pādottānāsana C

Note 1: There are two breaths in the 2nd and 4th *vinyāsas*
Note 2: The palms can be held (instead of turned outward) in in the 3rd *vinyāsa*.

Prasārita-pādottānāsana C flows directly from the 4th *vinyāsa* in *Prasārita-pādottānāsana* B.

1 Ekam
Inhale, extend the arms out to the side, palms facing down and shoulders relaxed. Gaze at the tip of the nose.

2 Dve
Exhale, bring the arms behind the back, interlace the fingers, draw the shoulders back and turn the palms outward. Inhale, stretch the arms and open the chest, sternum and collar bones. Gaze at the tip of the nose.

3 Trīṇi
Exhale, bend forward and press the crown of the head down into the floor with a straight neck, while you reach the hands around and overhead towards the floor. Keep the arms straight, shoulders relaxed and lengthened, fingers crossed, and palms turned outward. Release *mūla-bandha* slightly to relax through the hips. Straighten the legs, press the feet into the ground, and engage the thighs. This is the state of the *āsana*. Hold for five breaths, gazing at the tip of the nose.

4 Catvāri
Inhale and slowly come up to stand, keeping the fingers interlaced.

Exhale fully and hold this position, while keeping the fingers interlaced behind the back. Avoid releasing the hands before finishing the exhale completely. Gaze at the tip of the nose.

After the exhalation in the 4th *vinyāsa*, go directly to the next *āsana*. Place your hands on your hips while inhaling, and count this as the 1st *vinyāsa* in *Prasārita-pādottānāsana* D.

Benefits:
Refer to the list of benefits found at the end of the description for *Prasārita-pādottānāsana* D.

Vinyāsa	Prāṇa	Āsana	Dṛṣṭi	Bandha
Samasthitih		Stand straight		
1 Ekam	in	Jump 5 feet apart to the right, hands out to the sides		
2 Dve	out & in	Interlace fingers behind the back open the chest		
3 Trīṇi	out	Bend forward, lower the hands to the floor		
This is the state of the āsana, hold for 5 deep breaths				
4 Catvāri	In & out	Come up, hold the position		
5 Pañca	In	Extend hands out to the sides		
Samasthitih	out	Jump to the front of the mat		

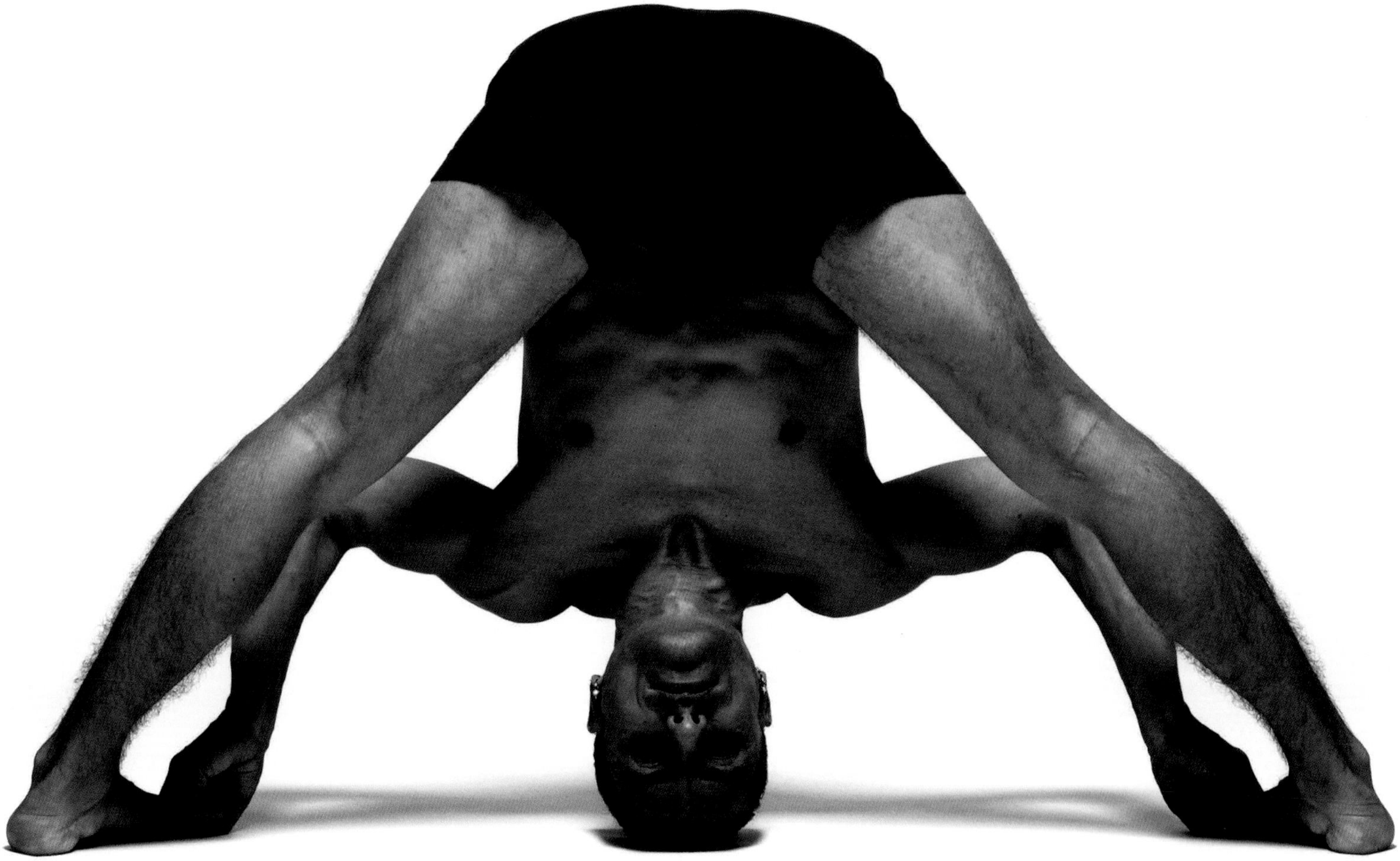

प्रसारितपादोत्तानासन घ

Prasārita-pādottānāsana D

Wide-foot forward bend pose D | 5 *vinyāsas*

1. *vinyāsa* 2. *vinyāsa* 3. *vinyāsa* 4. *vinyāsa* 5. *vinyāsa* Samasthitih

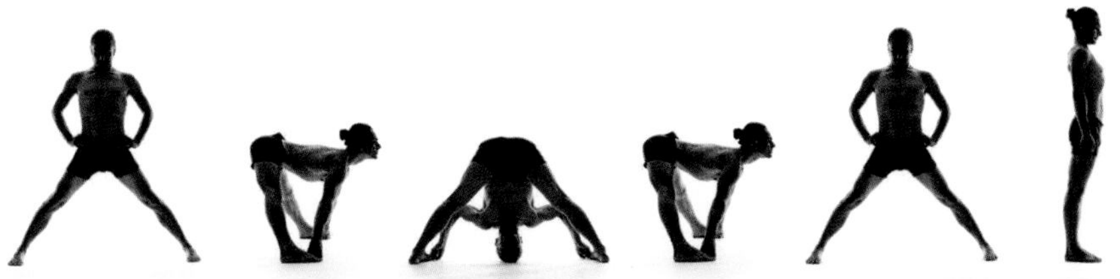

Prasārita-pādottānāsana D

Note: There are two breaths in the 2nd and 4th *vinyāsas*

Prasārita-pādottānāsana D follows directly after the 4th *vinyāsa* in *Prasārita-pādottānāsana* C.

<u>1 Ekam</u>
Inhale and place the hands on the hips and open the chest. Gaze at the tip of the nose.

<u>2 Dve</u>
Exhale and bend forward from the hips. Take hold of your big toes with the first two fingers and thumbs.

Inhale and pull slightly on the big toes to maintain the length in the arms, while simultaneously opening the chest and stretching the spine. Lift the head, and gaze at the tip of the nose.

<u>3 Trīṇi</u>
Exhale, lower the head, bending the upper body down in between the legs. Keep the neck straight and *uddīyana-bandha* pulled in. Pull on the big toes, and place the crown of the head on the floor, between the feet. This is the state of the *āsana*. Take five deep breaths here. Gaze at the tip of the nose.

<u>4 Catvāri</u>
Slowly inhale, pulling on the big toes and straightening the arms. Open the chest and lift the head, keeping the back of the neck relaxed. Gaze at the tip of the nose.

Exhale fully and hold this position.

<u>5 Pañca</u>
Inhale, place the hands on the hips and come to stand up. Gaze at the tip of the nose.

<u>Samasthitih</u>
Exhale while jumping back to the front of the mat, lowering the arms to the sides and bringing the feet together upon landing. Gaze at the tip of the nose.

<u>Benefits:</u>
While the variations in this group of positions, *Prasārita-pādottānāsana* A, B, C and D, do differ slightly, the overall benefits are very similar. All the poses:
• stretch and lengthen the hamstrings, feet, hips and back
• reverse blood flow and bring nourishment to the brain (when the head is inverted)
• dissolve excess fat from the hips and stomach
• increase the blood circulation of the upper body
C-variation:
• releases tension from the shoulders and shoulder blades
• stretches the wrists
• clears blockages in the air way.

Vinyāsa	Prāṇa	Āsana	Dṛṣṭi	Bandha
Samasthitih		Stand straight		
1 Ekam	in	Jump 5 feet apart to the right, hands on the hips, open the chest		
2 Dve	out & in	Take hold of the big toes, stretch out, head up		
3 Trīṇi	out	Bend forward		
This is the state of the āsana, breathe here for 5 breaths				
4 Catvāri	In & out	stretch out, head up, hold the pose		
5 Pañca	In	Hands to the hips, come up		
Samasthitih	out	Jump to the front of the mat		

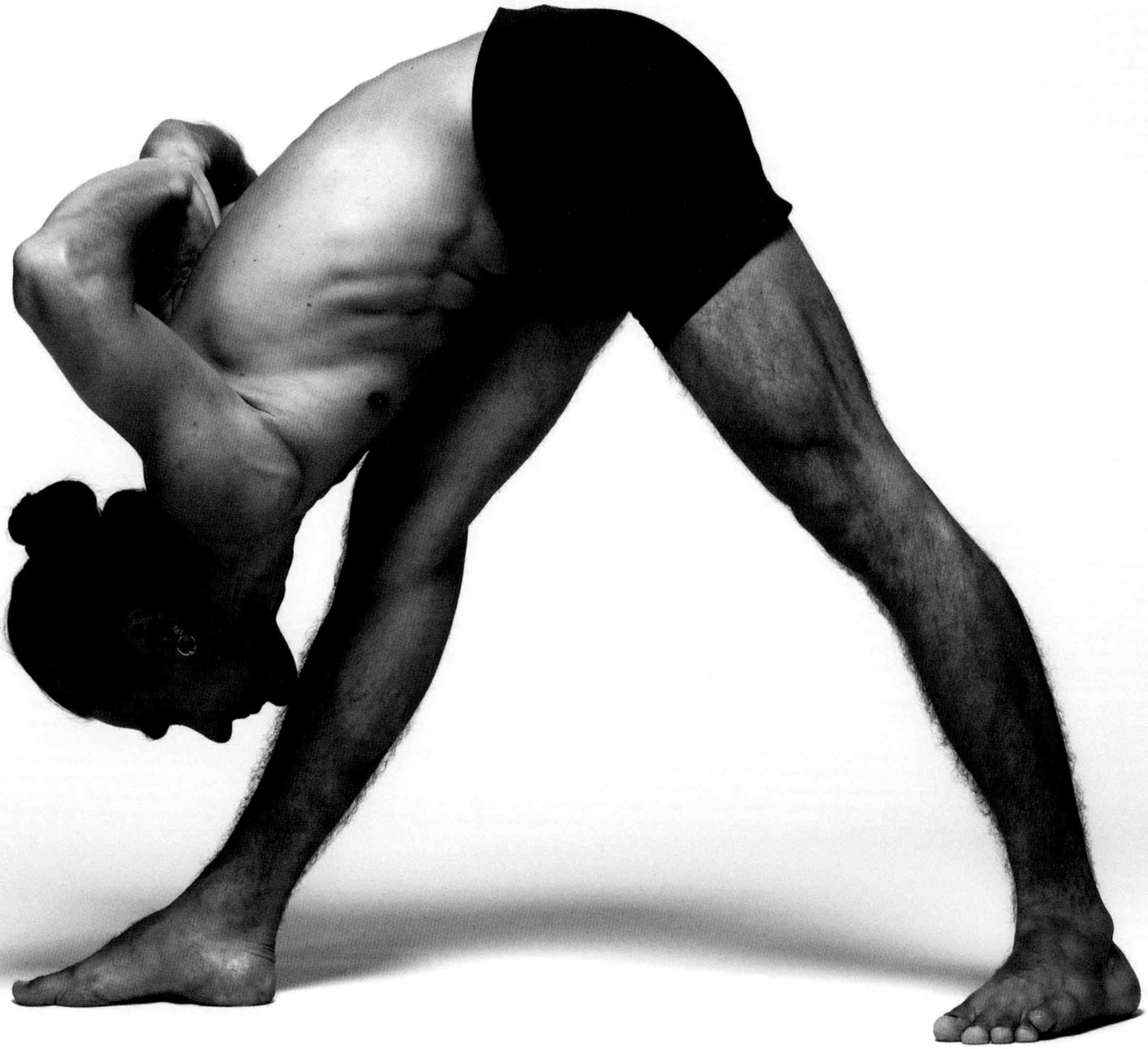

पार्श्वोत्तानासन

Pārśvottānāsana

Side stretch pose | 5 *vinyāsas*

Samasthitih | 1. *vinyāsa* | 2. *vinyāsa* | 3. *vinyāsa* | 4. *vinyāsa* | 5. *vinyāsa* | Samasthitih

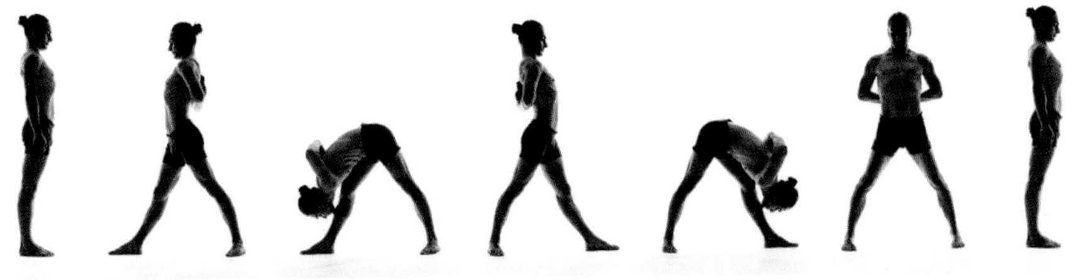

Pārśvottānāsana

Pārśva – side; ut – deep, strong, intense; tāna – stretch, extend, lengthen

Samasthiti
Stand straight with the feet together, arms by the sides, and gaze at the tip of the nose.

1 Ekam
Inhale, jump three feet out to the right. Turn the right foot 90 degrees out, so that it faces the back of the mat, keeping the left foot at an 85-90 degree angle. Place the hands behind the back and bring the palms together. Keep the hands facing upwards so that the little fingers touch the spine, and slide the hands up in between the shoulder blades. Turn the hips and chest towards the right leg, and lift the sternum while engaging the bandhas. Lift up from the left hip to relieve pressure in the left knee. Press the palms and fingers together in this inverted prayer position. Draw the shoulders back, open the chest and gaze at the tip of the nose.

2 Dve
Exhale, fold forward, and place the chest onto the right thigh and bring the chin to the shin. Engage the thigh muscles and keep the legs straight. Draw in *uddīyana-bandha* to open the chest and back while creating space for the stomach to sink into the thighs. This is the state of the *āsana* on the right side. Stay here for five breaths and gaze at the tip of the nose.

3 Trīṇi
Inhale, keep the legs straight and come up with an open chest. Keep the hands in the same position behind the back, face the feet to the front and change sides. Move the left foot 90 degrees out, so the toes face the front of the mat and leave the right foot at an 85-90 degree angle, with the toes facing the side of the mat. Bring the hips and chest to face the left leg, and lift the sternum up as you press the outer edge of the little fingers in towards the spine to open the chest further. Engage the bandhas, and gaze at the tip of the nose.

4 Catvāri
This fourth *vinyāsa* is the same as the second *vinyāsa*, but on the left side. This is the state of the *āsana*. Stay here for five breaths.

5 Pañca
Inhale, keep the legs straight and come up to stand. Apply the bandhas to support the back and hips. Keep the hands in the same position behind the back, and turn the feet forward to face the side of the mat. Gaze at the tip of the nose.

Samasthiti
Jump to the front of the mat while you exhale, and bring the arms down to the sides, gazing at the tip of the nose.

Benefits:
- increases flexibility in the hips, feet, and back
- releases tension through the shoulders and shoulder blades
- opens the chest and expands the breathing
- dissolves excess fat from the stomach and hips
- improves digestion and increases digestive fluids
- stabilizes the hips, feet, stomach and back.

Vinyāsa	Prāṇa	Āsana	Dṛṣṭi	Bandha
Samasthitih		Stand straight		
1 Ekam	in	Jump 3 feet apart to the right, turn right foot out, face the right leg, hands behind the back		
2 Dve	out	Bend forward		
This is the state of the āsana on the right side, breathe here for 5 breaths				
3 Trīṇi	in	Come up, turn to the left		
4 Catvāri	out	Bend forward		
This is the state of the āsana on the left side, breathe here for 5 breaths				
5 Pañca	in	Come up, turn the feet to the side of the mat		
Samasthitih	out	Jump to the front of the mat		

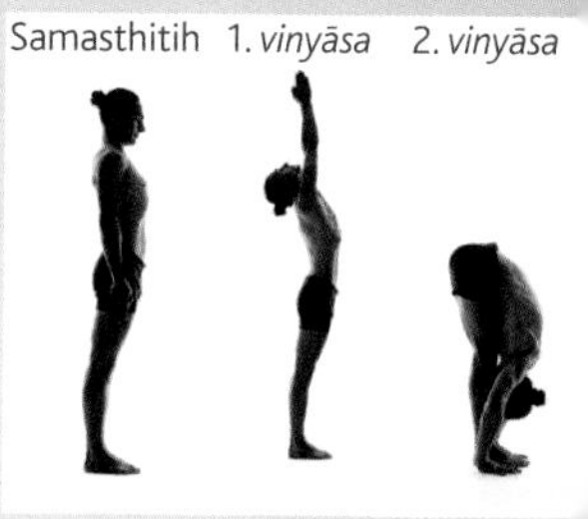

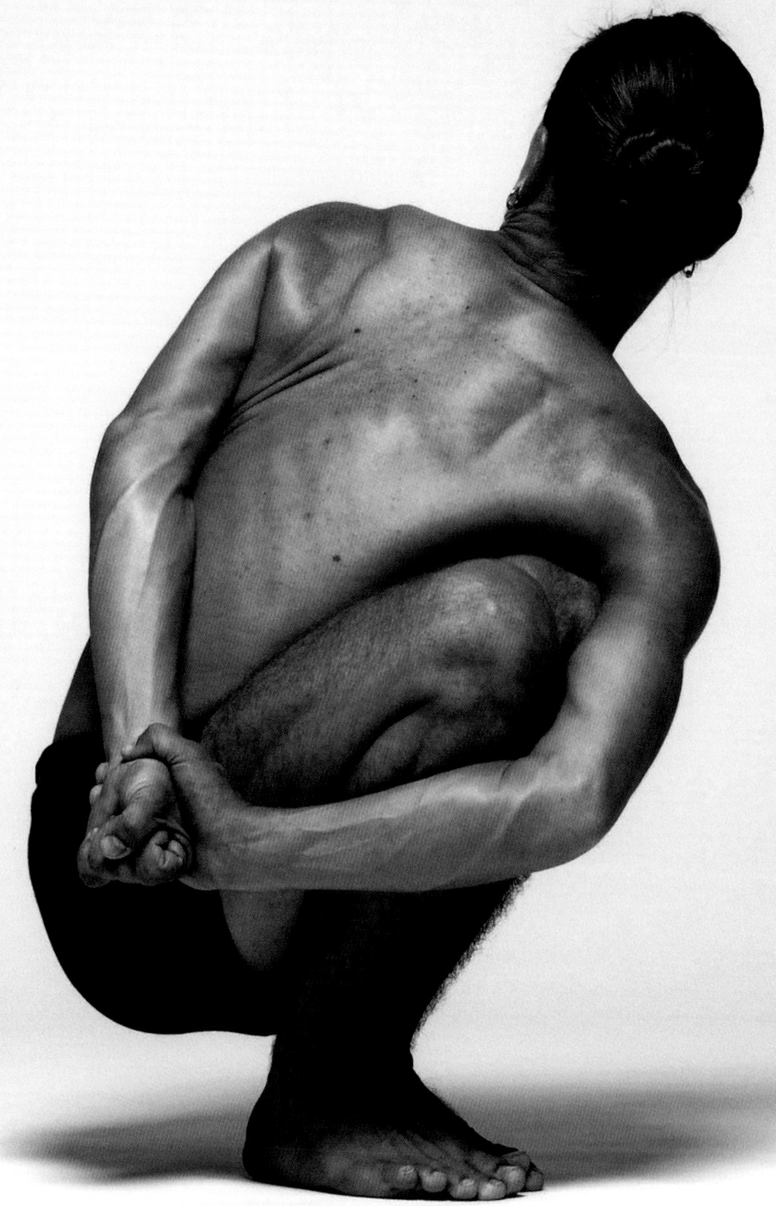

पाशासन

Pāśāsana

Noose pose | 14 *vinyāsas*

inyāsa 4. vinyāsa 5. vinyāsa 6. vinyāsa 7. vinyāsa 8. vinyāsa 9. vinyāsa 10. vinyāsa 11. vinyāsa 12. vinyāsa

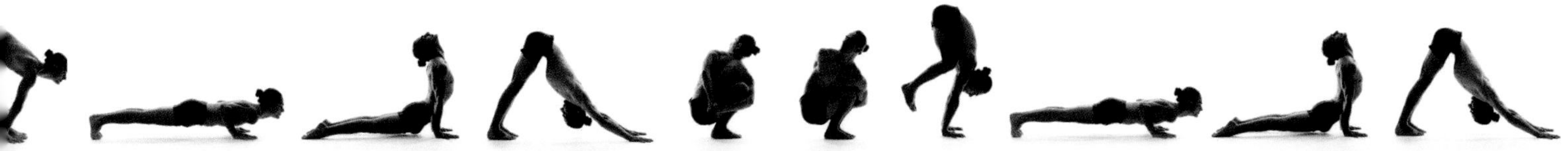

Pāśāsana

Pāśa – noose.

In *Pāśāsana*, the hands are similar to a rope tied in a tight noose around the legs.

Samasthitih
Stand straight with legs together, arms parallel to the body and look at the tip of the nose.

Vinyāsas 1-6 are the same as in *Sūryanamaskāra* A.

7 Sapta
Inhale and jump softly between the hands with bent knees. After jumping, stay in the squat pose, pressing the feet and knees evenly together with the heels on the ground. Rotate the torso far to the left, stretch your upper right arm and guide it gently, with an internal rotation, as far as possible to the left. Set the outer edge of the right armpit on the left thigh, slightly below the left knee. Then, twist the arm to the right, around the left knee to the front of the shins and guide it up towards the lower back. The right arm must remain firmly in place, as far down the left knee as possible. Avoid sliding the arm over the knee.

Bring the left arm behind the back and firmly grip either wrist. Lightly squeeze the free hand into a fist. Straighten the arms behind the back and twist the torso to the left. Press the heels down to the ground and keep the feet together. Keep the hips down and facing straight ahead (likewise with the knees) for the entire duration of the pose.

This is the state (sthiti) of the left side of the pose. Breathe deeply five times and look to the left side. The pose finishes on an exhalation.

8 Aṣṭau
Inhale, release the hands and repeat the position on the right side.This is the state (sthiti) of the right side of the pose. Look to the right side, breathe five times and finish the pose on an exhalation.

9 Nava
Inhale, release the hands and place the palms firmly on the ground besides each foot.

Using the strength of the arms and both *mūla* and *uddīyana-bandha*, lift the body up from the ground, keeping the legs is the same squat pose.

10 Daśa
Exhale, swing the body back, straighten the knees and land in *Catvāri* position, the 4th *vinyāsa* in *Sūryanamaskāra* A.

Vinyāsas 11 and 12 are the same as the 5th and 6th *vinyāsas* in *Sūryanamaskāra* A.

After the 12th *vinyāsa* in *Pāśāsana*, go directly to the 7th *vinyāsa* in Krauncāsana.

Practical tips
Keeping the heels on the ground throughout the posture may require long-term training. If the heels do not touch the ground, keep them in the air, but work them towards the ground as much as possible.

The position will develop faster if it is held for longer than five breathes while pressing the heels down strongly at the same time. Do not lift the hips up to ease the heels to the ground in the squat pose; rather, try to keep the hips down and facing straight forwards.

If the structural anatomy of the ankles and feet make it so that the heels cannot touch the ground even with the constant practice, it is better to roll the mat or fold a towel under the heels. That will help you to get a proper twist in the pose.

Benefits:
Pāśāsana belongs to the the group of *āsanas* involving back rotation. This pose:
- stretches the back, sides and stomach
- releases the nerves around the spine
- purifies the spinal cord
- purifies and releases the pathway of *suṣumnā-nāḍi*
- strengthens the leg muscles and stretches the ankles, calves and Achilles tendons.
- releases tension from the shoulders and upper back
- massages the liver, kidneys and gall bladder.

Vinyāsa	Prāṇa	Āsana	Dṛṣṭi	Bandha
Samasthitih		Stand straight		
Vinyāsas 1–6 according to Sūrya-namaskāra A				
7 Sapta	in	Jump into squat, left side		
This is the state of the left side āsana, hold for 5 deep breaths				
8 Aṣṭau	in	Switch to right side		
This is the state of the rigth side āsana, hold for 5 deep breaths				
9 Nava	in	hands on the floor, lift the body up		
10 Daśa	out	Catvāri position		
11 Ekādaśa	in	Upward-facing dog		
12 Dvādaśa	out	Downward-facing dog		
13 Trayodaśa	in	Jump forward, head up		
14 Caturdaśa	out	Bend forward		
Samasthitih	in & out	Come up, stand straight		

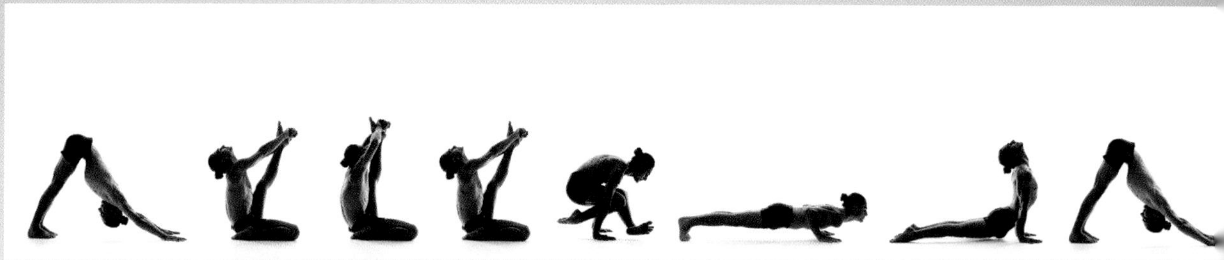

| continuing | 7. *vinyāsa* | 8. *vinyāsa* | 9. *vinyāsa* | 10. *vinyāsa* | 11. *vinyāsa* | 12. *vinyāsa* | 13. *vinyāsa* |

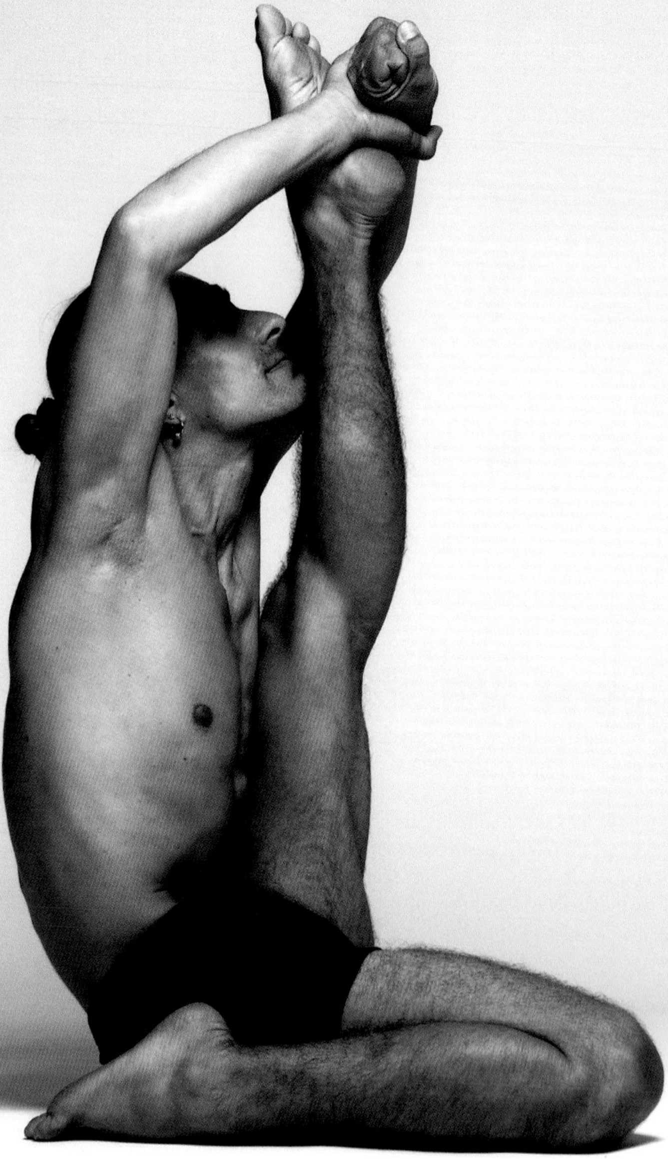

क्रौञ्चासन

Krauñcāsana

Crane pose | 22 *vinyāsas*

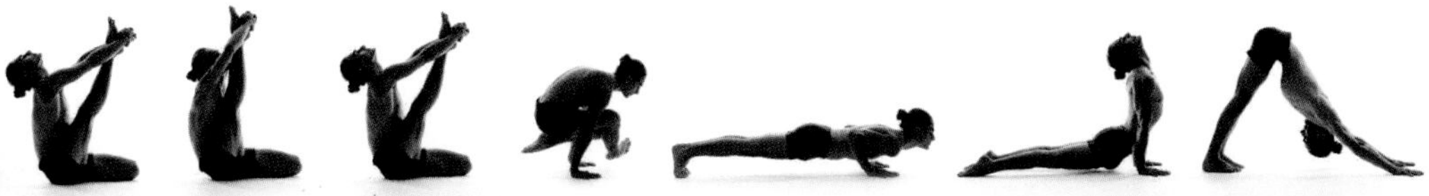

14. *vinyāsa* 15. *vinyāsa* 16. *vinyāsa* 17. *vinyāsa* 18. *vinyāsa* 19. *vinyāsa* 20. *vinyāsa*

Krauñcāsana

Kraunca – crane; mythical kraunca bird described in the Rāmāyaṇa epic

Note 1: There are two breaths in *vinyāsas* 9 and 16.
Note 2: From *vinyāsas* 10 and 17, one can jump back also with crossed legs.

Krauncāsana continues from the 12th *vinyāsa* in *Pāśāsana*.

7 Sapta
Inhale, jump through the arms to sitting, keeping the right leg bent back and take the left leg straight up and in front of you, to a diagonal. The right foot faces backwards and is placed next to the hip while the knee faces straight ahead, towards the front of the mat. Take hold of either wrist around the pointed, left foot. Keep the hip bones even on the ground, straighten the arms and the left leg and open the chest. Lift the head up and gaze at the tip of the nose. Gently pull on the foot to counterbalance the stretch.

8 Aṣṭau
Exhale and bend the upper body forward towards the left leg, while the hands are pulling the leg towards the torso. Both the left foot and upper body should settle in a position which faces straight up. Keep the chest and pelvis aligned straight ahead. *Mūla* and *uddīyana-bandhas* stabilize the pose and straighten the lower back. This is the state of the *āsana* on the right side. Place the chin onto the shin and gaze at the left big toe. Breathe deeply five times.

9 Nava
Inhale, return to the position of the 7th *vinyāsa* and hold the pose as you exhale.

10 Daśa
On the next inhalation, release the hands and place the palms down by either side of the pelvis. Bend the left leg and bring the foot toward the knee of the right leg, but not to the ground. Using the strength of the arms and both *mūla* and *uddīyana-bandha*, lift the body off the ground. Take the left foot through the arms next to the right foot. Both legs will now be in the air. Look at the tip of the nose.

11 Ekādaśa
Exhale, straighten the legs in the air and land into *Catvāri* pose, the 4th *vinyāsa* in *Sūryanamaskāra* A.

Vinyāsas 12 and 13 are the same as the 5th and 6th *vinyāsas* in *Sūryanamaskāra* A.

Repeat *vinyāsas* 7-11 on the left side, but count them as *vinyāsas* 14-18.

The 15th *vinyāsa* is the state of the pose on the left side. Breathe deeply five times.

Vinyāsas 19-20 are the same as the 5th and 6th *vinyāsas* in *Sūryanamaskāra* A.

From *Krauncāsana*'s 20th *vinyāsa*, take an extra inhalation and move directly to the 7th *vinyāsa* in *Śalabhāsana* A.

Benefits:
- purifies the kidneys
- stretches the hamstrings
- strengthens the abdominal muscles and straightens the back
- stimulates the lymph nodes
- purifies the small and large intestines
- cures sciatic pain and hemorrhoids.

Vinyāsa	Prāṇa	Āsana	Dṛṣṭi	Bandha
Samasthiti		Stand straight		
Vinyāsas 1–6 according to Sūrya-namaskāra A				
7 Sapta	in	Jump through, right leg folded back, left leg up, bind hands, head up		
8 Aṣṭau	out	Bend forward, chin to the shin		
This is the state of the right-side āsana, hold for 5 deep breaths				
9 Nava	in & out	Straighten arms, head up hold the pose		
10 Daśa	in	Hands on the floor, lift up		
11 Ekādaśa	out	Catvāri position		
12 Dvādaśa	in	Upward-facing dog		
13 Trayodaśa	out	Downward-facing dog		
14 Caturdaśa	in	Jump through, left leg folded back, right leg up, bind hands, head up		
15 Pañcadaśa	out	Bend forward, chin to the shin		
This is the state of the left-side āsana, hold for 5 deep breaths				
16 Ṣoḍaśa	in & out	Straighten arms, head up Hold the pose		
17 Saptadaśa	in	Hands on the floor, lift up		
18 Aṣṭadaśa	out	Catvāri position		
19 Ekonaviṃśatiḥ	in	Upward-facing dog		
20 Viṃśatiḥ	out	Downward-facing dog		
21 Ekaviṃśatiḥ	in	Jump forward, head up		
22 Dvāviṃśatiḥ	out	Bend forward		
Samasthitiḥ	in & out	Come up, stand straight		

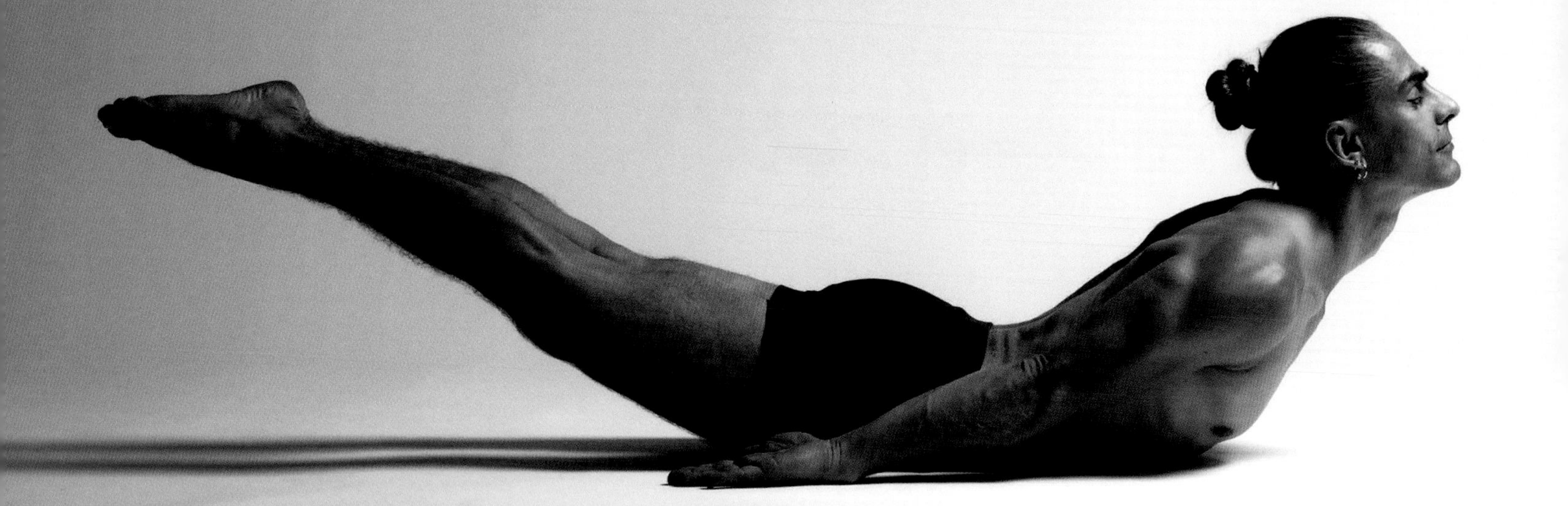

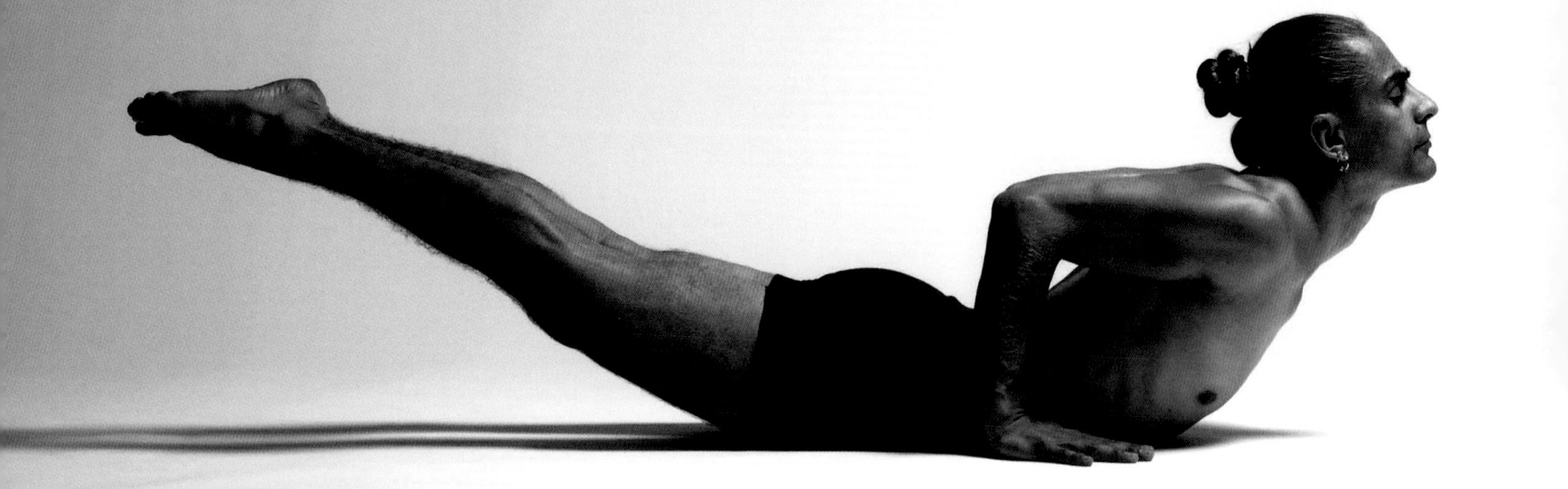

शलभासन क & ख

Śalabhāsana A & B

Locust pose A & B | 9 *vinyāsas*

continuing | 4. *vinyāsa* | 5A. *vinyāsa* | 5B. *vinyāsa* | 6. *vinyāsa* | 7. *vinyāsa*

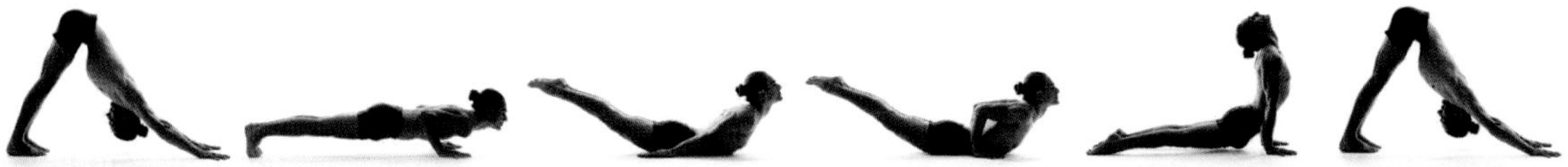

Śalabhāsana A & B

Śalabha – locust

Note 1: *Śalabhāsana* B is directly connected with *Śalabhāsana* A and both positions are counted as the 5th *vinyāsa*.
Note 2: Inhale on Krauncā*sanas* 20th *vinyāsa* (adho-mukha-śvanāsana) before continuing on to the 4th *vinyāsa* in *Śalabhāsana*.

Śalabhāsana continues from the 20th *vinyāsa* in Krauncāsana.

4 Catvāri
Exhale, bend the elbows by the sides, in line with the lower ribs and stay in *Catvāri* (*caturaṅga-daṇḍāsana*), as in the 4th *vinyāsa* in *Sūryanamaskāra* A. Stay lifted up off the ground and gaze at the tip of the nose.

5 Pañca
Śalabhāsana A
Inhale, lower the body to the ground and keep the navel as the center of gravity. Straighten the arms beside the thighs, palms facing up and fingers together. Press the backs of the palms towards the ground. Lift the head and feet up simultaneously. Keep the knees straight and feet together and pointed. Engage both *mūla* and *uddīyana-bandha* to stay supported in the posture.

The lower abdomen and *uddīyana-bandha* remains steady while breathing. The navel center (*nābhi*-cakra) operates as the body's fulcrum on the floor, keeping the position steady and avoiding the position to swing with the breath. Lift the chest up and relax the back muscles. This is the state (*sthiti*) of *Śalabhāsana* A. Gaze at the tip of the nose and breathe deeply five times. Stay in the pose until the end of the fifth breath, which is an exhalation.

Śalabhāsana B
Inhale and move the arms to the sides (at the lowest ribs). Press the palms firmly to the ground and spread the fingers. Keep the body in the same position as in *Śalabhāsana* A but lift the head, chest and legs up even higher. This is the state (*sthiti*) of *Śalabhāsana* B. Gaze at the tip of the nose and breathe deeply five times. Stay in the pose until the end of the fifth breath, which is an exhalation.

6 Ṣaṭ
On the next inhalation, lower the feet to the ground and spread them out about a foot's width apart. Lift the chest up, straighten the arms and take the head back, as in the 5th *vinyāsa* in *Sūryanamaskāra* A.

The 7th *vinyāsa* is the same as the 6th *vinyāsa* in *Sūryanamaskāra* A.

After the 7th *vinyāsa* in *Śalabhāsana* B, take an extra inhalation and move directly to the 4th *vinyāsa* in *Bhekāsana*.

Benefits:
In *Śalabhāsana*, the navel is pressed on the floor; the benefits of the pose occur in that same area. *Śalabhāsana*:
- relieves hernias
- cleanses maṇipura-cakra
- strengthens the digestive fire (agni)
- cleanses the large and small intestines
- strengthens the spine and back muscles.

Vinyāsa	Prāṇa	Āsana	Dṛṣṭi	Bandha
Samasthitih		Stand straight		
1 Ekam	in	Raise the arms		
2 Dve	out	Bend forward		
3 Trīṇi	in	Stretch back, head up		
4 Catvāri	out	Catvāri position		
5 Pañca	in	Stomach on the floor, A: arms straight back, palms up, head and feet up		
	in	B: hands to the sides, keep the head and feet up		
This is the state of the A & B āsanas, hold for 5 deep breaths				
6 Ṣaṭ	in	Upward-facing dog		
7 Sapta	out	Downward-facing dog		
8 Aṣṭau	in	Jump forward, head up		
9 Nava	out	Bend forward		
Samasthitih	in & out	Come up, stand straight		

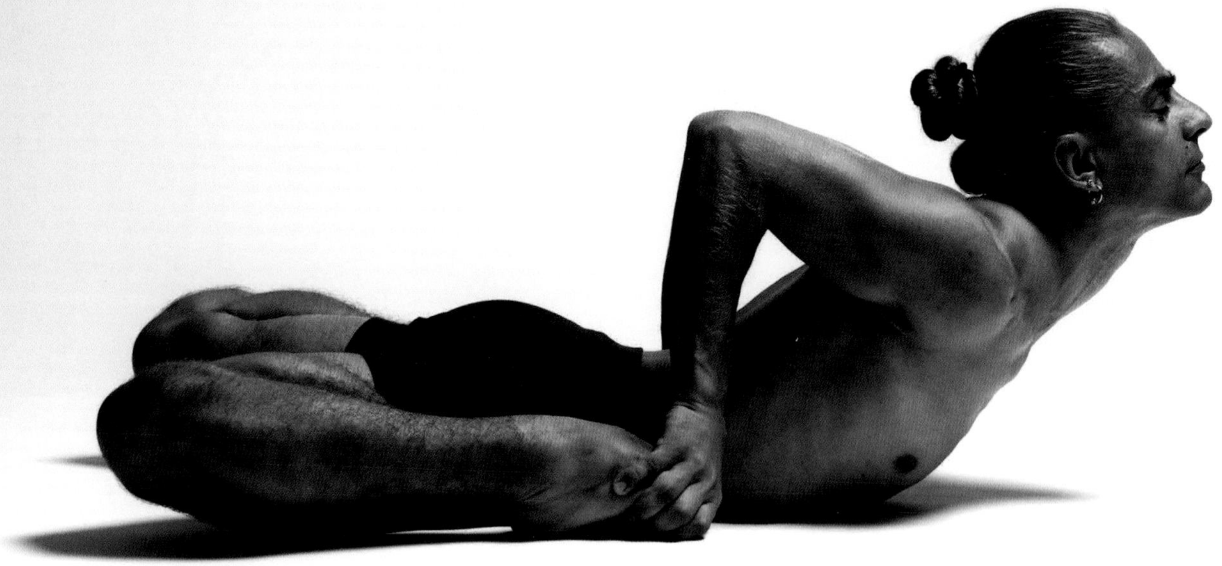

भेकासन

Bhekāsana

Frog pose | 9 *vinyāsas*

continuing | 4. *vinyāsa* | 5. in | 5. out | 6. *vinyāsa* | 7. *vinyāsa*

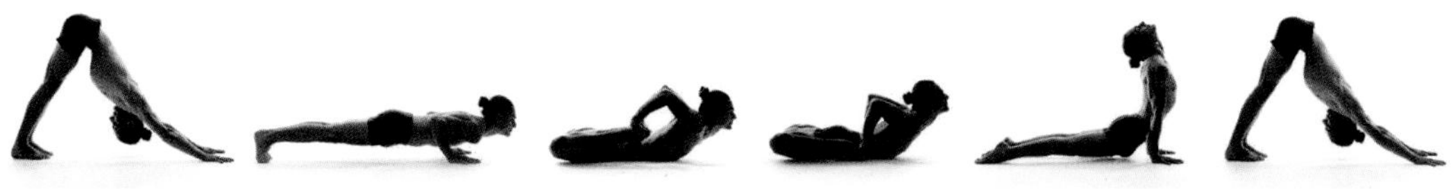

Bhekāsana

Bhekā – frog

Note 1: Take two breaths to get into the state of the pose in the 5th *vinyāsa*.

Note 2: Inhale in downward-facing dog (*adho-mukha-śvanāsana*) before continuing on to the 4th *vinyāsa*.

Bhekāsana continues from the 7th *vinyāsa* in *Śalabhāsana*.

4 Catvāri

Exhale, bend the elbows by the sides of the ribs and stay in *Catvāri* (caturaṅga-daṇḍāsana) position, as in the 4th *vinyāsa* of *Sūryanamaskāra* A. Stay lifted up off the ground and gaze at the tip of the nose.

5 Pañca

Inhale, lower the body to the ground and keep the navel as the center of gravity.

Bend the knees and take hold of the middle part of the feet with the hands. Get a firm grip on the in-step of the foot, rather than reaching for the toes alone.

Exhale, press the soles of the feet to the ground right beside the hips. The elbows should be facing up. Keep the feet straight while pushing them down with the hands. Avoid twisting the knees or feet at any angle or off to the sides. The knees should face backwards and the inner tights are slightly pulled in. Avoid pushing the knees together.

Lift the chest and head up and relax the back muscles, to get more of a stretch in the upper body. The strength from engaging *mūla* and *uddīyana-bandha* maintains stability in the posture; avoid swinging with the breath here. The navel area stays on the ground throughout the entire *āsana*. This is the state of the pose. Gaze at the tip of the nose and breathe deeply five times. The last breath is an exhalation.

The first inhalation and exhalation of this *vinyāsa* are preparation breaths for the pose. They are not included in the five-breath count of the state of the pose. Inhale and exhale to get into the pose, as described in this *vinyāsa*, and then breathe five times once you are in the state of the pose

6 Ṣaṭ

Inhale and release the legs about a foots-width apart, placing the balls of the feet on the ground. Place the hands on the floor next to the ribs. Roll over the toes, lift the chest up, straighten the arms and take the head back, as in the 5th *vinyāsa* in *Sūryanamaskāra* A. Gaze at the tip of the nose.

The 7th *vinyāsa* is the same as the 6th *vinyāsa* in *Sūryanamaskāra* A.

After the 7th *vinyāsa* in *Bhekāsana*, take an extra inhalation and go directly to the 4th *vinyāsa* in *Dhanurāsana*.

Benefits:

In *Bhekāsana*, the navel is pressed on the floor, as in *Śalabhāsana* A & B. The benefits of these positions are similar:

- stretch the thighs and hips
- release tension from the knees and hips
- cleanse *maṇipura-cakra*.

Vinyāsa	Prāṇa	Āsana	Dṛṣṭi	Bandha
Samasthitih		Stand straight		
1 Ekam	in	Raise the arms		
2 Dve	out	Bend forward		
3 Trīṇi	in	Stretch back, head up		
4 Catvāri	out	Catvāri position		
5 Pañca	in & out	Stomach on the floor, take hold of the feet Press the soles of the feet down, lift head and chest up		
This is the state of the āsana, hold for 5 deep breaths				
6 Ṣaṭ	in	Release the feet upward-facing dog		
7 Sapta	out	Downward-facing dog		
8 Aṣṭa	in	Jump forward, head up		
9 Nava	out	Bend forward		
Samasthitih	in & out	Come up Stand straight		

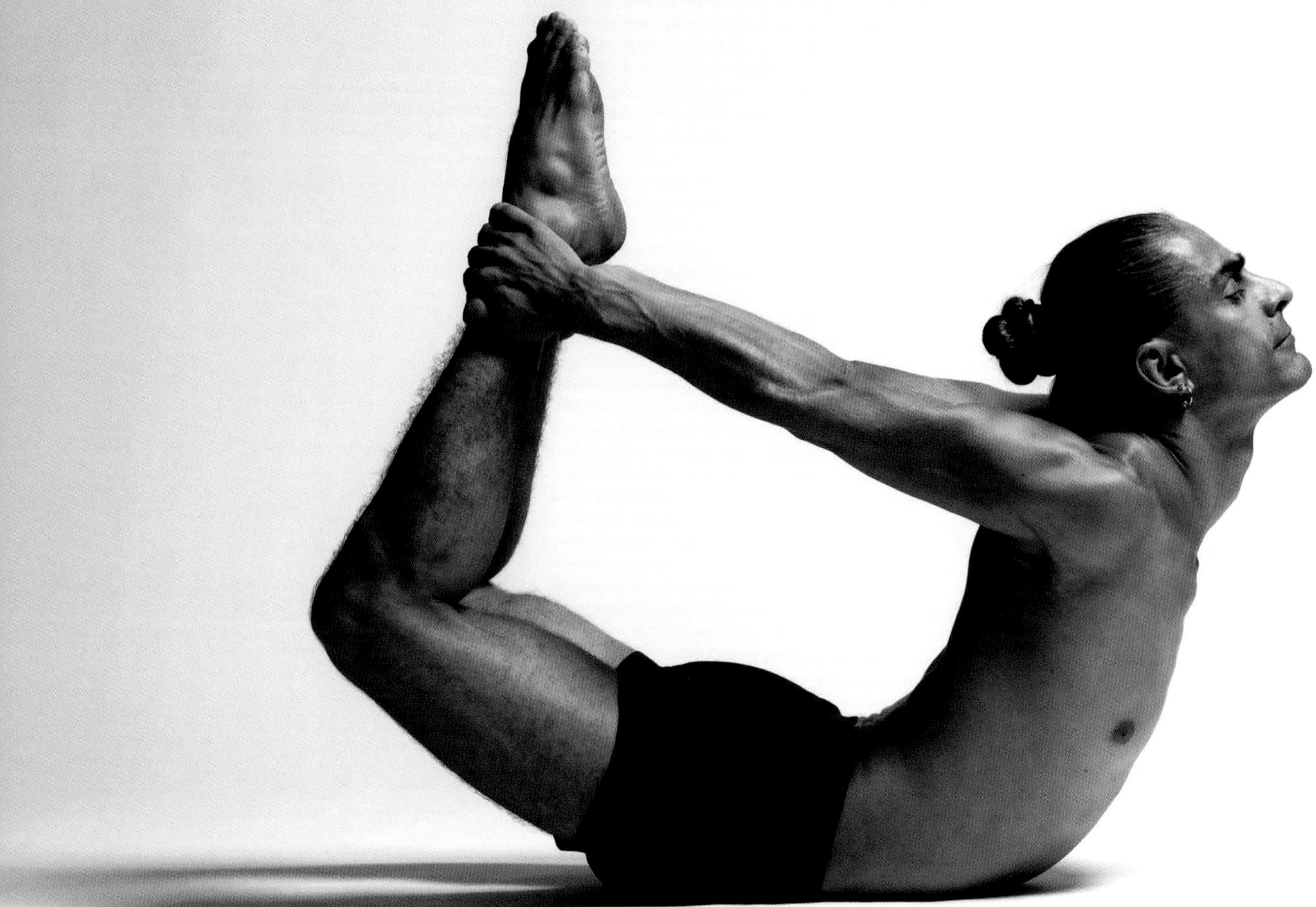

धनुरासन

Dhanurāsana

Bow pose | 8 *vinyāsas*

continuing | 4. *vinyāsa* | 5. *vinyāsa* | 6. *vinyāsa* | 7. *vinyāsa*

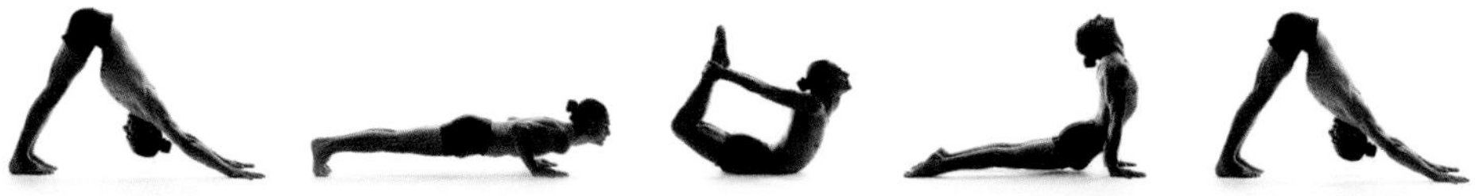

Dhanurāsana

Dhanuḥ – bow

Note: Inhale in downward-facing dog (*adho-mukha-śvanāsana*) before continuing onto the 4th *vinyāsa*.

Dhanurāsana continues from the 7th *vinyāsa* in *Bhekāsana*.

4 Catvāri
Exhale, bend the elbows by the sides of the ribs and stay in *Catvāri*, as in the 4th *vinyāsa* in *Sūryanamaskāra* A. Stay lifted up off the ground. Gaze at the tip of the nose.

5 Pañca
Inhale, lower the body to the ground and keep the navel as the center of gravity. Bend the knees, take hold of the ankles and straighten the arms. Keep the feet together and press the knees and inner thighs gently in towards each other. Lift the chest, head and legs simultaneously off the ground, keeping the navel area on the ground. Relax the back for more of a stretch in the upper body.

Straighten the legs up and keep a strong hold on the ankles; this straightening action deepens the stretch, particularly in the back and thighs. Strengthen both *mūla* and *uddīyana-bandha* to keep the position supported and avoid swinging the torso with the breath. Remember to keep the neck relaxed, even if the head is lifted up and tilted back. This is the state of the pose. Gaze at the tip of the nose and breathe deeply five times. Stay in the pose until the end of the fifth breath, which is an exhalation.

6 Ṣaṭ
Inhale and release the legs about a foots-width apart, placing the balls of the feet on the ground and the palms on the ground by the sides of the ribs. Roll over the toes, lift the chest up, straighten the arms and take the head back, as in the 5th *vinyāsa* in *Sūryanamaskāra* A. Gaze at the tip of the nose.

The 7th *vinyāsa* is the same as the 6th *vinyāsa* in *Sūryanamaskāra* A.

After the 7th *vinyāsa* in *Dhanurāsana*, take an extra inhalation and go directly to the 4th *vinyāsa* in *Pārśva-dhanurāsana*.

Benefits:
In *Dhanurāsana* the navel area stays firmly on the ground. The benefits of *Dhanurāsana* are similar to the two preceding *āsanas*:
- stretches the spine and the front side of the body
- stretches and strengthens the thighs
- strengthens and opens the chest
- cleanses *maṇipura-cakra*.

Vinyāsa	Prāṇa	Āsana	Dṛṣṭi	Bandha
Samasthitih		Stand straight		
1 Ekam	in	Raise the arms		
2 Dve	out	Bend forward		
3 Trīṇi	in	Stretch back, head up		
4 Catvāri	out	Catvāri position		
5 Pañca	in	Stomach on the floor, take hold of ankles, lift the head, chest and legs up		
This is the state of the āsana, hold for 5 deep breaths				
6 Ṣaṭ	in	Release the feet upward-facing dog		
7 Sapta	out	Downward-facing dog		
8 Aṣṭa	in	Jump forward, head up		
9 Nava	out	Bend forward		
Samasthitih	in & out	Come up Stand straight		

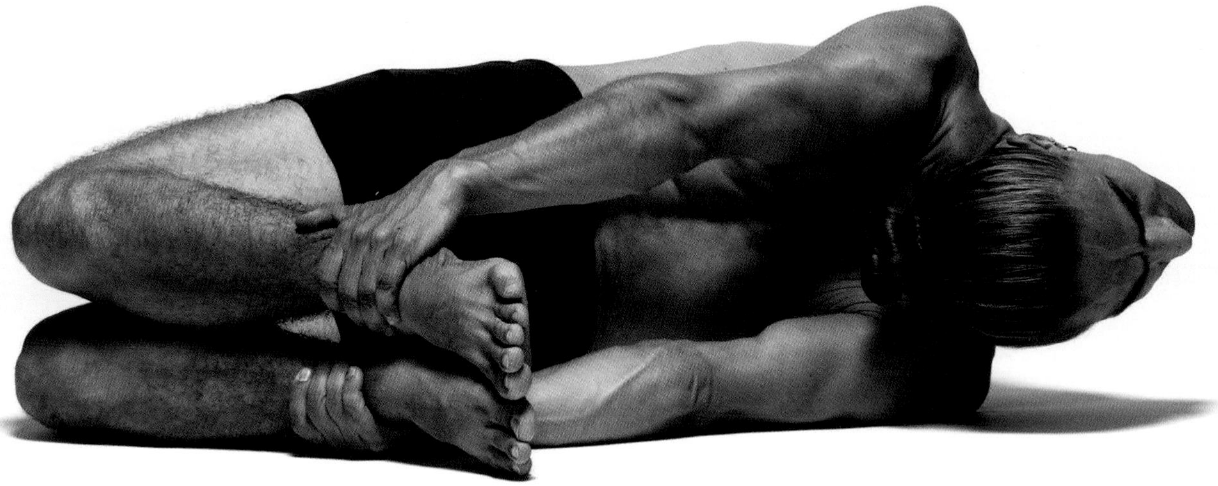

पार्श्वधनुरासन

Pārśva-dhanurāsana

Side bow pose | 13 *vinyāsas*

continuing | 4. *vinyāsa* | 5. *vinyāsa* | 6. *vinyāsa* | 7. *vinyāsa* | 8. *vinyāsa* | 9. *vinyāsa* | 10. *vinyāsa* | 11. *vinyāsa*

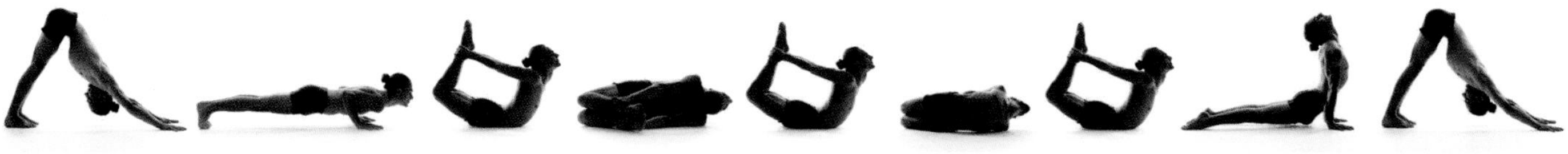

Pārśva-dhanurāsana

Pārśva – side, sivu; *dhanuḥ* – bow

Note: Inhale in downward-facing dog (*adho-mukha-śvanāsana*) before continuing on to the 4th *vinyāsa*.

Pārśva-dhanurāsana continues from the 7th *vinyāsa* in *Dhanurāsana*.

4 Catvāri
Exhale, bend the elbows by the sides of the ribs and stay in *Catvāri*, as in the 4th *vinyāsa* in *Sūryanamaskāra* A. Stay lifted up off the ground and gaze at the tip of the nose.

5 Pañca
Inhale, lower the body to the ground and keep the navel as the center of gravity. Bend the knees. Straighten the arms behind the back, and firmly take hold of both ankles. Keep the feet together and press the knees and inner thighs gently in towards each other. Lift the chest, head and feet simultaneously off the ground while keeping the navel area on the ground. This is the same position as the 5th *vinyāsa* in *Dhanurāsana*. Gaze at the tip of the nose.

6 Ṣaṭ
Exhale and roll the pose to the right side. Continue to lift and straighten the legs, relax the back and open the chest. Keep the head and neck in a straight line; avoid turning the head to the side. Press the knees and feet together. Stabilize the position on the right side, keeping the right shoulder, upper arm and top of the pelvis aligned. This is the state of the pose on the right side. Gaze at the tip of the nose and breathe deeply five times.

7 Sapta
Inhale and, keeping the feet together, roll back up into *Dhanurāsana*. Deepen the stretch of the spine into a bow, before moving directly into the next *vinyāsa*. Gaze at the tip of the nose.

8 Aṣṭau
On the next exhalation, directly roll onto the left side and hold onto the pose established in the previous *vinyāsa*. Continue according to the instructions in the 6th *vinyāsa*, but on the opposite side. This is the state of the pose on the left side. Gaze at the tip of the nose and breathe deeply five times.

9 Nava
Inhale, keep the feet together and roll back up into *Dhanurāsana*. Stretch the position gently upwards. Keep the navel area firmly on the ground, and gently press the knees and inner thighs closer together. Breathe deeply five times. Gaze at the tip of the nose. Stay in the pose until the end of the fifth breath, which is an exhalation.

10 Daśa
Inhale and release the legs about a foots-width apart, placing the balls of the feet on the ground and the palms on the ground by both sides of the ribs. Roll over the toes, lift the chest up, straighten the arms and tilt the head back, as in the 5th *vinyāsa* of *Sūryanamaskāra* A.

The 11th *vinyāsa* is the same as the 6th *vinyāsa* in *Sūryanamaskāra* A.

From *Pārśva-dhanurāsana*'s 11th *vinyāsa*, go directly to the 4th *vinyāsa* of *Uṣṭrāsana*.

Benefits:
Pārśva-dhanurāsana culminates the back-bending sequence, where the navel is pressed onto the floor. The benefits of *Pārśva-dhanurāsana* are similar to the preceding *āsanas*:
- stretches and strengthens the thighs
- removes tension in the pelvis (the side positions, in particular)
- cleanses *maṇipura-cakra*
- strengthens the digestive fire (*agni*).

Vinyāsa	Prāṇa	Āsana	Dṛṣṭi	Bandha
Samasthitih		Stand straight		
1 Ekam	in	Raise the arms		
2 Dve	out	Bend forward		
3 Trīṇi	in	Stretch back, head up		
4 Catvāri	out	Catvāri position		
5 Pañca	in	Stomach on the floor, take hold of ankles, lift the head, chest and legs up		
6 Ṣaṭ	out	Roll to the right side, feet and knees together		
This is the state of the right-side āsana, hold for 5 deep breaths				
7 Sapta	in	Roll back up to the center		
8 Aṣṭau	out	Roll to the left side, feet and knees together		
This is the state of the left-side āsana, hold for 5 deep breaths				
9 Nava	in	Roll back up to the center		
Hold for 5 deep breaths.				
10 Daśa	in	Release the feet, upward-facing dog		
11 Ekādaśa	out	Downward-facing dog		
12 Dvādaśa	in	Jump forward, head up		
13 Trayodaśa	out	Bend forward		
Samasthitih	in & out	Come up Stand straight		

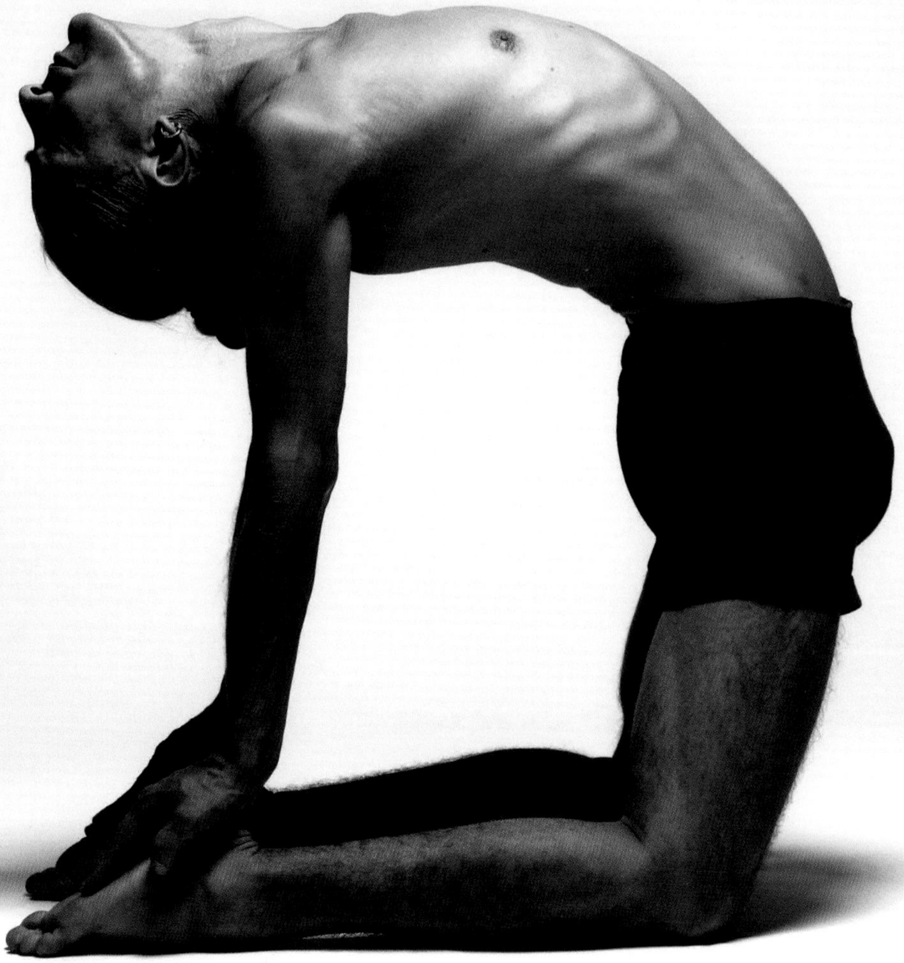

उष्ट्रासन

Uṣṭrāsana

Camel pose | 15 *vinyāsas*

continuing 7. *vinyāsa* 8. *vinyāsa* 9. *vinyāsa* 10. *vinyāsa* 11. *vinyāsa* 12. *vinyāsa* 13. *vinyāsa*

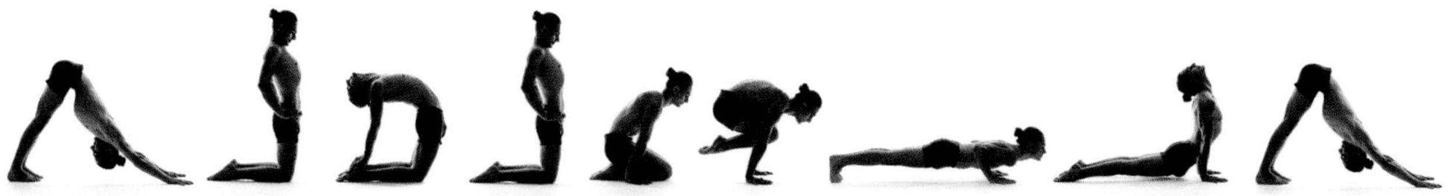

Uṣṭrāsana

Uṣṭra – camel

Note: There are two breaths in the 9th *vinyāsa*.

Uṣṭrāsana continues from the 11th *vinyāsa* in *Pārśva-dhanurāsana*.

7 Sapta
Inhale and jump softly forward, landing on the knees in between the hands. The knees and feet are hip-width apart. Place the hands on the hips, arch the chest open and expand the upper body. Gaze at the tip of the nose.

8 Aṣṭau
Exhale, keep stretching the chest up and lean slightly backward while pushing the hips forward. Lower the palms onto the heels and position the fingers along the feet so that they face towards the toes. Hold the heels with the palms.

Push the pelvis forward, stretch the front thighs and roll the shoulders back and down. Strengthen both bandhas, expand the arc of the chest upwards and tilt the head back, keeping it relaxed and controlled. This is the state of the pose. Gaze at the tip of the nose. Breathe deeply five times.

9 Nava
Inhale, come slowly up and place the hands on the hips, as in the 7th *vinyāsa*. Gaze at the tip of the nose.
Exhale and hold the posture.

10 Daśa
Inhale, release the hands from the hips and place the palms firmly on the ground, besides the middle part of the shins. Using the strength in the arms and *mūla* and uddīyana-bandhas, lift the body up from the ground with the legs hooked.

11 Ekādaśa
Exhale and swing the body back through the air. Straighten the legs and land into *Catvāri* position, the 4th *vinyāsa* in *Sūryanamaskāra* A.

Vinyāsas 12 and 13 are the same as the 5th and 6th *vinyāsas* in *Sūryanamaskāra* A.

From the 13th *vinyāsa* in *Uṣṭrāsana*, move directly to the 7th *vinyāsa* in *Laghu-vajrāsana*.

Benefits:
Uṣṭrāsana, and the following two postures, are part of the same back-bending group.
Back bends strengthen the spine, release the nervous system and prolong the yogi's life span. *Uṣṭrāsana* also:
- dissolves excess fat from the hips and waist
- strengthens the pelvis
- cleanses and opens mūlādhāra and *svādhiṣṭhāna-cakras*
- straightens the spine and improves posture
- releases the nerves around the spine.

Vinyāsa	Prāṇa	Āsana	Dṛṣṭi	Bandha
Samasthitih		Stand straight		
Vinyāsas 1–6 according to Sūrya-namaskāra A				
7 Sapta	in	Jump onto the knees, hands on the waist		
8 Aṣṭau	out	Hands on the heels, head back		
This is the state of the āsana, hold for 5 deep breaths				
9 Nava	in & out	Come up, hands on the waist Hold the pose		
10 Daśa	in	Hands on the floor, lift up		
11 Ekādaśa	out	Catvāri position		
12 Dvādaśa	in	Upward-facing dog		
13 Trayodaśa	out	Downward-facing dog		
14 Caturdaśa	in	Jump forward, head up		
15 Pañcadaśa	out	Bend forward		
Samasthitih	in & out	Come up Stand straight		

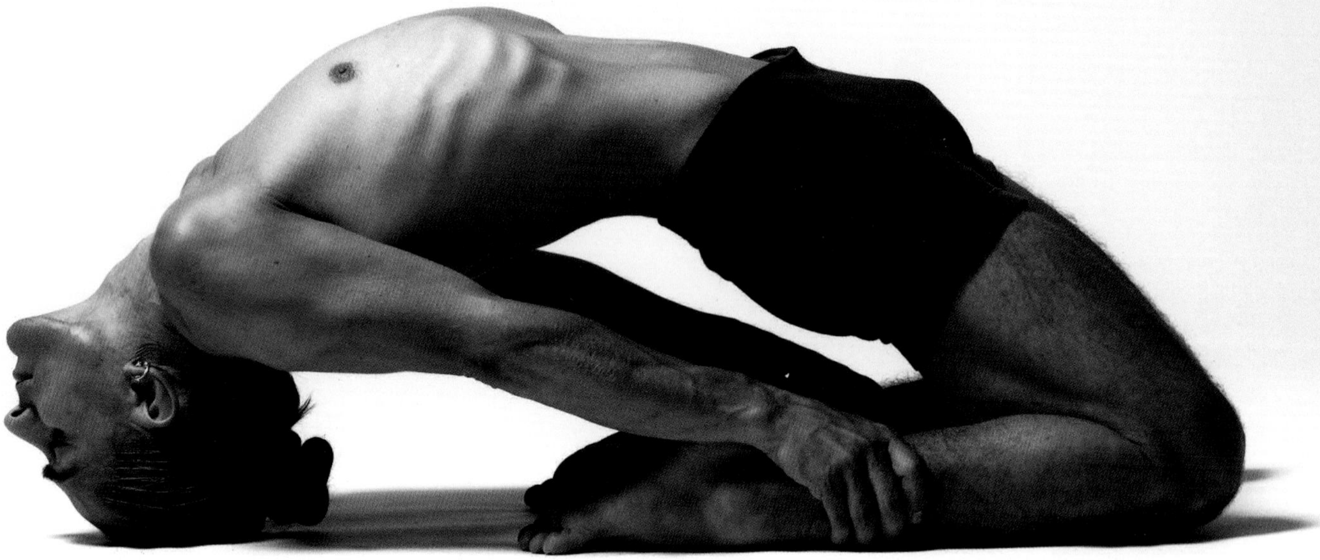

लघुवज्रासन

Laghu-vajrāsana

Light thunderbolt pose | 15 *vinyāsas*

continuing 7. *vinyāsa* 8. *vinyāsa* 9. *vinyāsa* 10. *vinyāsa* 11. *vinyāsa* 12. *vinyāsa* 13. *vinyāsa*

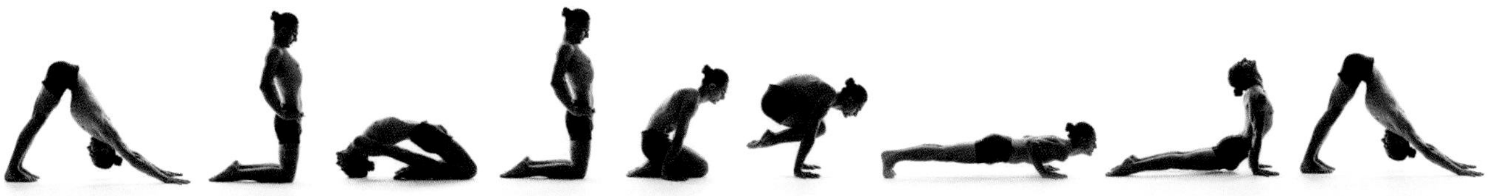

Laghu-vajrāsana

Laghu – light, little; *vajra* – thunderbolt

Note: There are two breaths in the 9th *vinyāsa*.

Laghu-vajrāsana continues from the 13th *vinyāsa* in *Uṣṭrāsana*.

7 Sapta

Inhale and jump softly forward, landing on the knees in between the hands. The knees and feet are hip-width apart. Place the hands on the hips, arch the chest open and expand the upper body. Gaze at the tip of the nose.

8 Aṣṭau

Exhale, open up from the chest and arch the back, while pushing the hips forward. At the same time, release the hands from the waist and lower them onto the ankles (not the calves or the knees), so that the thumbs are on the inside of the ankle and the other fingers are on the outside. The grip of the hand supports the position on the ankles, but the main strength for the pose comes from both *mūla* and *uddīyana-bandha*.

Push and lift the hips forward, stretch the front thighs, arch the chest up and lower the upper body as far back until the top of the head touches the floor. Straighten the arms as soon as the head touches the ground, and keep the body supported by the *mūla* and *uddīyana-bandha*. Keep hold of the ankles throughout. This is the state of the pose. Gaze at the tip of the nose. Breathe deeply five times.

Note! Straightening the arms will largely depend upon the proportions of one's body. If the arms cannot completely straighten, bend the elbows outward as much as necessary, but keep them off the ground. Try to keep the muscles engaged during the posture by lifting the pelvis and rib cage and constantly pulling up and lightly touching the head onto the ground.

9 Nava

Inhale, let the hips and chest guide the body back up and place the hands on the hips, as in the 7th *vinyāsa*. Keep the back and neck relaxed while moving up, and straighten the head up last. Gaze at the tip of the nose.

Exhale and hold the same position.

10 Daśa

Inhale, place the hands on either side of the shins, as in *Uṣṭrāsana*. Strengthen both *mūla* and *uddīyana-bandha* and lift the body off the ground with the legs hooked together.

11 Ekādaśa

Exhale, swing the body back through the air. Straighten the legs and land in *Catvāri* position, the 4th *vinyāsa* of *Sūryanamaskāra* A.

Vinyāsas 12 and 13 are the same as the 5th and 6th *vinyāsas* in *Sūryanamaskāra* A.

From *Laghu-vajrāsana*'s 13th *vinyāsa*, move directly to the 7th *vinyāsa* of *Kapotāsana*.

Benefits:

The benefits in *Laghu-vajrāsana* are the same as in *Uṣṭrāsana*, but *Laghu-vajrāsana* strengthens more the tights, hips and upper body.

Vinyāsa	Prāṇa	Āsana	Dṛṣṭi	Bandha
Samasthitih		Stand straight		
Vinyāsas 1–6 according to Sūrya-namaskāra A				
7 Sapta	in	Jump onto the knees, hands on the waist		
8 Aṣṭau	out	Hands on the ankles, head to the ground		
This is the state of the āsana, hold for 5 deep breaths				
9 Nava	in & out	Come up, hands on waist Hold the pose		
10 Daśa	in	Hands on the floor, lift up		
11 Ekādaśa	out	Catvāri position		
12 Dvādaśa	in	Upward-facing dog		
13 Trayodaśa	out	Downward-facing dog		
14 Caturdaśa	in	Jump forward, head up		
15 Pañcadaśa	out	Bend forward		
Samasthitih	in & out	Come up Stand straight		

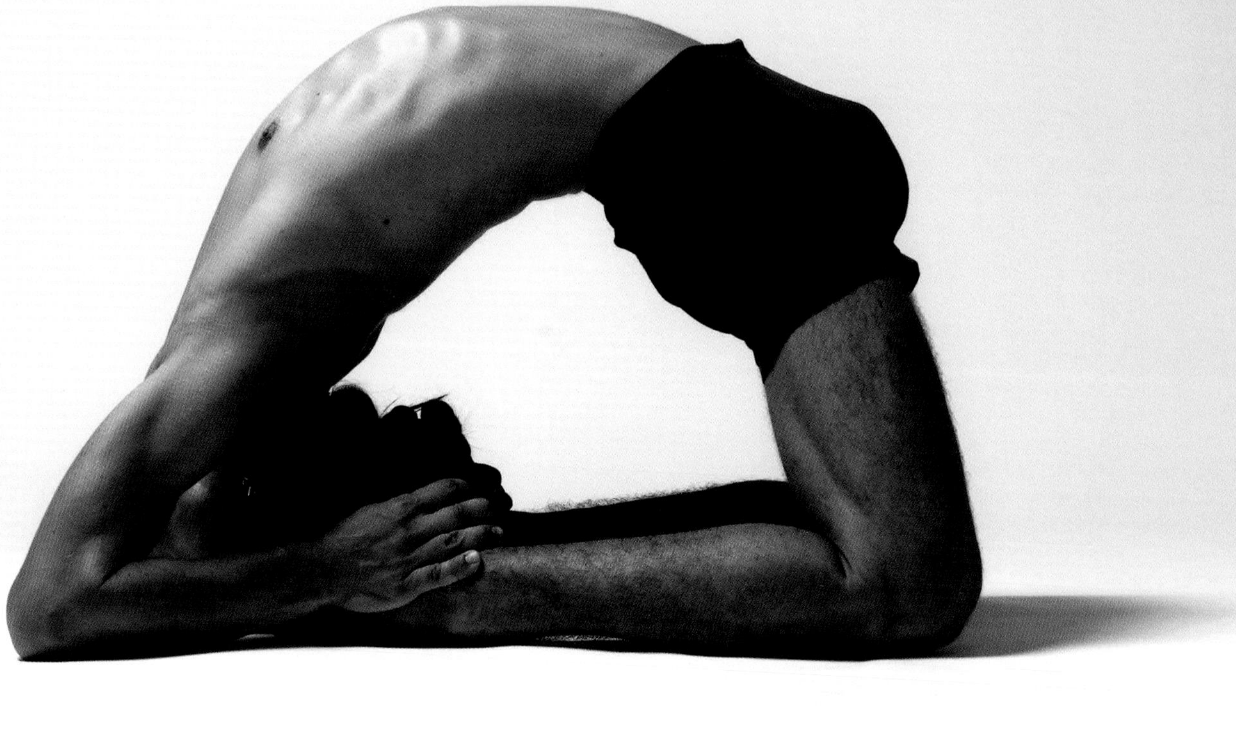

कपोतासन

Kapotāsana

Pigeon pose | 15 *vinyāsas*

continuing 7. *vinyāsa* 8. *vinyāsa* 9. *vinyāsa* 10. *vinyāsa* 11. *vinyāsa* 12. *vinyāsa* 13. *vinyāsa*

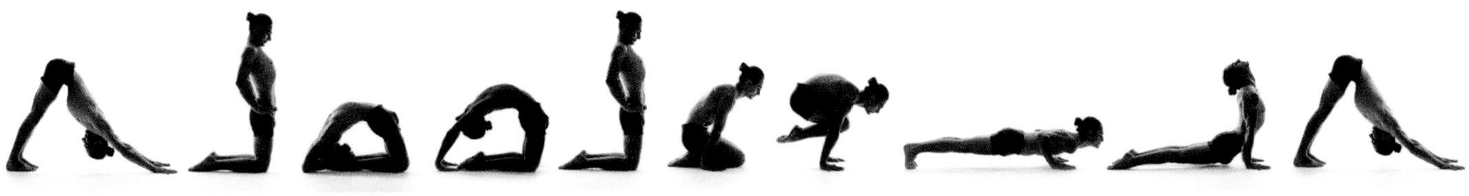

Kapotāsana

Kapota – pigeon, dove

Note 1: There are two poses which are each held for five breaths in the 8th *vinyāsa*.
Note 2: There are two breaths in the 9th *vinyāsa*.

Kapotāsana continues from the 13th *vinyāsa* in *Laghu-vajrāsana*.

7 Sapta
Inhale and jump softly forward, landing on the knees in between the hands. The knees and feet are hip-width apart. Place the hands on the hips, arch the chest open and expand the upper body. Gaze at the tip of the nose.

8 Aṣṭau
Exhale, open up from the chest and arch the back, while pushing the hips forward. Release the hands from the hips, place the palms together in front of the chest and, arching the upper body, stretch the arms back and take a firm grip of both heels with the palms.

Note: The hands can be placed onto the heels in a variety of ways.

The hands are usually placed at chest level in *kara-mudrā* (with the palms together, as in the opening *mantra* position). They can be placed onto the heels simultaneously, or one at a time. If the back is more rigid, one can first set the palms down onto the floor and then move or step them as close to the heels as they can naturally go. The elbows are placed on the floor facing straight back from the shoulders and the crown of the head (brahma-randhra) is between the feet. Push and lift the hips forward, focusing on *mūla-bandha*. Stretch the front thighs and push the chest outwards in an arch, focusing on *uddīyana-bandha*.

Do not let the muscles collapse in the posture; rather, lift the hips and chest continually upwards and touch the head lightly on the ground. This is the state of the pose. Gaze at the tip of the nose. Breathe deeply five times.

Inhale, place the palms of the hands on the ground behind the feet, fingers toward the toes. Straighten the arms and lift the chest in an arch. Keep the neck relaxed and head down. Try to relax the entire spine. Gaze at the tip of the nose. Breathe deeply five times.

9 Nava
Inhale, let the hips and chest guide the body up and place the hands on the hips, as in the 7th *vinyāsa*. Keep the back and neck relaxed while moving up and straighten the head last. Gaze at the tip of the nose.
Exhale and hold the same position.

10 Daśa
Inhale, place the hands on the either side of the shins, as in *Uṣṭrāsana*. Strengthen *mūla* and *uddīyana-bandha* and lift the body off the ground onto the arms, legs hooked together.

11 Ekādaśa
Exhale and swing the body back through the air. Straighten the legs and land in *Catvāri* position, the 4th *vinyāsa* in *Sūryanamaskāra* A.

Vinyāsas 12 and 13 are the same as the 5th and 6th *vinyāsas* in *Sūryanamaskāra* A.

From the 13th *vinyāsa* in *Kapotāsana*, move directly to the 7th *vinyāsa* of *Supta-vajrāsana*.

Benefits:
Kapotāsana has the same benefits as the two preceding *āsanas*, but in this pose, there is a deeper arch in the back and it stretches and opens more the upper arms and shoulders.

Vinyāsa	Prāṇa	Āsana	Dṛṣṭi	Bandha
Samasthitih		Stand straight		
Vinyāsas 1–6 according to Sūrya-namaskāra A				
7 Sapta	in	Jump onto the knees, hands on the waist		
8 Aṣṭa	out	Grab hold of the heels, elbows and head on the floor		
This is the state of the āsana, hold for 5 deep breaths				
	in	place hands on the ground behind the feet, straighten arms		
Hold for 5 deep breaths				
9 Nava	in & out	Come up, hands on the waist Hold the pose		
10 Daśa	in	Hands on the floor, lift up		
11 Ekādaśa	out	Catvāri position		
12 Dvādaśa	in	Upward-facing dog		
13 Trayodaśa	out	Downward-facing dog		
14 Caturdaśa	in	Jump forward, head up		
15 Pañcadaśa	out	Bend forward		
Samasthitih	in & out	Come up, Stand straight		

Assisted

8. *vinyāsa* | 9. out | 9. out | 9. out | 9. in | 9. in | 9. in

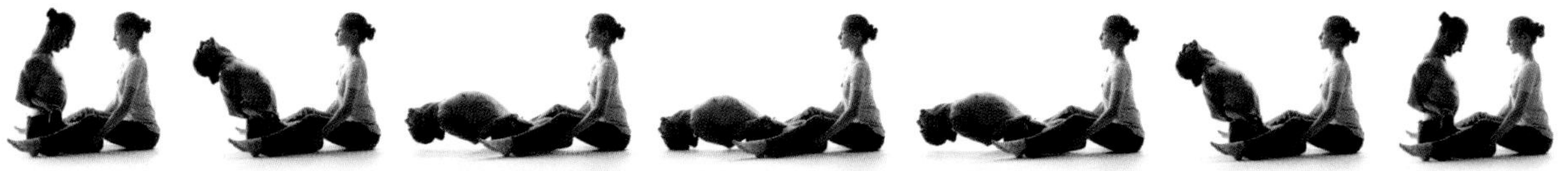

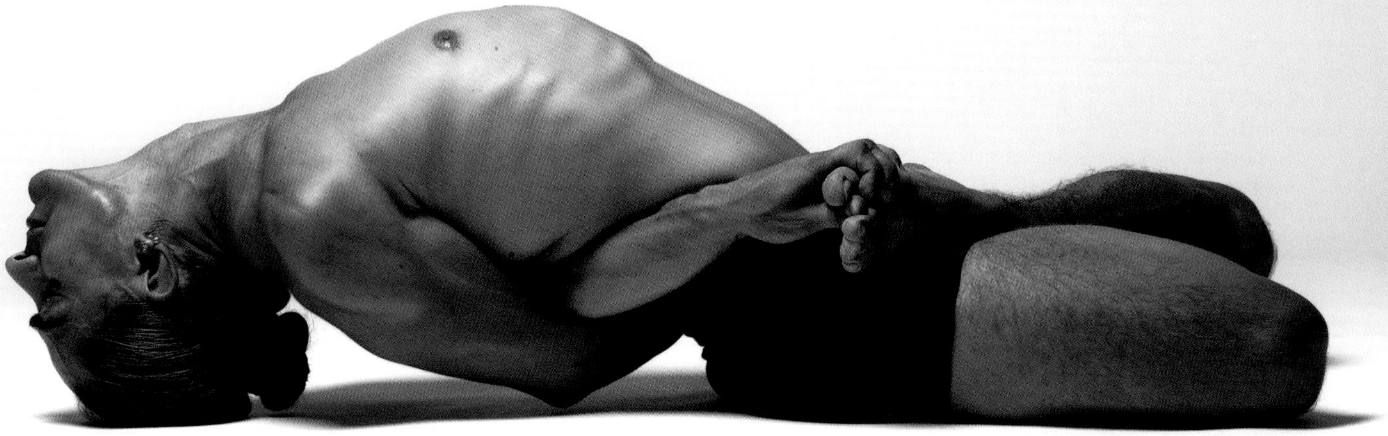

सुप्तवज्रासन

Supta-vajrāsana

Sleeping thunderbolt pose | 15 *vinyāsas*

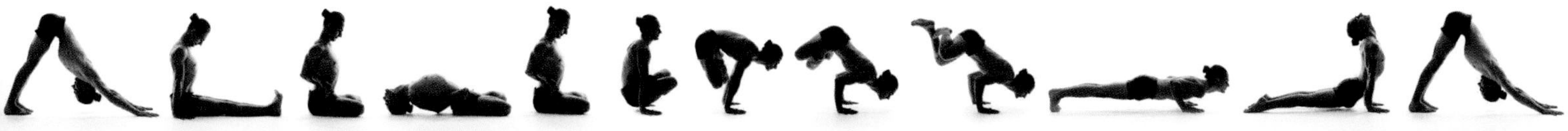
continuing
7. vinyāsa
8. vinyāsa
9. out
9. in
10. vinyāsa
11. vinyāsa
11. continuing
12. vinyāsa
13. vinyāsa

Supta-vajrāsana

Supta – sleeping; *vajra* – thunderbolt

Note 1: This posture is usually done with some assistance, as shown at the top of page 76.
Note 2: There are two breaths in *vinyāsa* 8 and many breaths in *vinyāsa* 9.
Note 3: The pose has three states, two still states and one moving state. All of them are included in the 9th *vinyāsa*.
Supta-vajrāsana continues from the 13th *vinyāsa* in *Kapotāsana*

7 Sapta

Inhale, jump through to sitting and straighten the legs in front of you.

8 Aṣṭau

Exhale and bring the feet and legs into lotus pose, placing the right foot first and then the left foot on top of the right. Take the left hand behind the back and bring it around to firmly grip the left big toe. Repeat the same on the right side. Keep the feet lightly flexed throughout the entire pose. Inhale, lift the chest up and lengthen the upper body. Press knees evenly toward the floor as in Baddha padmāsana, one of the last of the finishing postures. Gaze at the tip of the nose.

9 Nava

Asennon perustila

Inhale, keep a firm hold on the big toes, push the knees down to the ground, curve the thorax upwards and bend the upper body as far back so that the top of the head touches the floor. Strengthen both *mūla* and *uddīyana-bandha* to support the pose. Push the crossed arms down towards the lumbar area of the back to make more space for the arms and back to move. This will also make it easier to hold the big toes throughout the pose. Touch the head to the floor. This is the state of the pose. Gaze at the tip of the nose. Breathe deeply five times.

After the fifth exhalation, inhale and lift the body and head all the way up to sitting. On the next exhalation, bend the back and head down onto the floor; repeat this rhythmic movement at an even and controlled pace four times. Avoid jerking up and down forcefully. Keep the gaze at the tip of the nose throughout the pose. On the fifth time down, keep the crown of the head on the ground, as in the state of the pose in the beginning, and breathe deeply five times.

After the fifth exhalation, inhale and come up to the position in the 8th *vinyāsa*.

Exhale and hold the pose.

Please note that this position is usually done with assistance, but it is also possible to do individually. The assistant will keep his or her hands or feet on the practitioner's knees and hold the knees down while keeping the hands bound. When you move backwards, touch the floor with the crown of the head and keep the chest deeply arched. When moving up, inhale and lift up so that the head comes up last, keeping a firm grip on the big toes. Use the pelvic muscles and the thighs, along with the *mūla* and *uddīyana-bandha*, to support and facilitate the upward lift.

10 Daśa

Inhale, release the big toes and place the palms firmly on the ground on both sides of the thighs. With the strength of the arms and *mūla* and *uddīyana-bandha*, raise the body off the ground and through the arms by lifting the hips up strongly. Gaze at the tip of the nose.

11 Ekādaśa

Exhale and swing the body back through the air. Release the lotus position and land in *Catvāri* position, the 4th *vinyāsa* in *Sūryanamaskāra* A.

Vinyāsas 12 and 13 are the same as the 5th and 6th *vinyāsas* in *Sūryanamaskāra* A.

From *Supta-vajrāsana*'s 13th *vinyāsa*, move directly to the 4th *vinyāsa* of *Bakāsana* A.

Benefits:

- dissolves excess fat from the hips and waist
- strengthens and limbers up the hips
- removes tension in the shoulder blades and shoulder area
- releases the nerves around the spine
- opens the chest and straightens the back
- stretches the knees, ankles and joints.

Vinyāsa	Prāṇa	Āsana	Dṛṣṭi	Bandha
Samasthitih		Stand straight		
Vinyāsas 1–6 according to Sūrya-namaskāra A				
7 Sapta	in	Jump through to sitting		
8 Aṣṭau	out	lotus pose, grab hold of the big toes, baddha-padmāsana		
	& in	open chest up		
9 Nava	out	lean back, head to the floor		
Hold for five breaths				
	in	come up to sitting		
Repeat x 4				
	out in	head to the floor up to sitting		
	out	lean back one more time		
Hold for five breaths				
	in out	come up to sitting hold the pose		
10 Daśa	in	hands on the floor, lift up		
11 Ekādaśa	out	Open the lotus pose, Catvāri position		
12 Dvādaśa	in	Upward-facing dog		
13 Trayodaśa	out	Downward-facing dog		
14 Caturdaśa	in	Jump forward, head up		
15 Pañcadaśa	out	Bend forward		
Samasthitih	in & out	Come up, Stand straight		

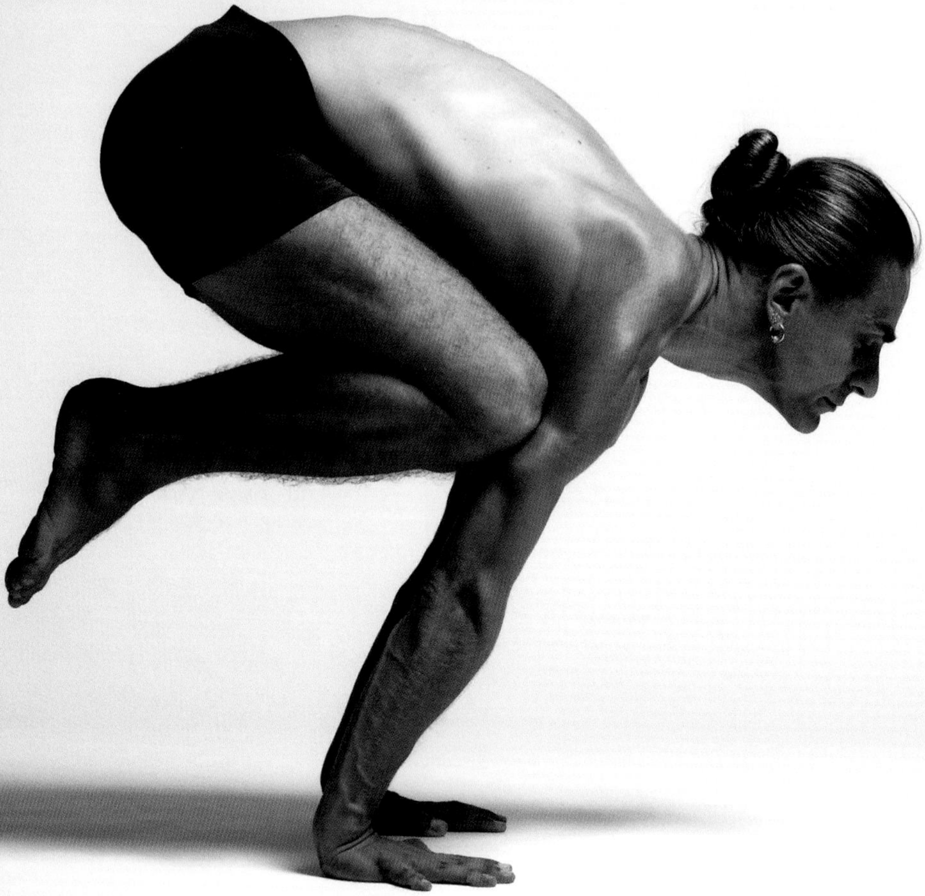

बकासन क

Bakāsana A

Crow pose | 13 *vinyāsas*

continuing 7. in 7. out 8. *vinyāsa* 9. *vinyāsa* 10. *vinyāsa* 11. *vinyāsa*

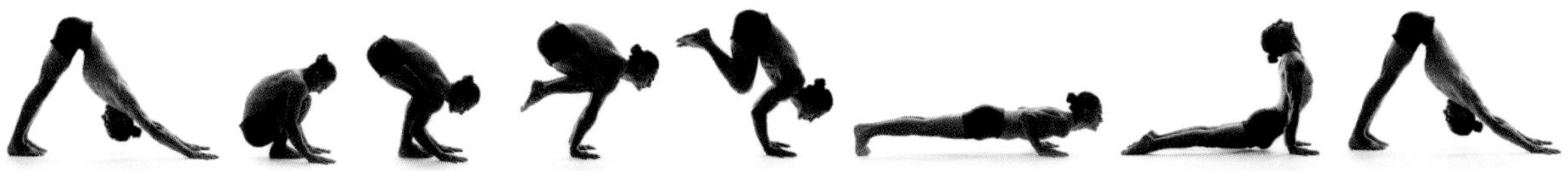

Bakāsana A

Baka – crow

Note: There are two breaths in the 7th *vinyāsa*.

Bakāsana A continues from the 13th *vinyāsa* in *Supta-vajrāsana*.

7 Sapta

Inhale and jump softly between the hands (like in *Pāśāsana*), keeping the knees bent and feet together. Stay in the squat and complete the inhalation.

Exhale, place the knees on the upper arms by the armpits and grip the ground firmly with the hands. Gaze at the tip of the nose.

8 Aṣṭau

Inhale, lift the feet off the ground, keeping the heels together, toes pointed and straighten the arms. Hold the *mūla* and *uddīyana-bandha* tightly throughout the lift and in the state of the posture. Lift the hips, feet and head up. This is the state of the pose. Gaze at the tip of the nose and breathe deeply five times.

9 Nava

Exhale, swing the body back through the air, straighten the legs and land into *Catvāri* position, the 4th *vinyāsa* in *Sūryanamaskāra* A.

Vinyāsas 10 and 11 are the same as the 5th and 6th *vinyāsas* in *Sūryanamaskāra* A.

From the 10th *vinyāsa*, move onto the next posture, the 7th *vinyāsa* in *Bakāsana* B.

Benefits:

Bakāsana strengthens the upper body, arms and shoulders.

Note: The shoulders need to be strong enough for *Bakāsana* A in order to be able to do the more demanding poses that come later on in the Intermediate series.

Vinyāsa	Prāṇa	Āsana	Dṛṣṭi	Bandha
Samasthitih		Stand straight		
Vinyāsas 1–6 according to Sūrya-namaskāra A				
7 Sapta	in & out	Jump into squat, feet together, heels on the ground Knees on the upper arms		
8 Aṣṭau	in	Lift into the pose, feet together, arms straight		
This is the state of the āsana, hold for 5 deep breaths				
9 Nava	out	Jump back into Catvāri position		
10 Daśa	in	Upward-facing dog		
11 Ekādaśa	out	Downward-facing dog		
12 Dvādaśa	in	Jump forward, head up		
13 Trayodaśa	out	Bend forward		
Samasthitih	in & out	Come up Stand straight		

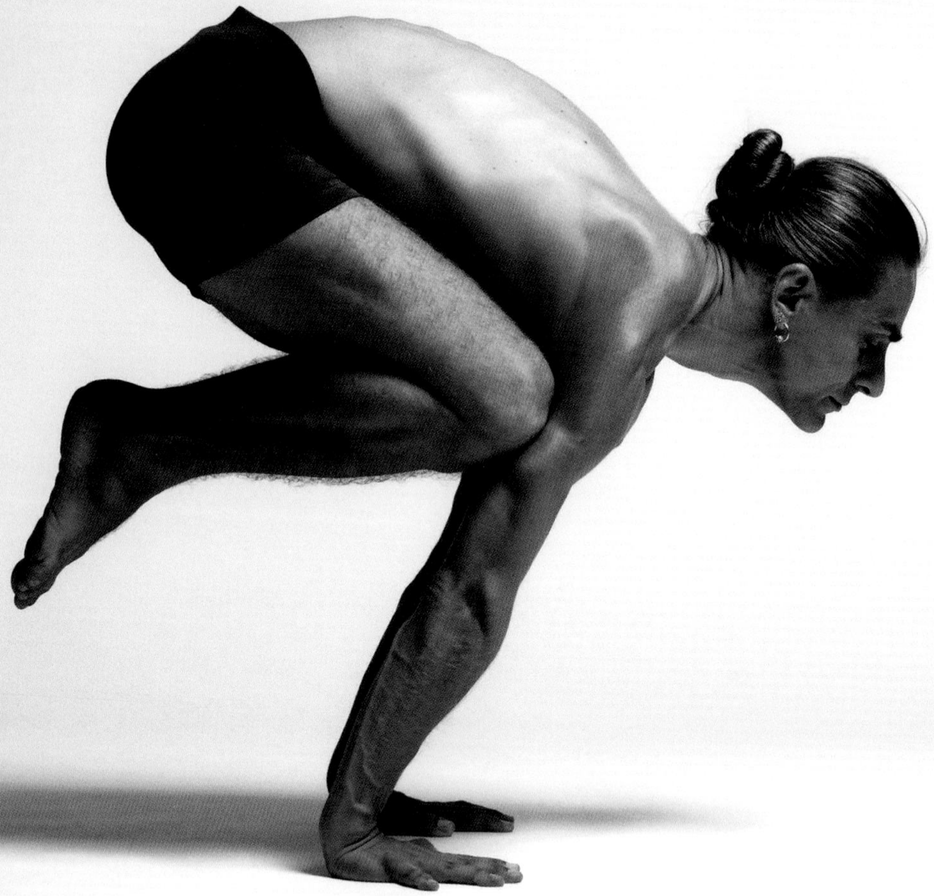

बकासन ख

Bakāsana B

Crow pose | *12 vinyāsas*

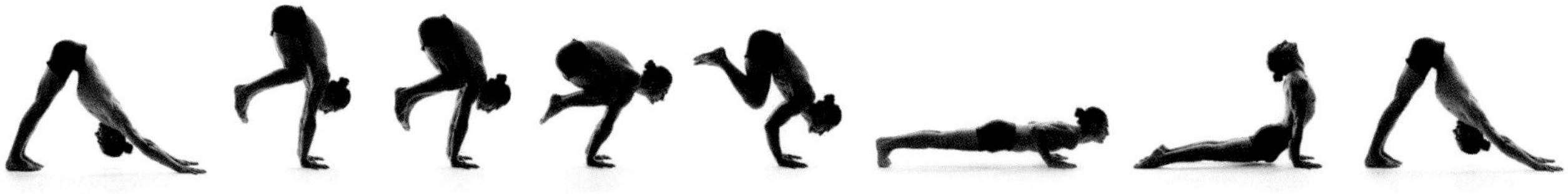

Bakāsana B

Baka – crow

Bakāsana B continues from the 11th *vinyāsa* in *Bakāsana* A.

7 Sapta

Inhale and jump smoothly and directly into *Bakāsana* B, supported by the arms and *mūla* and *uddīyana-bandha*, without touching the feet onto the ground during the jump. Place the knees high up, on the upper arms close to the armpits, keeping the feet together and straighten the arms. Lift the hips, feet and head up. This is the state of the pose. Gaze at the tip of the nose. Breathe deeply five times.

    During the jump, focus the mind on keeping a strong arm position and resolve not to touch the feet to the floor.

8 Aṣṭau

Exhale, swing the body back in the air, straighten the knees and land in *Catvāri* position, the 4th *vinyāsa* in *Sūryanamaskāra* A.

Vinyāsas 9 and 10 are the same as the 5th and 6th *vinyāsas* in *Sūryanamaskāra* A.

From the 10th *vinyāsa*, move onto the next posture, the 7th *vinyāsa* in *Bharadvājāsana*.

Benefits:

Bakāsana strengthens the upper body, arms and shoulders.

Note: The shoulders need to be strong enough for *Bakāsana* B in order to be able to do the more demanding poses that come later on in the intermediate series.

Vinyāsa	Prāṇa	Āsana	Dṛṣṭi	Bandha
Samasthitih		Stand straight	🧍	▽ ⊙
Vinyāsas 1–6 according to Sūrya-namaskāra A				
7 Sapta	in	Jump straight into the pose, straighten the arms	🧍	▽ ⊙
This is the state of the āsana, hold for 5 deep breaths				
8 Aṣṭau	out	Jump back into Catvāri position	🧍	▽ ⊙
9 Nava	in	Upward-facing dog	🧍	▽ ⊙
10 Daśa	out	Downward-facing dog	🧍	▽ ⊙
11 Ekādaśa	in	Jump forward, head up	🧍	▽ ⊙
12 Dvādaśa	out	Bend forward	🧍	▽ ⊙
Samasthitih	in & out	Come up Stand straight	🧍	▽ ⊙

continuing | 7. *vinyāsa* | 8. *vinyāsa*

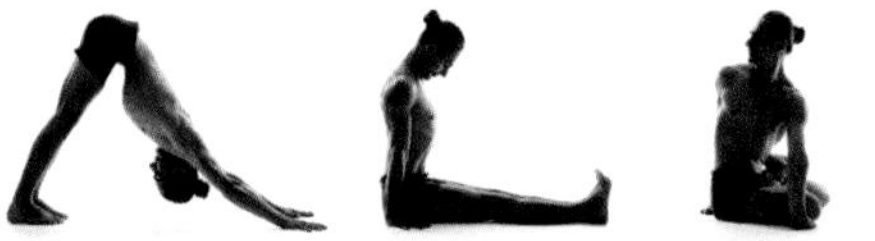

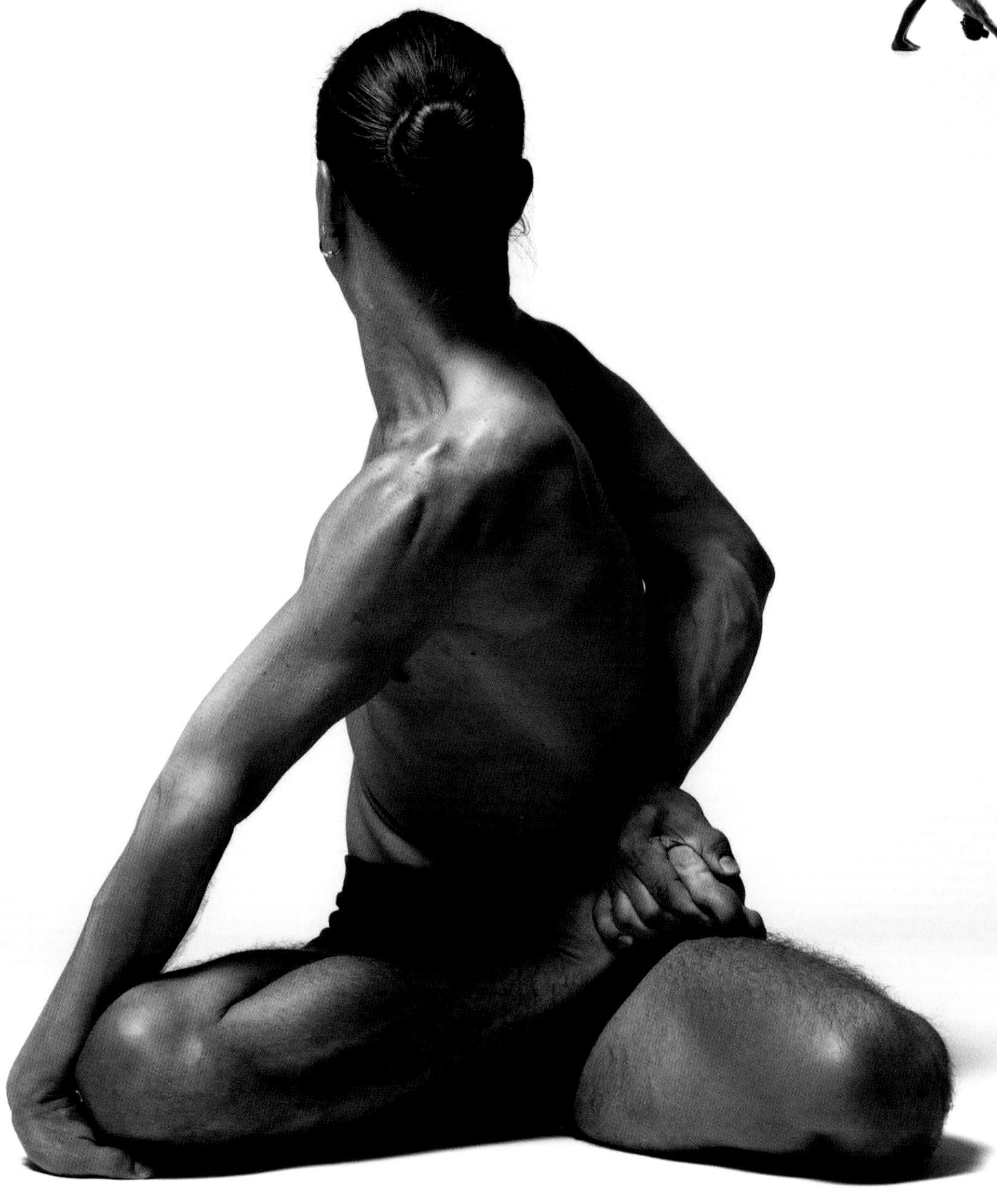

भरद्वाजासन

Bharadvājāsana

Bharadvaja's pose | 20 *vinyāsas*

9. *vinyāsa* 10. *vinyāsa* 11. *vinyāsa* 12. *vinyāsa* 13. *vinyāsa* 14. *vinyāsa* 15. *vinyāsa* 16. *vinyāsa* 17. *vinyāsa* 18. *vinyāsa*

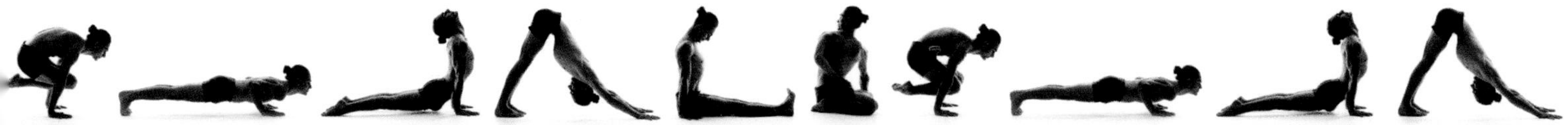

Bharadvājāsana

Bharadvāja – sage's name

Note: There are two breaths in the 7th and 13th *vinyāsas*.

Bharadvājāsana continues from the 10th *vinyāsa* in *Bakāsana* B.

7 Sapta
Inhale, jump through to sitting and straighten the legs in front of you. Gaze at the tip of the nose.
Exhale and hold the pose.

8 Aṣṭau
Inhale, bend the left knee and bring the foot beside the hip, pointing the foot backwards. Move the knee about 45 degrees out diagonally, so that the knee is on the edge of the *yoga* mat. The right foot comes into half-lotus by placing the foot into the left groin. The right knee is about 45 degrees out to the other edge of the *yoga* mat. The hips are pointing straight ahead and the hip bones are grounded on the floor. Take the right arm behind the back towards to right foot and grasp the big toe with the first two fingers and thumb. Flex the right foot.

Next, place the left hand under the right knee (or just above, between the knee and thigh) and press the palm completely to the ground. Rotate the torso to the right while simultaneously pressing the left palm into the ground and keeping the right thumb, index and middle fingers hooked onto the flexed big toe of the right foot. Engage the *mūla* and *uddīyana-bandha*, lift the chest and lengthen the torso. This is the state of the pose on the right side. Turn the head to look to the right, keeping the neck straight. Breathe deeply five times.

9 Nava
Follow the instructions for the jumping-back technique which works best for you.
First jump-back technique:
Inhale, release the hands and the position of the legs. Lift the crossed feet in the air and keep them in front of the body.
Second jump-back technique:
Inhale, release the hands and bring the left foot forward. Keep it bent in the air while the right foot stays in half-lotus.
Third jump-back technique:
Inhale, release the hands and bring the left foot into a full lotus-pose.
Fourth jump-back technique:
Inhale, release the hands and place them on the ground, on both sides of the hips, keeping the legs in the same position.
The pose then continues.

Strengthen *mūla* and *uddīyana-bandha* and press the hands firmly into the ground. Raise the whole body off the ground and move through the arms by lifting the hips up strongly. Gaze at the tip of the nose.

10 Daśa
Exhale and swing the body back through the air. Straighten the knees and land in *Catvāri* position, the 4th *vinyāsa* in *Sūryanamaskāra* A.

Vinyāsas 11–12 are the same as the 5th and 6th *vinyāsas* in *Sūryanamaskāra* A.
Repeat *vinyāsas* 7–10 on the left side, but count them as *vinyāsas* 13–16.
The 14th *vinyāsa* is the state of the pose on the left side. Breathe deeply five times.
Vinyāsas 17–18 are the same as the 5th and 6th *vinyāsas* in *Sūryanamaskāra* A.
From the 18th *vinyāsa* in *Bharadvājāsana*, move to the 7th *vinyāsa* in *Ardha-matsyendrāsana*.

Benefits:
Bharadvājāsana and the next posture, *Ardha-matsyendrāsana*, belong to the same group of rotation postures.
Bharadvājāsana:
- stretches the intercostal muscles
- opens the chest
- straightens scoliosis
- cleanses and strengthens the heart and anāhata-cakra (heart center) and improves heart conditions, i.e arrhythmia
- cleanses the liver and spleen
- strengthens and stretches the wrists
- in addition to a strong stretch in half-lotus, limbers up the knee and ankle joints.

Vinyāsa	Prāṇa	Āsana	Dṛṣṭi	Bandha
Samasthitih		Stand straight		
Vinyāsas 1–6 according to Sūrya-namaskāra A				
7 Sapta	in & out	Jump through to sitting Hold the pose		
8 Aṣṭau	in	Bend left leg, right leg to half lotus, left hand under the right knee, right hand holding the right big toe, rotate to the right		
This is the state of the right side āsana, hold for 5 deep breaths				
9 Nava	in	Hands on the floor, lift up		
10 Daśa	out	Catvāri position		
11 Ekādaśa	in	Upward-facing dog		
12 Dvādaśa	out	Downward-facing dog		
13 Trayodaśa	in	Jump through to sitting		
14 Caturdaśa	in	Bend right leg, left leg to half lotus, right hand under the left knee, left hand holding the left big toe, rotate to the left		
This is the state of the left side āsana, hold for 5 deep breaths				
15 Pañcadaśa	in	Hands on the floor, lift up		
16 Ṣoḍaśa	out	Catvāri position		
17 Saptadaśa	in	Upward-facing dog		
18 Aṣṭadaśa	out	Downward-facing dog		
19 Ekonaviṃ-śatiḥ	in	Jump forward, head up		
20 Viṃśatiḥ	out	Bend forward		
Samasthitih	in & out	Come up Stand straight		

अर्धमत्स्येन्द्रासन

Ardha-matsyendrāsana

Half Matsyendra's pose | 20 *vinyāsas*

continuing 7. *vinyāsa* 8. *vinyāsa*

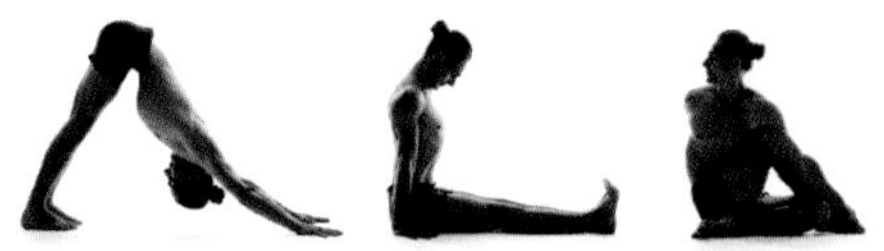

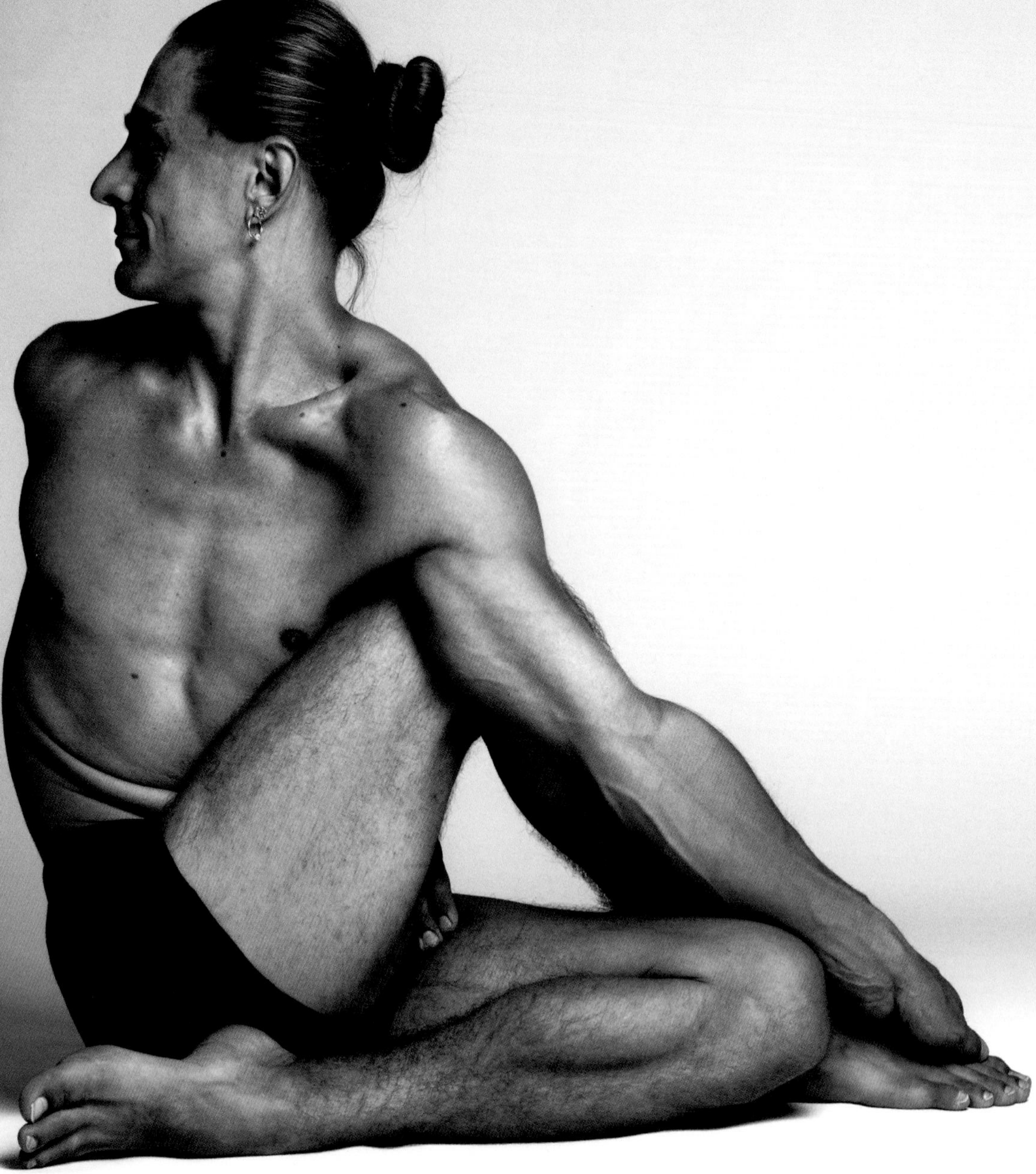

9. *vinyāsa* 10. *vinyāsa* 11. *vinyāsa* 12. *vinyāsa* 13. *vinyāsa* 14. *vinyāsa* 15. *vinyāsa* 16. *vinyāsa* 17. *vinyāsa* 18. *vinyāsa*

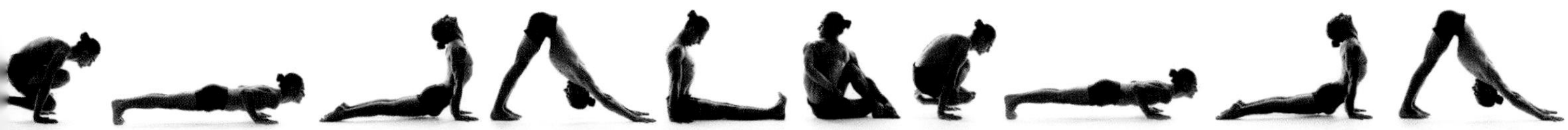

Ardha-matsyendrāsana

Ardha – half; *Matsyendra* – sage's name

Note: There are two breaths in the 7th and 13th *vinyāsas*.

Ardha-matsyendrāsana continues from the 18th *vinyāsa* in *Bharadvājāsana*.

7 Sapta
Inhale, jump through to sitting without touching the hips to the ground and straighten the legs in front of you. Gaze at the tip of the nose.
Exhale and hold the pose.

8 Aṣṭau
Inhale, bend the left knee and bring the foot next besides the right hip, pointing the foot backwards. Cross the right leg over the left thigh, placing the right foot on the ground besides the left knee. Keep the hips, left knee and right foot pointing straight ahead.

Rotate the torso to the right and place the left upper arm onto the right thigh. Continue the rotation by stretching the left arm towards the right foot and gripping the arch of the foot, with the fingertips holding the arch of the foot and the thumb on top. Straighten the spine and lift the chest up as you reach the right arm behind the back and towards the left groin.

Place the right hand into the groin, and lightly grab hold of the front thigh (sartorius muscle). Rotate the head and entire upper body to the right, staying upright. Keep the neck straight and relaxed. Both hip bones remain on the ground. This is the state of the pose on the right side. Look to the right and breathe deeply five times.

9 Nava
Follow the instructions for the jump-back technique which best applies to you.

First jump-back technique:
Inhale, release the hands and the position of the legs. Lift the feet in the air and cross them in front of the body.
Second jump-back technique:
Inhale, release the hands and place them on the ground on either side of the hips. Keep the feet in the same position.

The pose then continues.
Strengthen both *mūla* and *uddīyana-bandha* and press the hands, which are besides either side of the pelvis, firmly on the ground. Raise the whole body off the ground and bring the feet through the arms by lifting the hips up with strength and control. Gaze at the tip of the nose.

10 Daśa
Exhale and swing the body back through the air. Straighten the legs and land in *Catvāri* position, the 4th *vinyāsa* in *Sūryanamaskāra* A.

Vinyāsas 11-12 are the same as the 5th and 6th *vinyāsas* in *Sūryanamaskāra* A.

Repeat *vinyāsas* 7-10 on the left side, counting them as *vinyāsas* 13-16. The 14th *vinyāsa* is the state of the pose on the left side. Breathe deeply five times.

Vinyāsas 17-18 are the same as the 5th and 6th *vinyāsas* in *Sūryanamaskāra* A.

From *Ardha-matsyendrāsana*'s 18th *vinyāsa*, move to the 7th *vinyāsa* in *Ekapāda śīrṣāsana*.

Benefits:
The benefits are the same as the previous pose, *Bharadvājāsana*.

Vinyāsa	Prāṇa	Āsana	Dṛṣṭi	Bandha
Samasthitiḥ		Stand straight		
Vinyāsas 1–6 according to Sūrya-namaskāra A				
7 Sapta	in & out	Jump through to sitting Hold the pose		
8 Aṣṭau	in	Bend both knees, cross the right over the left, grab the right foot and left inner thigh with hands, rotate to the right		
This is the state of the right side āsana, hold for 5 deep breaths				
9 Nava	in	Hands on the floor, lift up		
10 Daśa	out	Catvāri position		
11 Ekādaśa	in	Upward-facing dog		
12 Dvādaśa	out	Downward-facing dog		
13 Trayodaśa	in & out	Jump through to sitting Hold the pose		
14 Caturdaśa	in	Bend both knees, cross the left over the right, grab the left foot and inner right thigh with hands, rotate to the left		
This is the state of the left side āsana, hold for 5 deep breaths				
15 Pañcadaśa	in	Hands on the floor, lift up		
16 Ṣoḍaśa	out	Catvāri position		
17 Saptadaśa	in	Upward-facing dog		
18 Aṣṭadaśa	out	Downward-facing dog		
19 Ekonaviṃśatiḥ	in	Jump forward, head up		
20 Viṃśatiḥ	out	Bend forward		
Samasthitiḥ	in & out	Come up Stand straight		

continuing | 7. *vinyāsa* | 8. *vinyāsa* | 9. *vinyāsa* 10. *vinyāsa* | 11. *vinyāsa* | 12. *vinyāsa* | 13. *vinyāsa*

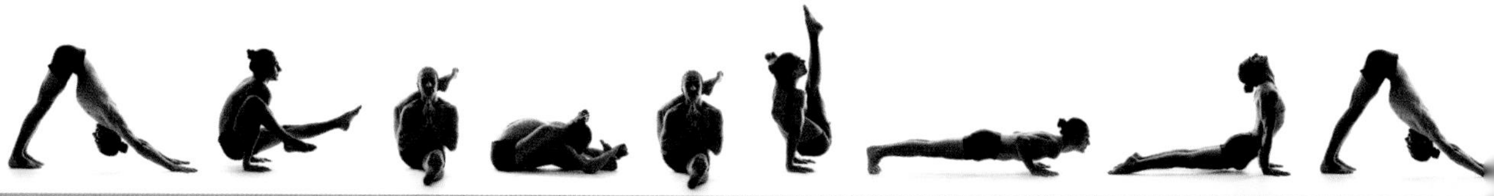

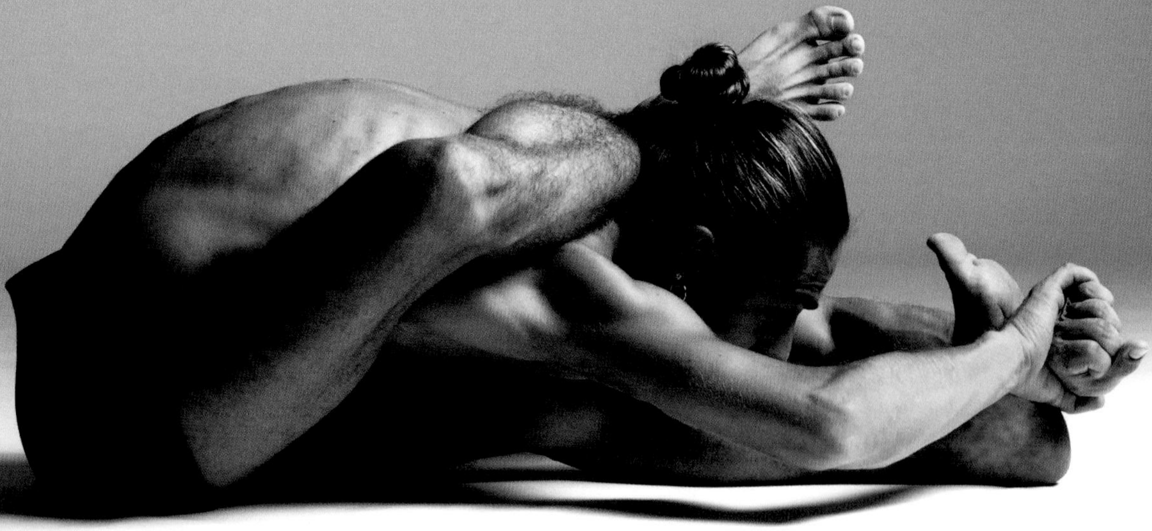

एकपादशीर्षासन

Ekapāda-śīrṣāsana

One foot behind the head | 22 *vinyāsas*

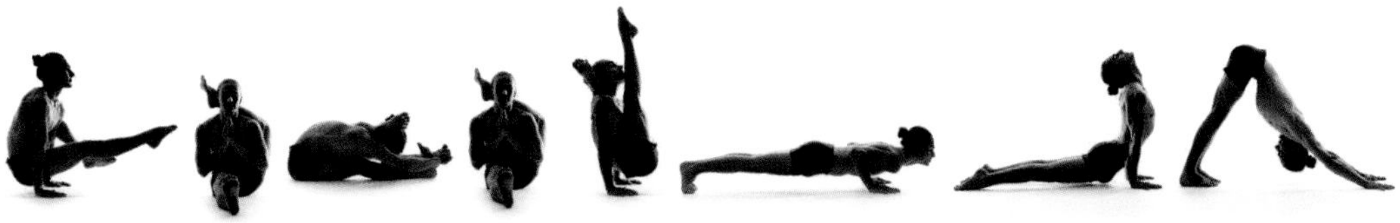

Ekapāda-śīrṣāsana

Eka – one; *pāda* – foot; *śīrṣā* – head

Note: There are two breaths in the 9th and 16th *vinyāsas*.

Ekapāda-śīrṣāsana continues from the 18th *vinyāsa* in *Ardha-matsyendrāsana*.

7 Sapta

Inhale and jump forward to sitting. The left leg floats through the arms while the right leg is landing on the right upper arm. Straighten the left leg out in front of you. Hold the right leg behind the right upper arm and take hold with one or both hands of the right shin and ankle. Extend the bent right knee out to the side and back, allowing the hip to open up. Pull the right leg behind the right shoulder, place the right ankle behind the neck and point the foot.

Take the hands, palms together, towards the chest in *kara-mudrā* (also called añjali-mudra). Using the muscles in the tights and hips, press the right leg back and down to avoid building too much pressure in the neck. Lift the head up and back to help the foot stay behind the neck. Straighten the back and expand the upper body. Gaze at the tip of the nose.

8 Aṣṭau

Exhale, strengthen the *mūla* and *uddīyana-bandha* and lean forward onto the left leg. Press the head back and move the chin forward while bending down to keep the right foot firmly placed on the back of the neck. Place the chin onto the left shin and take a firm grip of either wrist behind the left foot. This is the state of the pose on the right side. Gaze at the left big toe and breathe deeply five times.

9 Nava

Inhale and return to the position of the 7th *vinyāsa*, where the back is straight. Place the hands in *kara-mudrā*. Hold the pose for an exhalation as well.

10 Dasa

Inhale, release the hands onto the ground on either side of the pelvis. Using the strength of the *mūla* and *uddīyana-bandha* and arms, lift the body off the ground with the foot still behind the neck. Lift the left leg straight up in the front of the face or touch the chin onto the left leg. Gaze at the left big toe.

11 Ekādaśa

Exhale, bend the left leg in the air and take it in between the hands, towards the back while the right foot slides off the back of the neck. Straighten the legs in the air behind you and land in *Catvāri* position, like in the 4th *vinyāsa* in *Sūryanamaskāra* A.

Vinyāsas 12 and 13 are the same as the 5th and 6th *vinyāsas* in *Sūryanamaskāra* A.

Repeat *vinyāsas* 7–11 from the right side, counting them as *vinyāsas* 14–18 on the left side.

The 15th *vinyāsa* is the state of the pose on the left side. Breathe deeply five times.

Vinyāsas 19–20 are the same as the 5th and 6th *vinyāsas* in *Sūryanamaskāra* A.

From the 20th *vinyāsa* in *Ekapāda-śīrṣāsana*, move to the 7th *vinyāsa* in *Dvipāda-śīrṣāsana*.

Benefits:

Ekapāda-śīrṣāsana is the first of the three consecutive postures where one, or both, legs are behind the head.Therefore, effects of these three positions are similar, in that, they:

- cleanse the liver
- relieve the rectum and anus of such problems like constipation, hemorrhoids and fistulas
- open and strengthen the hips
- strengthen the neck and spine
- straighten the back and improve posture.

Vinyāsa	Prāṇa	Āsana	Dṛṣṭi	Bandha
Samasthitih		Stand straight		
Vinyāsas 1–6 according to Sūrya-namaskāra A				
7 Sapta	in	Jump right leg on the right arm, left leg through the arms, right leg behind the head, hands to kara-mudra		
8 Aṣṭau	out	Bend forward, chin to the shin		
This is the state of the right side āsana, hold for 5 deep breaths				
9 Nava	in & out	Come up to sitting, hold the pose		
10 Daśa	in	Hands on the floor, lift up		
11 Ekādaśa	out	Catvāri position		
12 Dvādaśa	in	Upward-facing dog		
13 Trayodaśa	out	Downward-facing dog		
14 Caturdaśa	in	Jump left leg on the left arm, right leg through the arms, left leg behind the head, hands to kara-mudra		
15 Pañcadaśa	out	bend forward, chin to the shin		
This is the state of the left side āsana, hold for 5 deep breaths				
16 Ṣoḍaśa	in & out	Come up to sitting, hold the pose		
17 Saptadaśa	in	Hands on the floor, lift up		
18 Aṣṭadaśa	out	Catvāri position		
19 Ekonaviṃśatiḥ	in	Upward-facing dog		
20 Viṃśatiḥ	out	Downward-facing dog		
21 Ekaviṃśatiḥ	in	Jump forward, head up		
22 Dvāviṃśatiḥ	out	Bend forward		
Samasthitih	in & out	Come up, Stand straight		

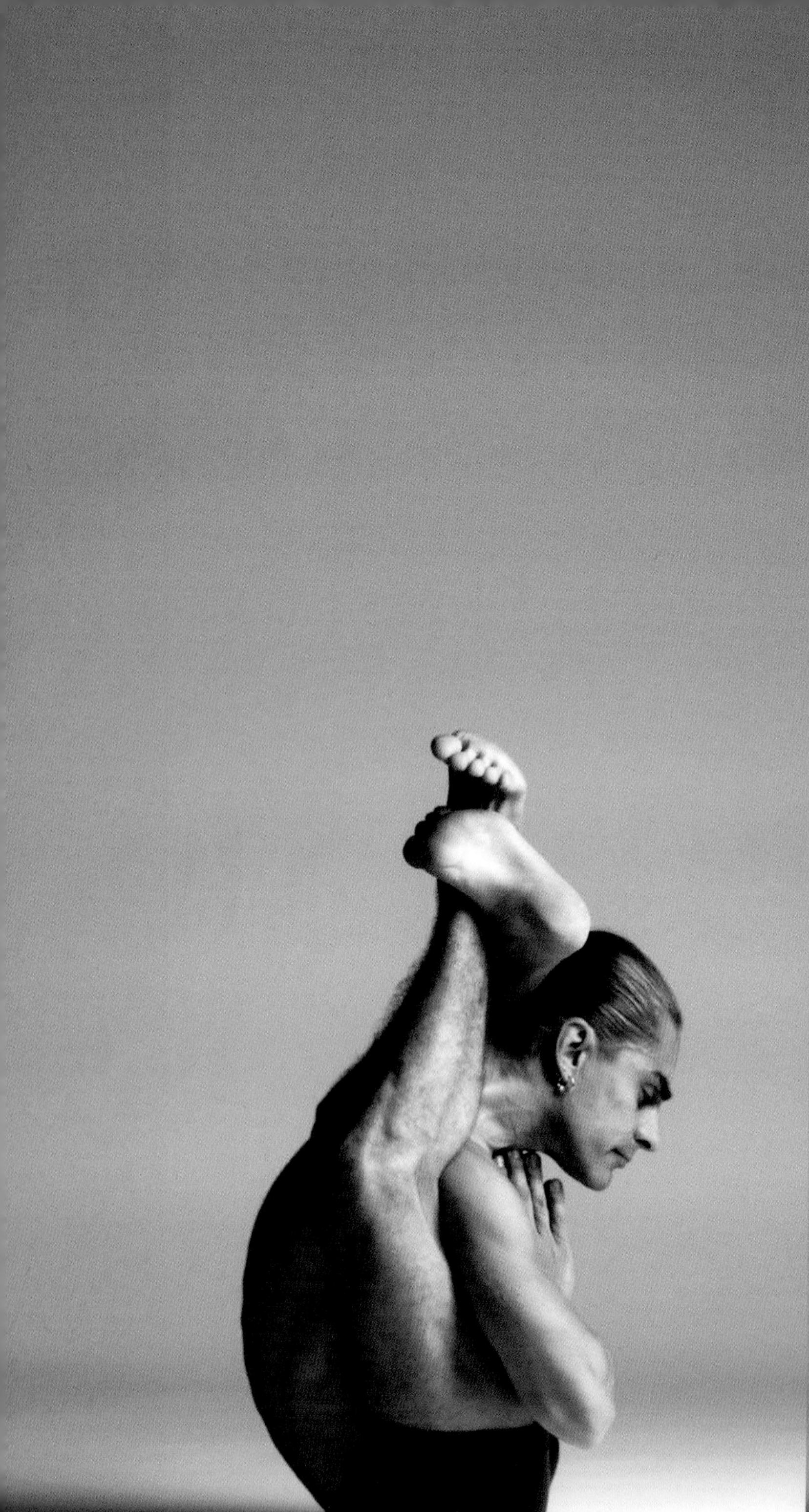

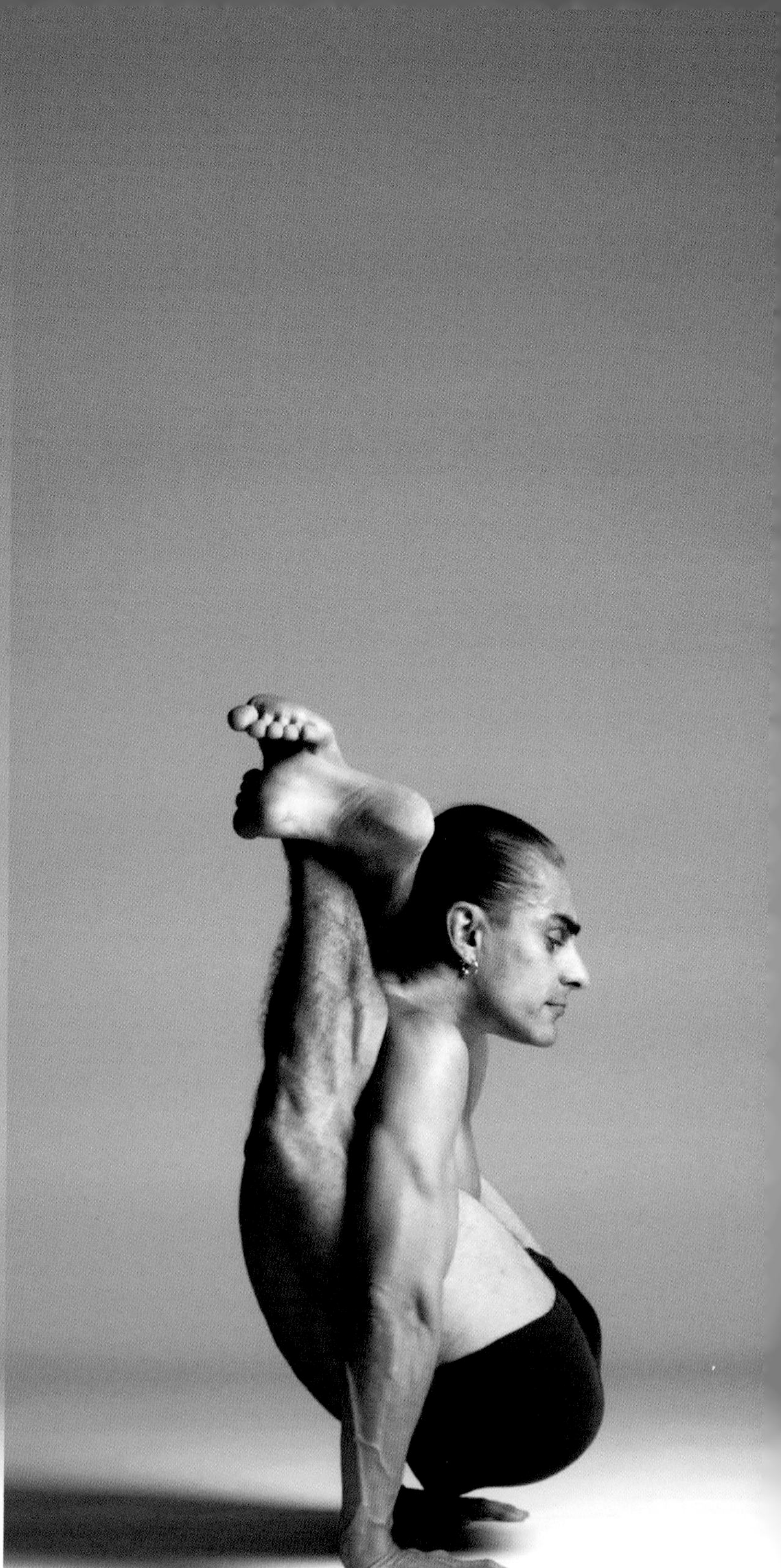

द्विपादशीर्षासन

Dvipāda-śirṣāsana

Both feet behind the head | 14 *vinyāsas*

continuing 7. *vinyāsa* 7. continuing 8. *vinyāsa* 9. *vinyāsa* 10. *vinyāsa* 11. *vinyāsa* 12. *vinyāsa*

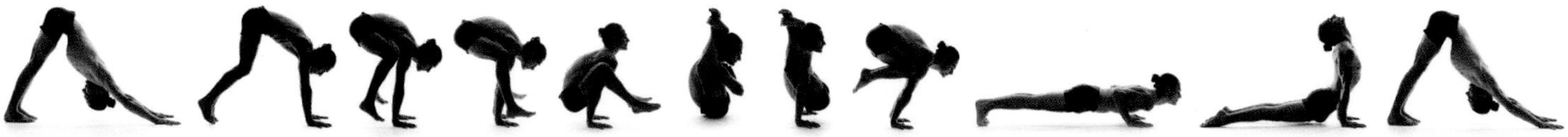

Dvipāda-śirṣāsana

Dvi – two; *pāda* – foot; *śirṣā* – head

Note 1: There can be five breaths in the 8th and 9th *vinyāsas*.

Note 2: Guruji said that the feet are hooked in the pose, but nowadays they supposed to be pointed.

Dvipāda-śīrṣāsana continues from the 20th *vinyāsa* in *Ekapāda-śīrṣāsana*.

7 Sapta

Inhale and jump the legs onto the upper arms, in the same way as in the primary series pose, Bhuja-pīḍāsana, but keep the feet and ankles uncrossed. Sit down and slide the right arm out from under the right leg, which you can then straighten out onto the floor.

Take both hands or just the left hand onto the left leg, as in *Ekapāda-śīrṣāsana*. Direct the bent left knee sideways and backwards, allowing the hip to open. Pull the left leg behind the left shoulder, place the ankle behind the neck and point the foot. Raise the head and straighten the back so that it is lighter to keep the left leg in place behind the neck.

Next, with the right hand, pull the right foot behind the head, setting it on top of the left ankle. For students with a good amount of mobility in the hips, the feet can be placed behind the neck without the help of the hands. In this case, the arms keep the balance on the floor in front of the body.

Hook the feet together by flexing them (older form). The feet can also be pointed as long as they remain securely in place (newer form). Straighten the back and lift the chest up. Place the hands in *kara-mudrā* at the level of the heart and keep the head straight. This is the state of the pose. Gaze at the tip of the nose. Breathe deeply five times.

8 Aṣṭau

Inhale and release the hands onto the ground on either side of the pelvis. With the strength of the *mūla* and *uddīyana-bandha* and arms, lift the body up from the ground keeping the legs behind the neck. Keep gazing at the nose tip.

Exhale and hold the pose (Guruji sometimes held this pose even for five breaths for strengthening the body).

9 Nava

Inhale, release the feet behind the head and slide the legs back into *Bakāsana*. Place the knees on the upper arms, feet together, and straighten the arms. Lift the head up and gaze at the tip of the nose (Guruji sometimes held also this pose for five breaths).

10 Daśa

Exhale, jump from *Bakāsana* into *Catvāri* position, like in the 4th *vinyāsa* in *Sūryanamaskāra* A. Straighten the legs in the air during the jump. Gaze at the tip of the nose.

Vinyāsas 11 and 12 are the same as the 5th and 6th *vinyāsas* in *Sūryanamaskāra* A.

From the *Dvipāda-śīrṣāsanas* 20th *vinyāsa*, move to the 7th *vinyāsa* in *Yoganidrāsana*.

Benefits:

The effects in *Dvipāda-śīrṣāsana* are the same as in *Ekapāda-śīrṣāsana*; however, by placing both legs behind the neck, the hips and lower back are stretched and opened on a much deeper level.

Vinyāsa	Prāṇa	Āsana	Dṛṣṭi	Bandha
Samasthitih		Stand straight		
Vinyāsas 1–6 according to Sūrya-namaskāra A				
7 Sapta	in	jump both legs over the upper arms, sit down; left leg behind head, right leg follows, hands in kara-mudra		
This is the state of the āsana, hold for 5 deep breaths				
8 Aṣṭau	in & out	Hands on the floor, lift the body up Hold the pose		
9 Nava	in	Move back into Bakāsana		
10 Daśa	out	Jump back into Catvāri position		
11 Ekādaśa	in	Upward-facing dog		
12 Dvādaśa	out	Downward-facing dog		
13 Trayodaśa	in	Jump forward, head up		
14 Caturdaśa	out	Bend forward		
Samasthitih	in & out	Come up Stand straight		

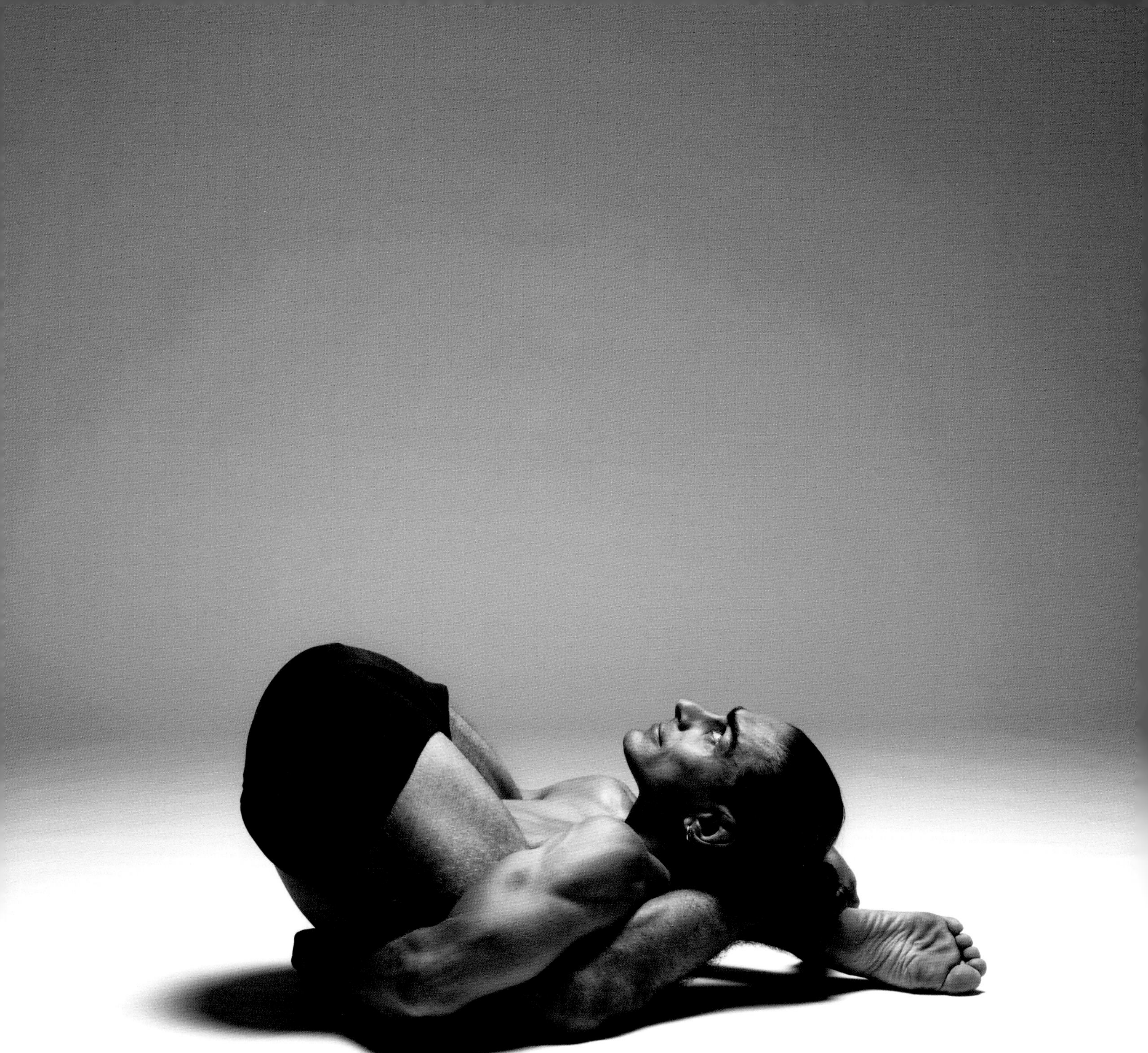

योगनिद्रासन

Yoganidrāsana

Yogi's sleep pose | 13 *vinyāsaa*

continuing | 7. *vinyāsa* | 8. *vinyāsa* | 9. in | 9. out | 10. *vinyāsa* | 11. *vinyāsa*

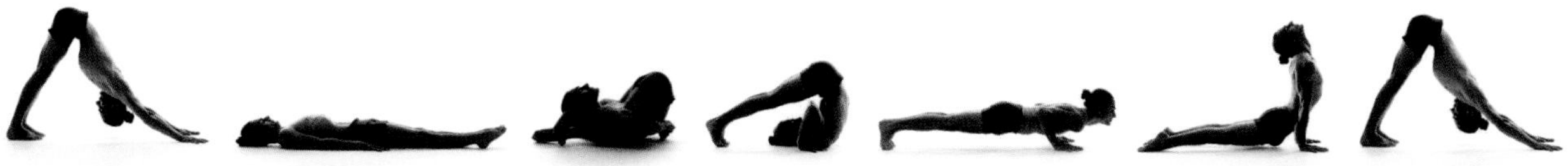

Yoganidrāsana

Yoga – path to liberation; *nidrā* – yogic meditative sleep

Note: There are two breathes in the 7th and 9th *vinyāsas*.

Yoganidrāsana continues from the 12th *vinyāsa* in *Dvipāda-śīrṣāsana*.

7 Sapta

Inhale and jump through to sitting without touching the legs to the ground. Lie down on the same inhalation. Gaze at the tip of the nose.

Exhale and hold the position.

8 Aṣṭau

Inhale, lift the left leg off the ground and bring it back toward the left shoulder. Take hold of the left leg as in *Ekapāda-śīrṣāsana*. Direct the left knee sideways and backwards, allowing the hip to open. Pull the left leg behind the left shoulder, place the ankle behind the neck and point the foot. Raise the head and straighten the back which should make it easier to keep the left leg behind the neck.

Next, raise the right leg towards the right shoulder. With the help of the right hand, first open the right leg sideways and backwards and then pull the leg behind the right shoulder. Set the right foot on top of the left ankle and point the foot.

For students with a good amount of mobility in the hips, the feet can be placed behind the neck without the help of the hands.

The feet act as a cushion on which the head can settle softly onto, as a meditative pose. Take the hands behind the back and grip firmly with either wrist.

Push the feet downwards with the back of the head, while the pelvis presses towards the floor. Open the chest and straighten the back. This is the state of the pose. Gaze between the eyebrows and breathe deeply five times.

9 Nava

Inhale, release the feet and take them over the head to the ground about a foot away from each other. Place the palms to the ground on both sides of the head and, with the strength of the arms, push the body into *cakrāsana*, without pressing the head on the ground during the roll. Exhale and take *Catvāri* position, as in the 4th *vinyāsa* in *Sūryanamaskāra* A. Gaze at the tip of the nose.

The 10th and 11th *vinyāsas* are the same as the 5th and 6th *vinyāsas* in *Sūryanamaskāra* A.

From the 11th *vinyāsa* in *Yoganidrāsana*, move to the 7th *vinyāsa* in *Ṭiṭṭibhāsana* A.

Benefits:

The benefits and effects of *Yoganidrāsana* are similar to the two preceding *āsanas*.

Vinyāsa	Prāṇa	Āsana	Dṛṣṭi	Bandha
Samasthitih		Stand straight		
Vinyāsas 1–6 according to Sūrya-namaskāra A				
7 Sapta	in & out	Jump to sitting, lie down Hold the pose		
8 Aṣṭau	in	Left leg behind the head, then the right		
This is the state of the āsana, hold for 5 deep breaths				
9 Nava	in & out	Release the legs, Cakrāsana, back-roll Into Catvāri position		
10 Daśa	in	Upward-facing dog		
11 Ekādaśa	out	Downward-facing dog		
12 Dvādaśa	in	Jump forward, head up		
13 Trayodaśa	out	Bend forward		
Samasthitih	in & out	Come up Stand straight		

टिट्टिभासन क & ख & ग

Ṭiṭṭibhāsana A, B and C

Tittibha bird pose | 16 *vinyāsas*

A

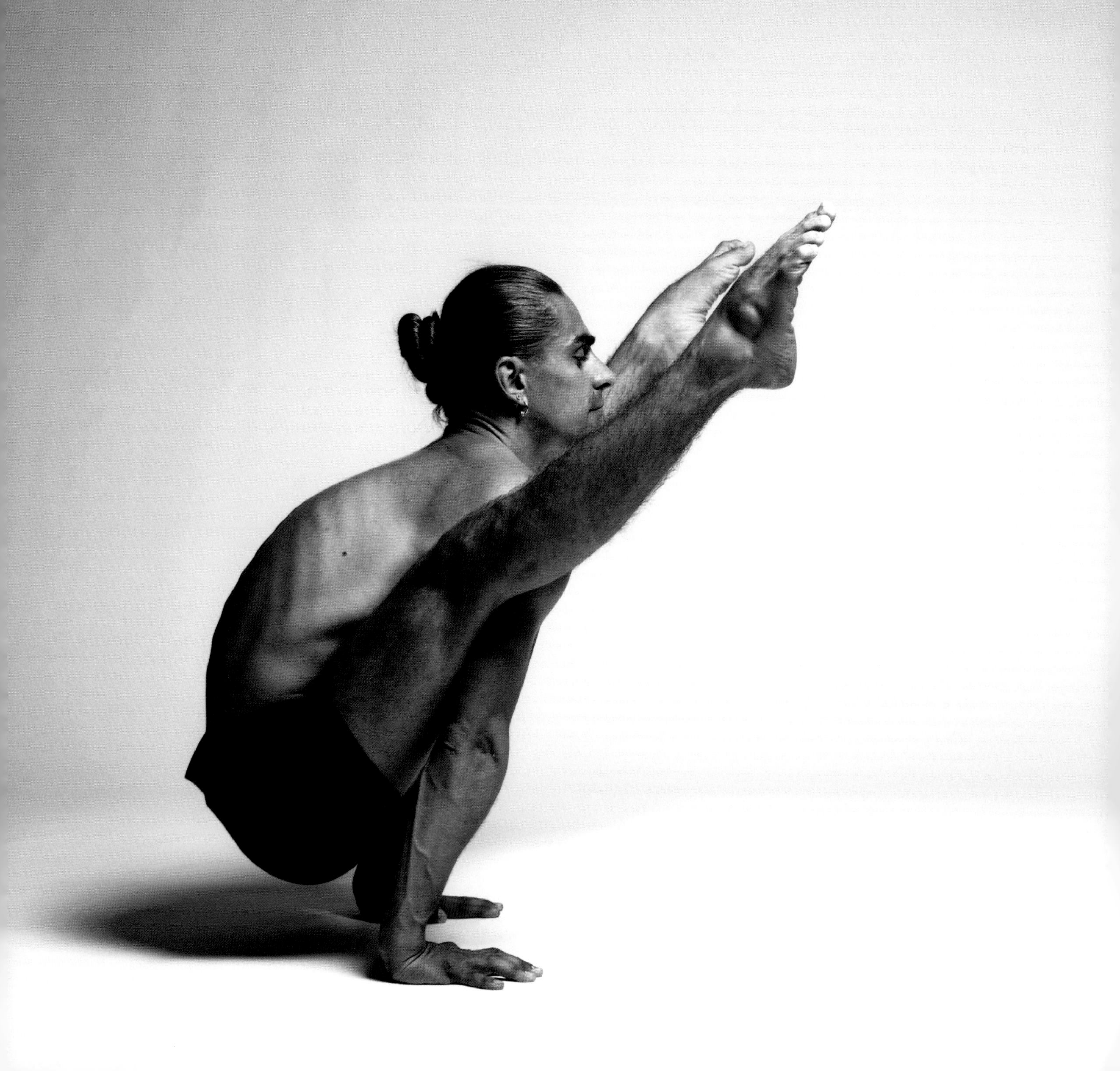

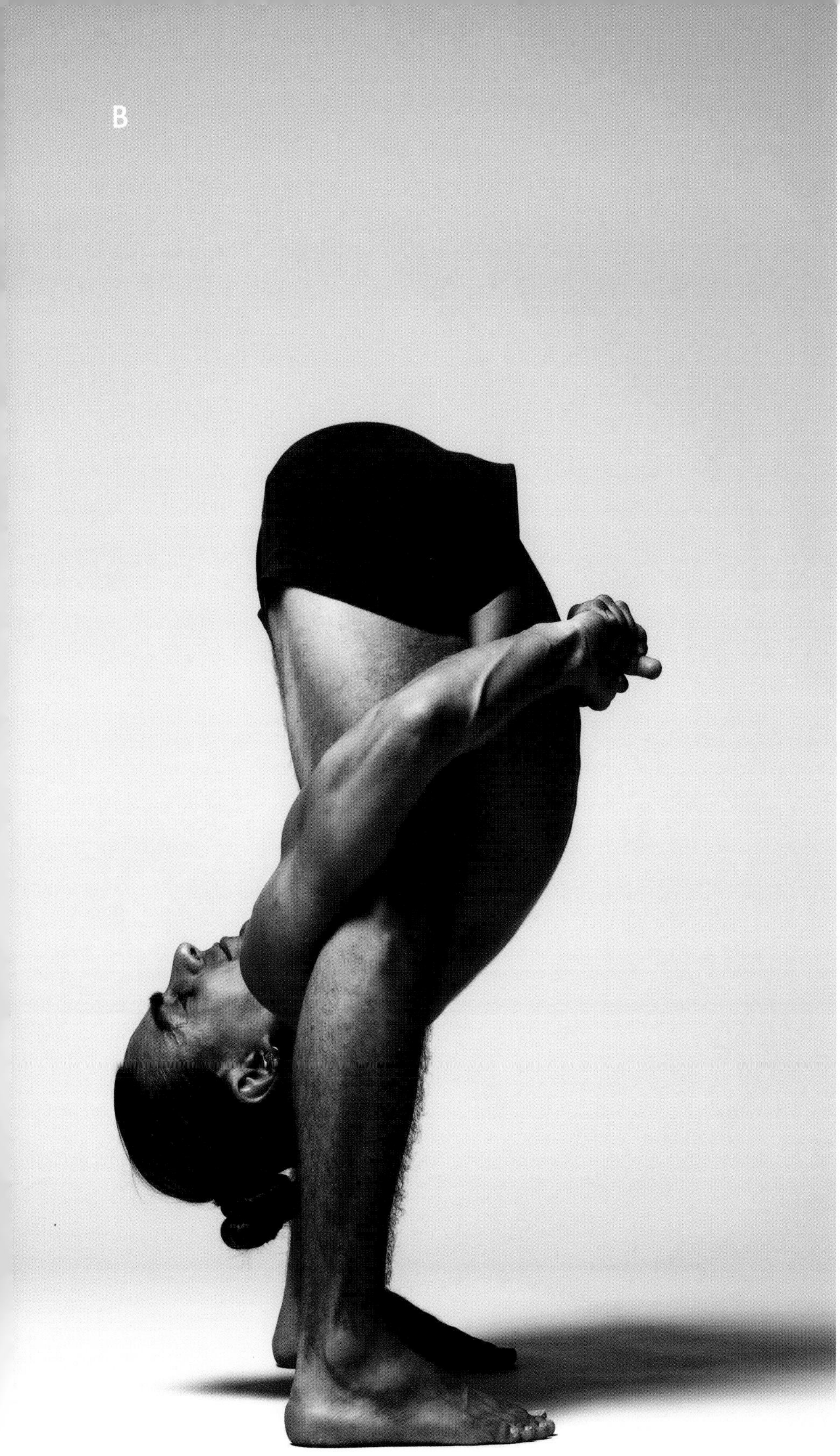

Vinyāsa	Prāṇa	Āsana	Dṛṣṭi	Bandha
Samasthitih		Stand straight		
Vinyāsas 1–6 according to Sūrya-namaskāra A				
7 Sapta	in	jump both legs onto the upper arms, straighten the legs and point the feet		
This is the state of Ṭiṭṭibhāsana A, hold for 5 deep breaths				
8 Aṣṭau	out	Feet on the floor, 2 feet apart, hands behind the back, lift the head, straighten the legs		
This is the state of Ṭiṭṭibhāsana B, hold for 5 deep breaths.				
9 Nava	in & out	Head down, look down to the floor Walk five steps forward and five steps back		
First state of Ṭiṭṭibhāsana C, walk 5 + 5 steps				
	in	Feet 1/2 foot apart, fingers crossed		
Second state of Ṭiṭṭibhāsana C, hold for 5 deep breaths				
10 Daśa	in & out	Hands to the floor, legs up into Ṭiṭṭibhāsana A Hold the pose		
11 Ekādaśa	in	Legs into Bakāsana		
12 Dvādaśa	out	Jump back into Catvāri position		
13 Trayodaśa	in	Upward-facing dog		
14 Caturdaśa	out	Downward-facing dog		
15 Pañcadaśa	in	Jump forward, head up		
16 Ṣoḍaśa	out	Bend forward		
Samasthitih	in & out	Come up Stand straight		

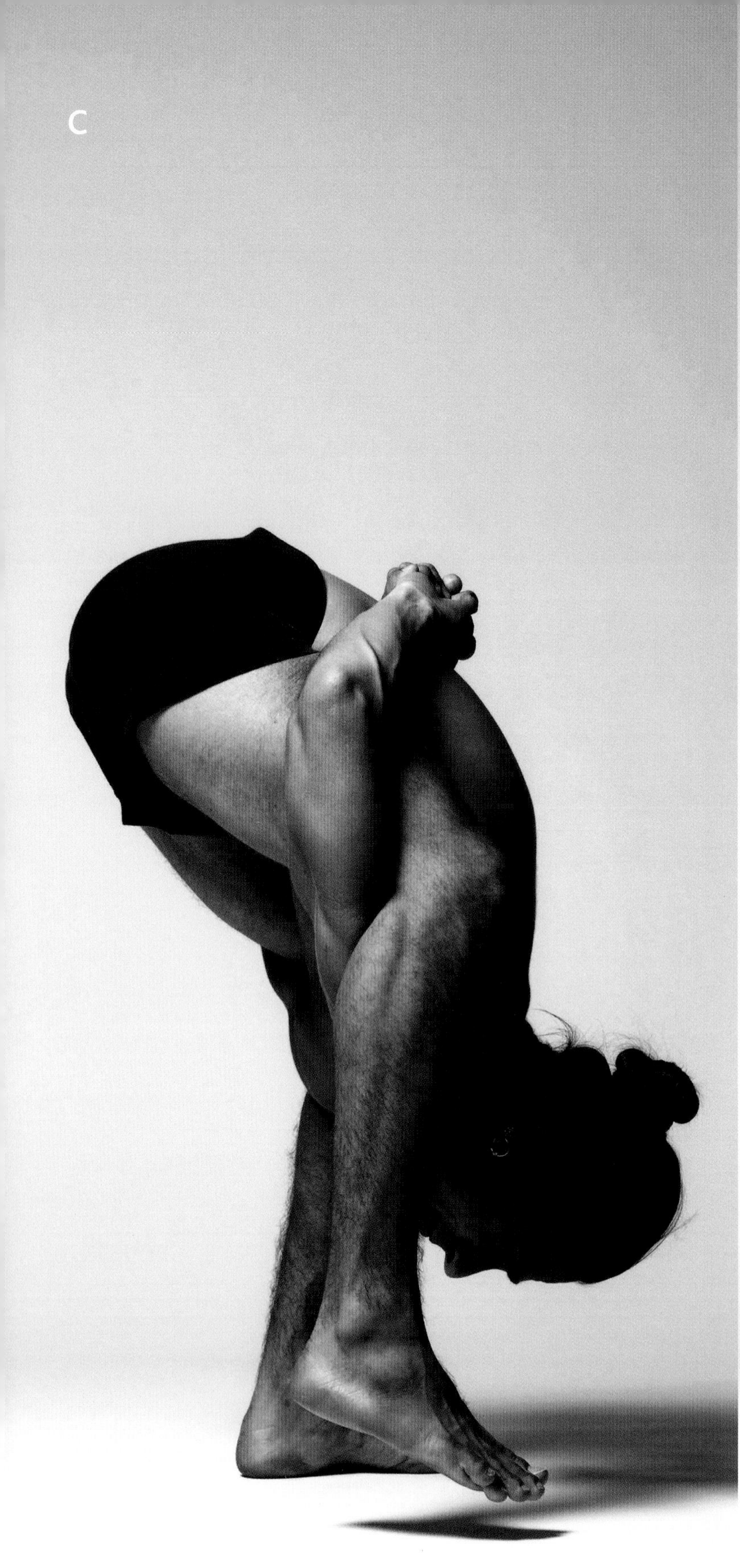
C

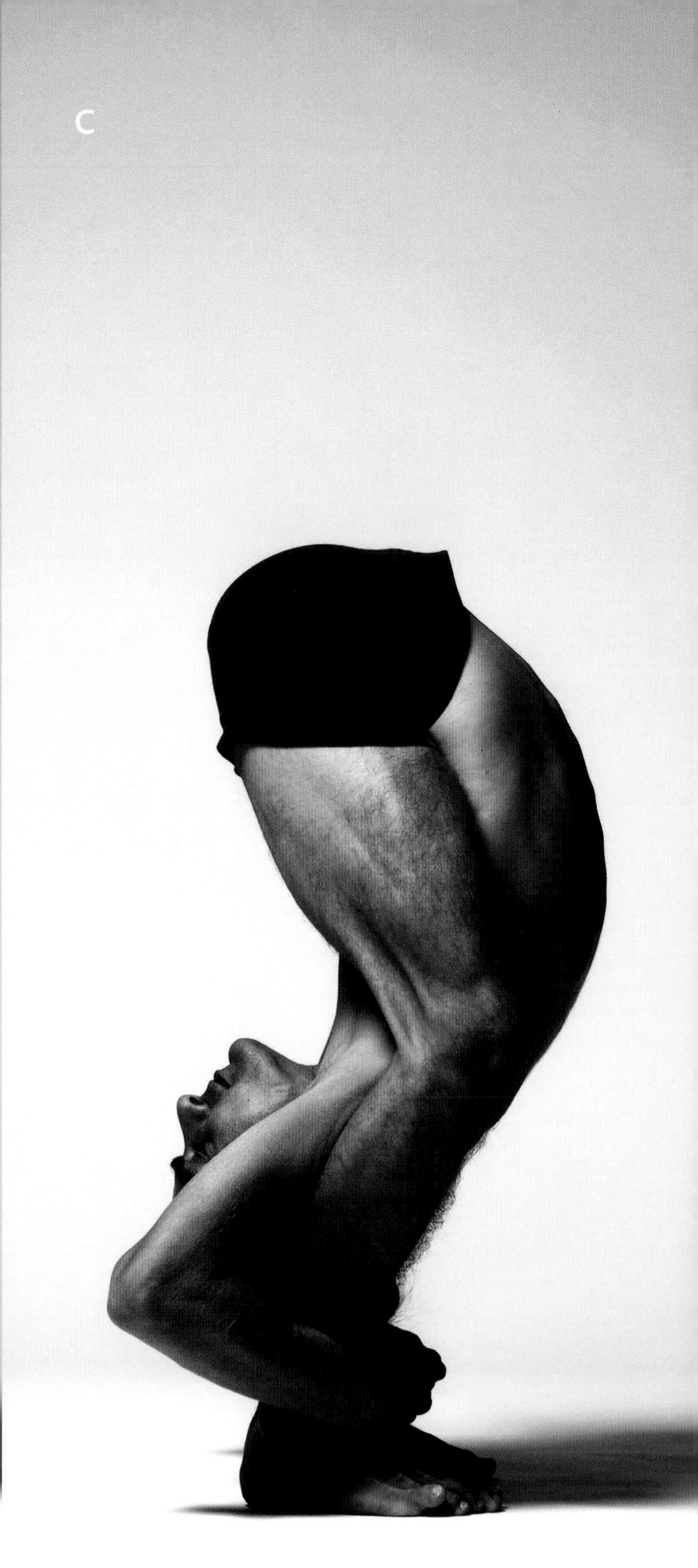
C

continuing 7. *vinyāsa* 7. continuing 8. *vinyāsa*

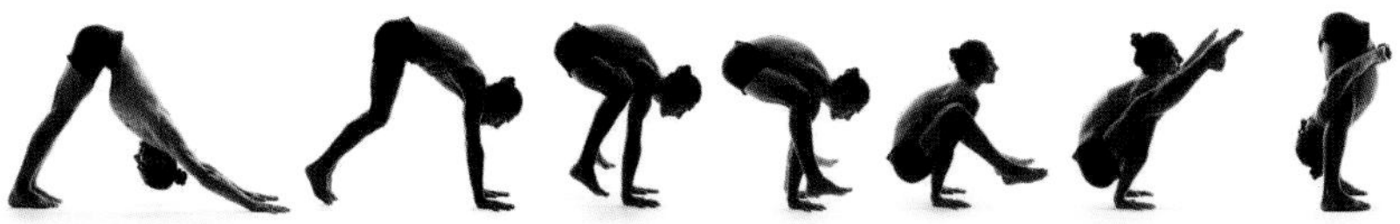

9. *vinyāsa* 9. continuing 10. *vinyāsa* 11. *vinyāsa* 12. *vinyāsa* 13. *vinyāsa* 14. *vinyāsa*

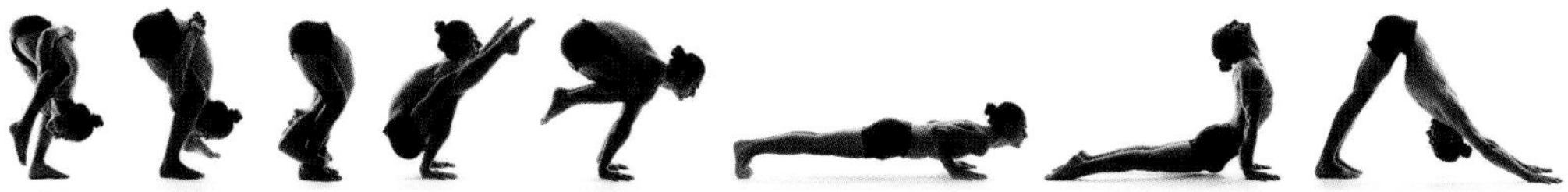

Ṭiṭṭibhāsana A, B and C

Tiṭṭibha – a long-tailed, jacana bird (Latin; *parra jacana*) which makes a 'tit-tit' sound; also translated as firefly

Note 1: The 9th *vinyāsa* includes both the walking and static positions in *Ṭiṭṭibhāsana* C.
Note 2: There are two different dṛṣtis in the 9th *vinyāsa*.
Note 3: There are two breaths in the 10th *vinyāsa*.
Note 4: There are two options for walking in the *Ṭiṭṭibhāsana* C.

Ṭiṭṭibhāsana continues from the 11th *vinyāsa* of *Yoganidrāsana*

7 Sapta
Inhale and jump the legs onto the upper arms, in the same manner as in *Bhuja-pīḍāsana*; only, straighten the legs out to the front, in the same angle as *Navāsana* (in the primary series) and point the feet. Straighten the arms and neck. This is the state of the pose in *Ṭiṭṭibhāsana* A. Gaze at the tip of the nose and breathe deeply five times.

8 Aṣṭau
Exhale and lower the feet to the ground with about a two-foot distance in between. Bend the torso down between the legs, so that the shoulders come through to the back sides of the legs. Take the hands around the lower back and grab either one of the wrists or the fingers. Straighten the legs and lift the head up, so that the chin is close to the collarbones. This is the state of the pose in *Ṭiṭṭibhāsana* B. Gaze at the tip of the nose and breathe deeply five times.

9 Nava
Inhale, lower the head down and gaze at the floor (Adho-mukha-*dṛṣṭi*), keeping hold of the hands around the back, and with the feet still separated about two feet apart. Start walking five steps forward and five steps backwards. The right leg steps first about the length of one foot forward.
There are two options for the walking.

Option 1:
Lift the foot up during the same inhalation, which starts on the ninth *vinyāsa*, and lower the foot down on an exhalation. This is the first step forward. Take the same step with the left foot. Walk forward three more steps, always lifting the foot with an inhalation and landing on the same foot on the exhalation. After finishing the forward steps, walk back five steps, in the same way as when you walked forward.
Option 2:
Inhale, take a step forward with the right leg and as you exhale, step with the left leg. This way you will alternate the legs, taking five steps with the right leg (on the inhalation) and five steps with the left leg (on the exhalation).
After finishing the steps forward, take five steps back with each leg, in the same way as when you walked forward.

Continue...
After the last exhalation of the last step, inhale and bring the feet 1/2 foot wide. The feet are parallel to each other, facing straight towards the front (the feet do not form a V-position, with the heels touching together and the feet out at an angle). Bend the torso and shoulders down between the legs, like in the 8th *vinyāsa*, but now take the hands around and in front of the ankles and clasp the fingers firmly. Both *āsanas*, the walking state and the stationary state (with the fingers clasped around the ankles) are different states of the same pose, *Ṭiṭṭibhāsana* C. Straighten the legs and the neck, gaze at the tip of the nose and breathe deeply five times.

10 Daśa
Inhale, place the palms firmly on the ground and lift the legs back into *Ṭiṭṭibhāsana* A. Gaze at the tip of the nose.
Exhale and hold the pose (Guruji sometimes held this pose for five breaths for strengthening the body).

11 Ekādaśa
Inhale and with a strong upward motion, lift up from the pelvis and slide the legs one at a time, or simultaneously, onto the back of the upper arms into *Bakāsana* (Guruji sometimes held also this pose for five breaths for strengthening the body). Gaze at the tip of the nose.

12 Dvādaśa
Exhale and jump back from *Bakāsana* into *Catvāri* position.

The 13th and 14th *vinyāsas* are the same as in the 5th and 6th *vinyāsas* in *Sūryanamaskāra* A.

From the 14th *vinyāsa* in *Ṭiṭṭibhāsana*, move to the 7th *vinyāsa* in *Piñcha-mayurāsana*.

Benefits:
Ṭiṭṭibhāsana is an effective purifier, cleansing and gradually removing all impurities from the nervous system.

पिञ्छमयूरासन

Pińcha-mayūrāsana

Peacock tail pose | 13 *vinyāsas*

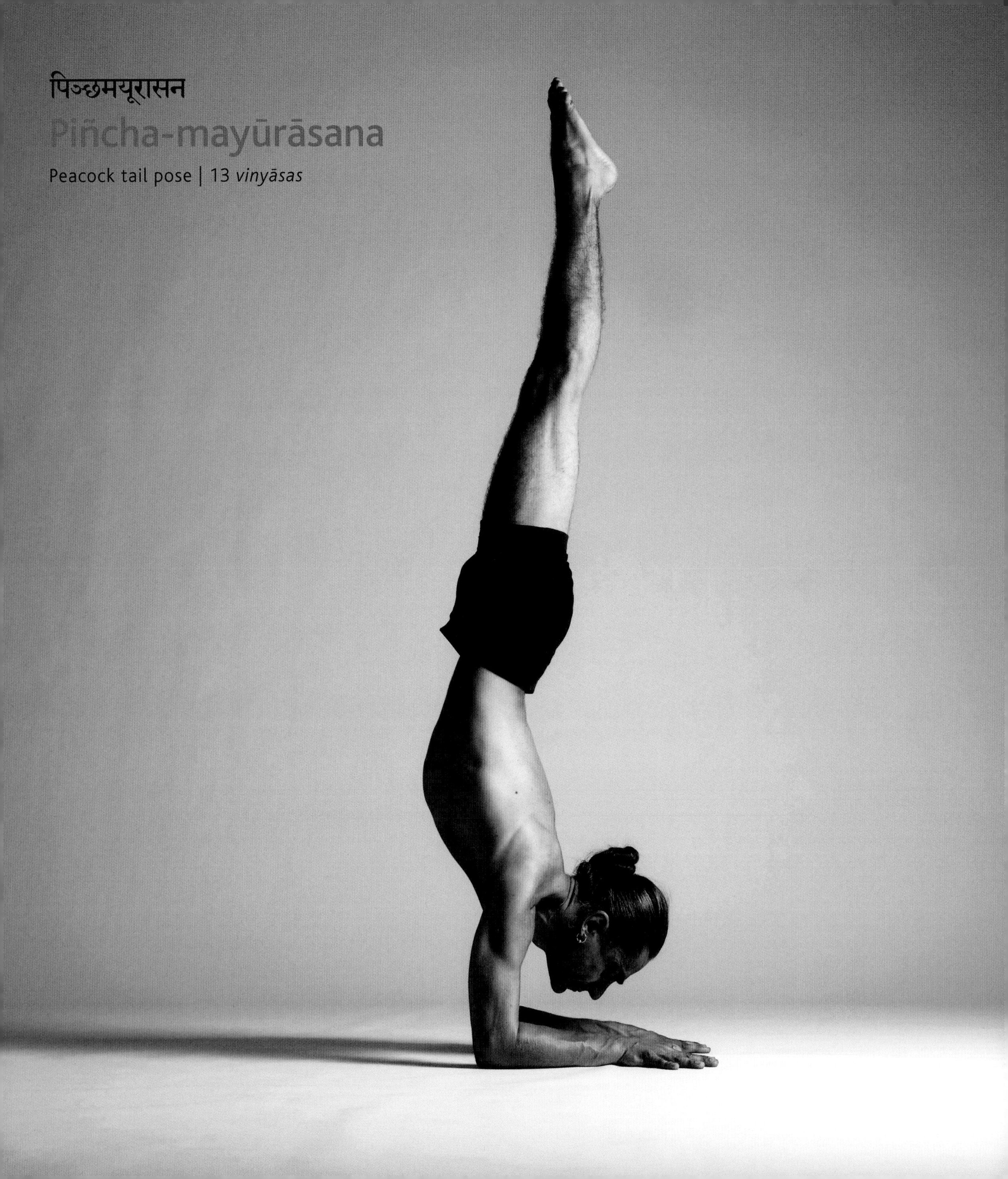

continuing 7. *vinyāsa* 8. *vinyāsa* 9. *vinyāsa* 10. *vinyāsa* 11. *vinyāsa*

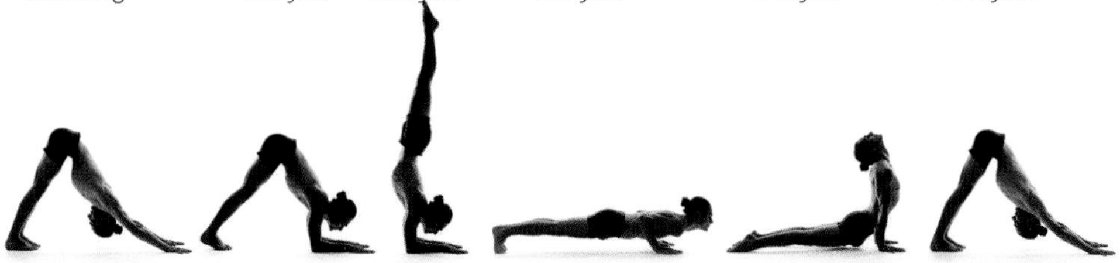

Piñcha-mayūrāsana

Piñcha – tail; *mayūrā* – peacock

Note: There are two breathes in the 7th *vinyāsa*.

Piñcha-mayurāsana continues from the 14th *vinyāsa* in *Ṭiṭṭibhāsana*.

7 Sapta

Inhale and lower the knees to the ground. Place the arms, shoulder-width apart, onto the ground in front of the knees, facing straight forward. Spread the fingers wide and press the palms and fingers firmly onto the floor. The elbows, forearms and palms will keep the position stable.

Exhale, straighten the legs and get ready to lift the body vertically up and onto the forearms.
Gaze at the tip of the nose.

8 Aṣṭau

Inhale, press the forearms and palms firmly into the ground and stabilize the shoulders. Raise the head up and keep the chin forward. Strengthen both *mūla* and *uddīyana-bandha*. Lift (or jump) the legs one at a time or simultaneously. Straighten the posture, point the feet and press them together. Keep the arms aligned with the shoulders, facing straight ahead. Avoid sliding the elbows out to the side and bringing the hands or thumbs together. This is the state of the pose. Gaze at the tip of the nose and breathe deeply five times.

9 Nava

Exhale and fall down into *Catvāri* position.

On the way down, push with the arms and jump slightly up. The elbows will then raise up and the palms will replace the forearms and land down next to the sides. Reduce effort by always keeping the *mūla* and *uddīyana-bandha* engaged, lightening and strengthening the body. Keep the feet flexed while falling down and let the balls of the feet touch the floor first. Descend onto the ground into *Catvāri* position as smoothly as possible. Gaze at the tip of the nose.

The 10th and 11th *vinyāsas* are the same as the 5th and 6th *vinyāsas* in *Sūryanamaskāra* A.

From the 11th *vinyāsa* in *Piñcha-mayurāsana*, move to the 7th *vinyāsa* in *Kāraṇḍavāsana*.

Benefits:

Piñcha-mayūrāsana and the following pose, *Kāraṇḍavāsana*, have similar effects:

- *Piñcha-mayurāsana* and *Kāraṇḍavāsana* clean and free the anāhata-cakra, heart cakra
- strengthen the sides, shoulders and arms
- improve digestion and cleanse the liver and spleen.

To succeed in both *Piñcha-mayurāsana* and Karandavāsana, both *mūla* and *uddīyana-bandha* must remain strong. According to Śrī Pattabhi Jois, the *rudrasi-nāḍi* (sciatic nerve), which moves throughout the body, is the key to succeed in these positions. Weakness of the sciatic nerve creates difficulty in doing these two poses; however, patient practice of *Piñcha-mayurāsana* and *Kāraṇḍavāsana* will strengthen the *rudrasi-nāḍi*.

Vinyāsa	Prāṇa	Āsana	Dṛṣṭi	Bandha
Samasthitih		Stand straight		
Vinyāsas 1–6 according to Sūrya-namaskāra A				
7 Sapta	in & out	Kneel down, prepare the hands and legs		
8 Aṣṭau	in	Lift the pose up		
This is the state of the āsana, hold for 5 deep breaths				
9 Nava	out	Fall down into Catvāri position		
10 Daśa	in	Upward-facing dog		
11 Ekādaśa	out	Downward-facing dog		
12 Dvādaśa	in	Jump forward, head up		
13 Trayodaśa	out	Bend forward		
Samasthitih	in & out	Come up Stand straight		

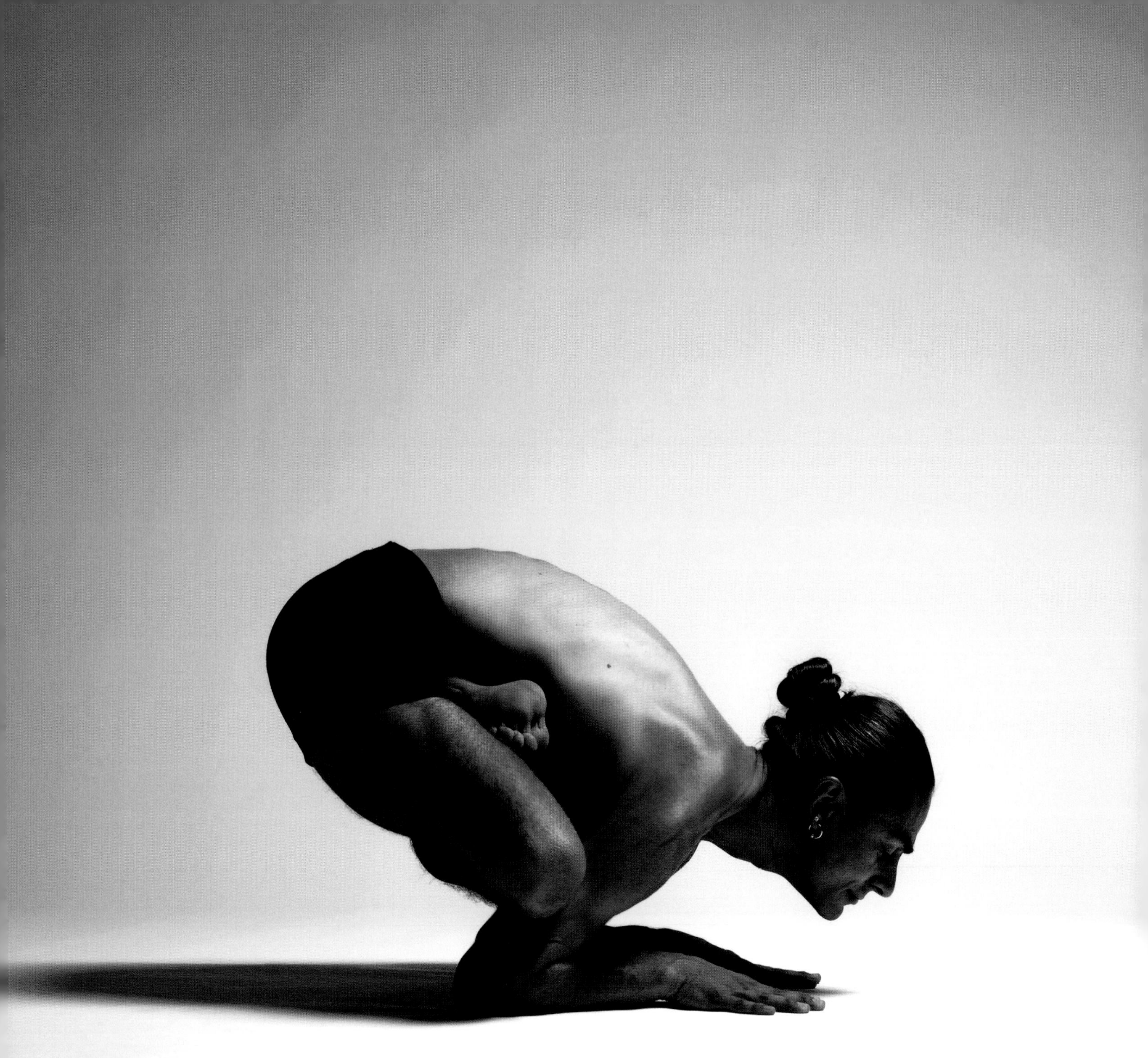

कारण्डवासन

Kāraṇḍavāsana

Goose pose | 15 *vinyāsas*

continuing 7. *vinyāsa* 8. *vinyāsa* 9. *vinyāsa* 9. continuing 10. *vinyāsa* 10. continuing 11. *vinyāsa* 12. *vinyāsa* 13. *vinyāsa* 14. *vinyāsa* 15. *vinyāsa* *Samasthitih*

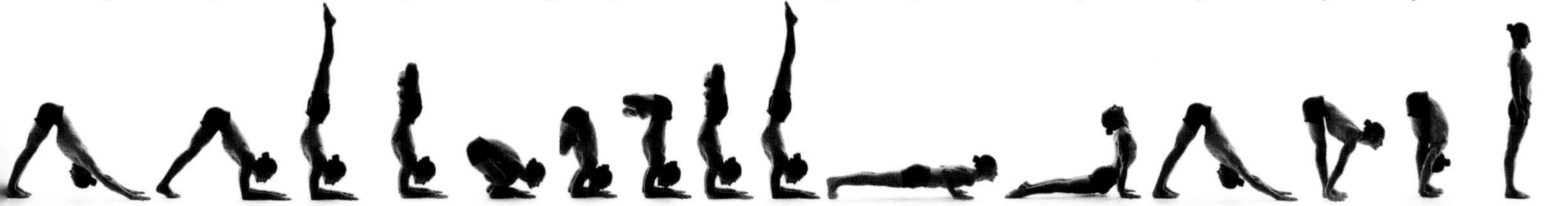

Kāraṇḍavāsana

Kāraṇḍavā – goose

Note: There are two breaths in the 7th *vinyāsa*.

Kāraṇḍavāsana continues from the 11th *vinyāsa* in *Piñcha-mayurāsana*.

7 Sapta

Inhale and lower the knees to the ground. Place the arms, shoulder-width apart, onto the ground in front of the knees, facing straight forward. Spread the fingers wide and press the palms and fingers firmly onto the floor. The elbows, forearms and palms will keep the position stable.

Exhale, straighten the legs and get ready to lift the body vertically up and onto the forearms. Gaze at the tip of the nose.

8 Aṣṭau

Inhale, press the forearms and palms firmly into the ground and stabilize the shoulders. Raise the head up and keep the chin forward. Strengthen both *mūla* and *uddīyana-bandha*. Lift (or jump) the legs up, one at a time, or simultaneously. Straighten the posture, point the feet and press them together. Keep the arms aligned with the shoulders, facing straight ahead. Avoid sliding the elbows out to the side and bringing the hands or thumbs together. Gaze at the tip of the nose.

9 Nava

Exhale, bend the knees and bring the feet into full lotus pose. The right foot goes into the left groin and the left foot goes on top of the right leg. Keep the head up and the arms faced straight ahead, aligned with the shoulders. Avoid sliding the elbows outwards and bringing the thumbs together. Strengthen the *mūla* and *uddīyana-bandha*. Round the back and lower the upper body by slowly bringing the lotus pose down onto the upper arms close to the armpits. Keep the lotus pose strong by pressing the feet inwards and deeper into the position and close to the body. Keep the body strong and pelvis lifted up, avoiding the upper arms and pelvis to move too close to the ground. Hold the head up and keep the chin forward. This is the state of the pose. Gaze at the tip of the nose and breathe deeply five times.

10 Daśa

Inhale, lift the lotus pose up with the strength of both *mūla* and *uddīyana bandha* and the arms. The lifting technique is the same as how you came down, keeping the back rounded and legs close to the body. After balancing in the position at the top, release the lotus and straighten the legs up, without tilting backwards or falling down to the front. Gaze at the tip of the nose.

11 Ekādaśa

Exhale and fall down into *Catvāri* position. On the way down, push with the arms and jump slightly up. The elbows will then raise up and the palms will replace the forearms and land down next to the sides. Keep the feet flexed while falling down and let the balls of the feet touch the floor first. Descend onto the ground into *Catvāri* position as smoothly as possible. Gaze at the tip of the nose.

The 12th to 15th *vinyāsas* are the same as the 5th to 8th *vinyāsas* in *Sūryanamaskāra A*.

Samasthitih

Come up from the 15th *vinyāsa* and move directly into *Samasthitiḥ*, hands by the sides.

Benefits:

The therapeutic effects of *Kāraṇḍavāsana* are the same as in *Piñcha-mayurāsana*, but the lotus pose and the down/up movement deepens the impact of the position.

Kāraṇḍavāsana:

- opens the back, hips, knees and ankles
- increases the metabolism and speeds digestion
- purifies and strengthens the internal organs and the lower cakras
- strengthens the upper arms and shoulders
- strengthens the *rudrasi-nāḍi*, sciatic nerve
- cleans and releases the *anāhata-cakra*, heart cakra.

Vinyāsa	Prāṇa	Āsana	Dṛṣṭi	Bandha
Samasthiti		Stand straight		
Vinyāsas 1–6 according to Sūrya-namaskāra A				
7 Sapta	in & out	Kneel down, prepare the hands and legs		
8 Aṣṭau	in	Lift the pose up		
9 Nava	out	Legs into lotus-pose, lower the lotus pose onto the upper arms		
This is the state of the āsana, hold for 5 deep breaths				
10 Daśa	in	Come back up, straighten the legs		
11 Ekādaśa	out	Fall down into Catvāri position		
12 Dvādaśa	in	Upward-facing dog		
13 Trayodaśa	out	Downward-facing dog		
14 Caturdaśa	in	Jump forward, head up		
15 Pañcadaśa	out	Bend forward		
Samasthitih	in & out	Come up Stand straight		

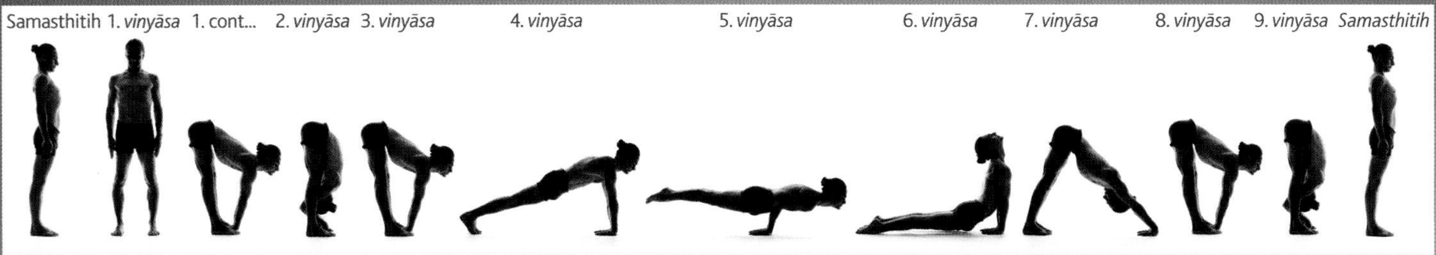

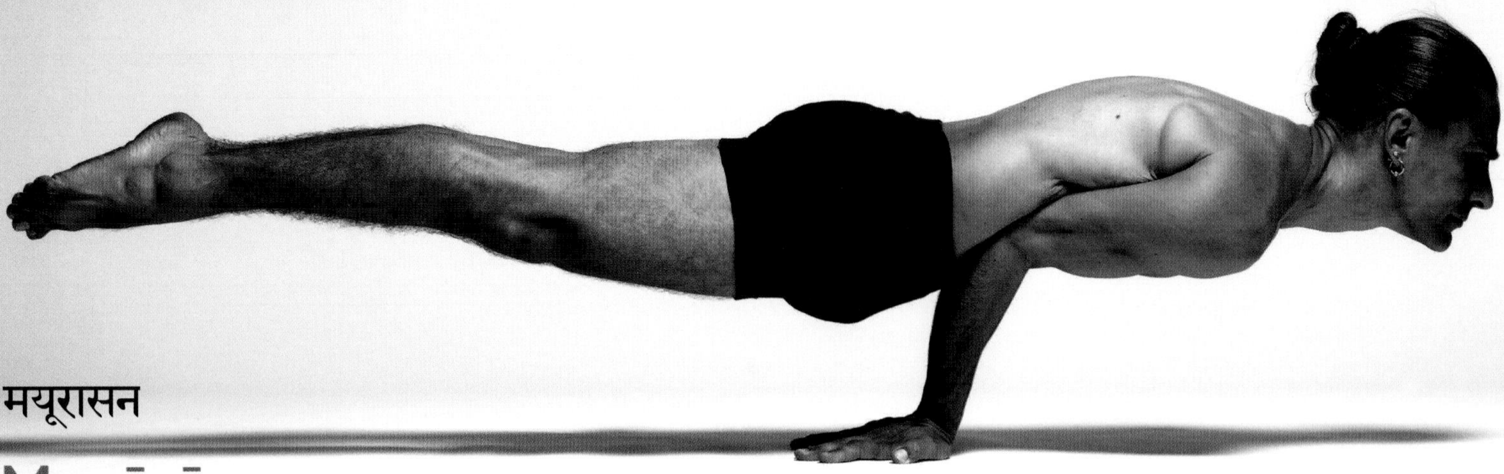

मयूरासन

Mayūrāsana

Peacock pose | 9 *vinyāsas*

Mayūrāsana

Mayūra – peacock

Mayūrāsana continues after *Kāraṇḍavāsana*.

Note: At this stage in the interview, Śrī Pattabhi Jois chanted *ślokas* from *Haṭha-yoga-pradīpikā* (1.30, 1.32 and 1.33) to show the link between the *Aṣṭāṅga* system and the ancient text of *Haṭha-yoga*.

Samasthitih
Stand straight with the feet together and hands down by the sides. Gaze at the tip of the nose.

1 Ekam
Inhale, jump the feet one foot apart and bend forward. Place the palms on the ground between the legs with the fingers facing backwards and the little fingers touching. Lift the head up and open the chest, while pressing the palms to the ground. This is the same pose as the 3rd *vinyāsa* in *Sūryanamaskāra* A, only the fingers are facing backwards. Gaze at the tip of the nose.

2 Dve
Exhale, release the head down and bend the elbows slightly to the side so that you can take the head between the arms and legs. Gaze at the tip of the nose.

3 Trīṇi
Inhale, lift the head back up and keep the palms on the ground like at the end of the 1st *vinyāsa*. Gaze at the tip of the nose.

4 Catvāri
Exhale and jump back, as in the 4th *vinyāsa* in *Sūryanamaskāra* A, but now the fingers point backwards, with the little fingers touching. The body and arms stay straight up, without bending into *Catvāri* position.

5 Pañca
Inhale...

Dharam avaṣṭabhya kara-dvayena tat kūrpara-sthāpita-nābhi-pārśvaḥ uccāsano daṇḍavatutthitaḥ khe/ (Haṭha-yoga-pradīpikā 1.30)

Inhale, bend the elbows (kūrpara) and place them firmly on both sides of the navel (*nābhi*). Strengthen the *mūla* and *uddīyana-bandha*. Keep the head up and chin forward throughout the *āsana*. Tilt the body slightly forward, lift the legs up and find the balance in this horizontal line. Avoid touching the ground with the head or feet. Keep the legs straight and feet pointed back. Actively engage the stomach and press the elbows inwards, so that they do not slip out to the sides.This is the state of the pose. Gaze at the tip of the nose and breathe deeply five times.

6 Ṣaṭ
Inhale and release the feet (still pointed, no need to roll over the toes) onto the ground about one foot apart.

Straighten the arms and bend the body backwards as in the 5th *vinyāsa* in *Sūryanamaskāra* A (upward dog), with the palms on the floor and the fingers still facing backwards. Gaze at the tip of the nose.

7 Sapta
Exhale and move as in the the 6th *vinyāsa* in *Sūryanamaskāra* A, but slide the head, at the end, through the arms and gaze at the navel. Keep the palms pressed on the ground throughout.

8 Aṣṭau
Inhale, lift the head up to the front of the arms and jump forwards, as in the 7th *vinyāsa* in *Sūryanamaskāra* A; only, bring the legs to the outsides of the hands with the fingers still facing backwards. Gaze at the tip of the nose.

9 Nava
Exhale, bend forward, open the elbows slightly out to the side and take the head between the arms and legs. Gaze at the tip of the nose.

Samasthitih
Inhale, come up to standing and jump the feet together, leaving the hands by the sides of the body. Gaze at the tip of the nose.

Benefits:
In *Mayūrāsana*, the elbows are pressed strongly on both sides of the navel. This action cleanses the liver and spleen and massages the internal organs. Weight on the stomach area stimulates the metabolism and speeds up the removal of toxins from the body.

"Māyūram etet pravadanti pīṭham//harati sakala-rogān āśu gulmodarādīn abhibhavati ca doṣān āsana śrī-mayūram/ bahu kadaśana-bhukta bhasma kuryād aśeṣa janayati jaṭharāgni jārayet kālakūtam" (Haṭha-*yoga*-pradīpikā 1.32-33)

Mayūrāsana cleanses the liver and spleen and makes the body so strong that it can resist the kālakūta poison (hālāhala) of the monstrous Vasuki nāga (serpent).

It is said that once the gods and demons were churning the ocean to extract the nectar of immortality from it. Before the nectar was extracted, snake poison, which was so strong that all living beings could be killed from it, came to the surface. Lord Shiva saved the world by drinking the poison, which turned his neck into its characteristic blue color.

In this *āsana*, when the elbows are placed on both sides of the navel, all diseases will vanish and the body's internal problems will be removed. Diseases caused by bad food or food poisoning will also vanish. This is a particularly important *āsana*.

"Harati sakala-rogān āśu gulmodarādin"
Gulma means the liver and spleen, which are especially difficult to purify completely by any other *āsana* or technique besides *Mayūrāsana*.

"Abhibhavati ca doṣān āsana śrī-mayūram"
All disease will be improved and prevented through *Mayūrāsana*.

"Bahu kadaśana-bhukta bhasma kuryād aśeṣa janayati jaṭharāgni jārayet kālakūtam"
It improves discomfort caused by contaminated food or food poisoning.

Vinyāsa	Prāṇa	Āsana	Dṛṣṭi	Bandha
Samasthitih		Stand straight		
1 Ekam	in	jump a foot apart, hands on the floor, fingers pointed back, head up		
2 Dve	out	Bend forward, head down between the arms		
3 Trīṇi	in	Stretch back, head up		
4 Catvāri	out	Jump back, straighten the arms		
5 Pañca	in	Elbows on both sides of the navel, balance the body up on the elbows		
This is the state of the āsana, hold for 5 deep breaths				
6 Ṣaṭ	in	feet on the floor, upward-facing dog		
7 Sapta	out	Downward-facing dog		
8 Aṣṭau	in	Jump forward, head up		
9 Nava	out	Bend forward, head between the arms		
Samasthitih	in & out	Come up to standing jump the feet together		

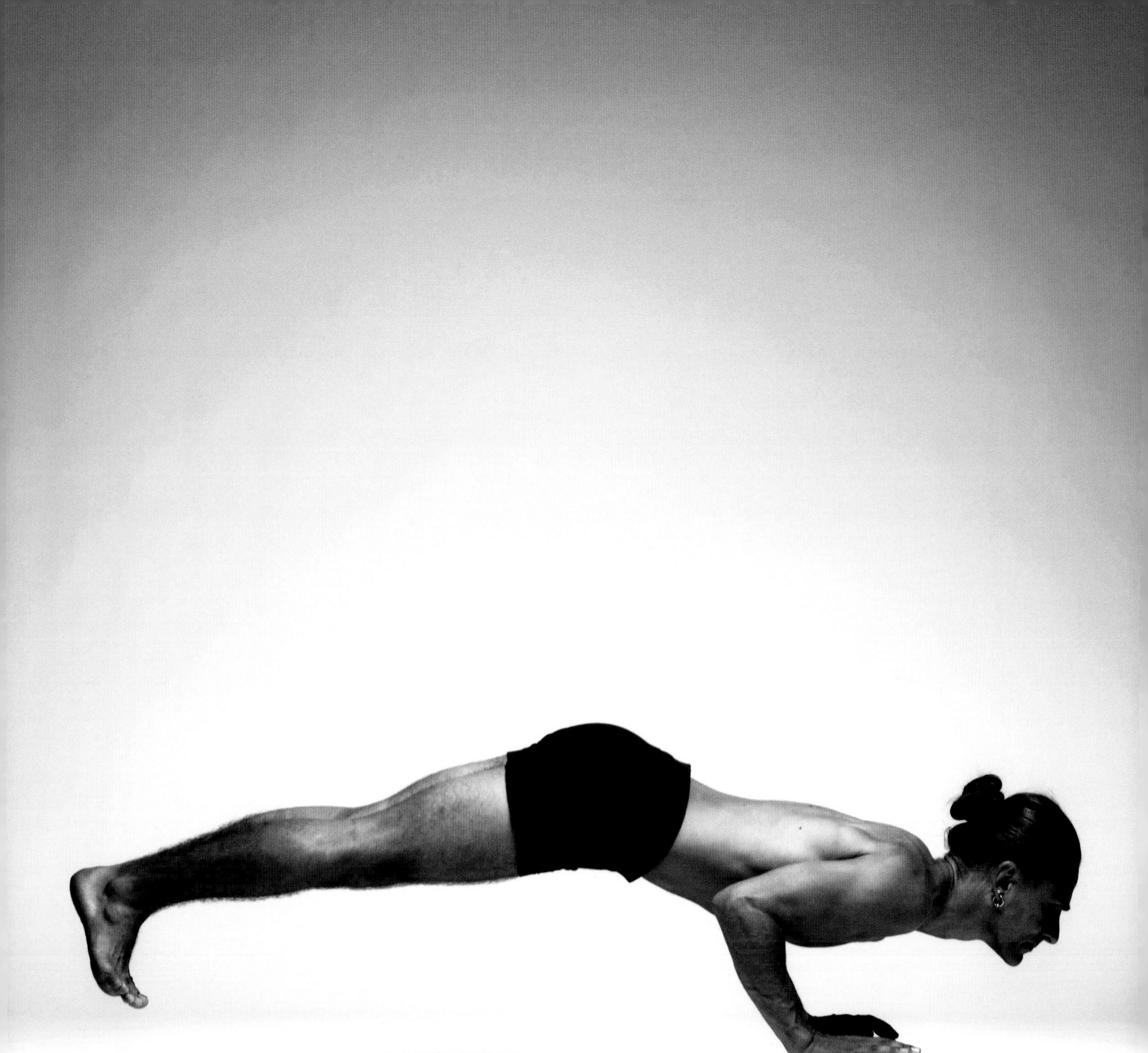

नक्रासन

Nakrāsana

Crocodile pose | 9 *vinyāsas*

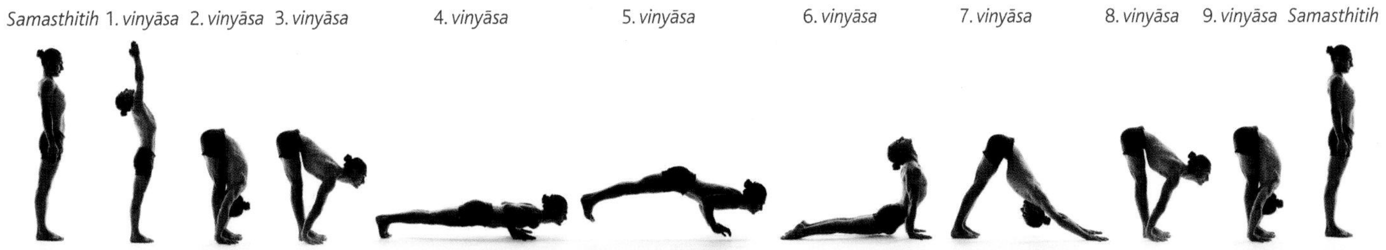

Nakrāsana

Nakra – crocodile

Samasthitih
Stand straight with the feet together and hands down by the sides. Gaze at the tip of the nose.

Vinyāsas 1–4 are the same as the first four *vinyāsas* in *Sūryanamaskāra* A. When jumping back into *Catvāri*, the 4th *vinyāsa*, bring the feet together. Stay in *Catvāri*, keeping the body straight and finish the exhalation. Do not touch the upper body or knees onto the ground. Keep the palms firmly on the ground, approximately at the level of the diaphragm and the elbows at a 90 degree angle. Lift the head up, so that the chin faces forward diagonally.

5 Pañca
Inhale, strengthen the *mūla* and *uddīyana-bandha* and keep the entire body in a straight line. Push off strongly with the hands and balls of the feet, so that the whole body "jumps" in the air and moves forward. The arms shouldn't straighten too much from the 90 degree angle for easier effort and the legs should move with the arms in one unit, rather than lifting up separately and landing at different times. Keep the feet together for the whole duration of the *āsana*. The jump starts on an inhalation and ends on an exhalation. In other words, the moment of lifting up is on an inhalation and coming down on an exhalation. Jump smoothly five times forward and five times backwards, ending at the same place as where you started. Jump clearly and breathe calmly. In between each jump, pause for a moment until the end of the exhalation. The state of *Nakrāsana* consists of these five forward jumps and five backward jumps. Gaze at the tip of the nose while jumping.

Vinyāsas 6–9 are the same as the *vinyāsas* 5–8 in *Sūryanamaskāra* A.

Samasthitih
Inhale and come up from the 9th *vinyāsa*, leaving the hands by the sides of the body.

Benefits:
Nakrāsana is designed specifically to strengthen the shoulders and arms, as well as the entire upper body and *mūla* and *uddīyana-bandha*. The whole body should remain strong while jumping.

Vinyāsa	Prāṇa	Āsana	Dṛṣṭi	Bandha
Samasthitih		Stand straight		
1 Ekam	in	Raise the arms		
2 Dve	out	Bend forward		
3 Trīṇi	in	Stretch back, head up		
4 Catvāri	out	Catvāri position, do not descend to the ground		
5 Pañca	in & out	Jump five times forward and five times backward		
This is the state of the āsana				
6 Ṣaṭ	in	Upward-facing dog		
7 Sapta	out	Downward-facing dog		
8 Aṣṭau	in	Jump forward, head up		
9 Nava	out	Bend forward		
Samasthitih	in & out	Come up Stand straight		

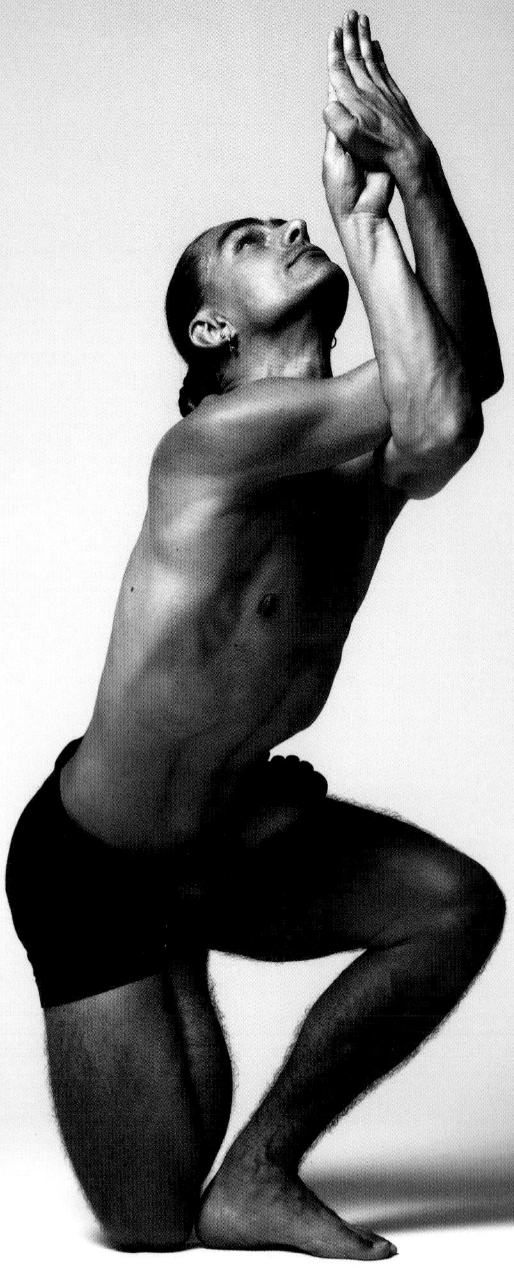

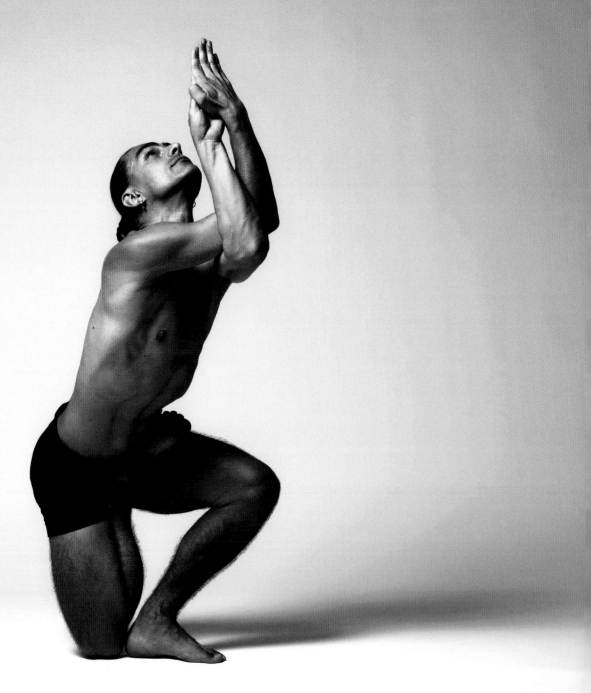

वातायनासन

Vātāyanāsana

Window (air) pose | 20 *vinyāsas*

Vātāyanāsana

Vāta – air; *Vātāyana* – window (opening the window to let air in)

According to Guruji, *Vātāyana* means window, from which air (*vāta*) can flow into the room (body). Many sources state that *Vātāyana* signifies the head of a horse, as *Vātāyana* can signify either a window or the head of a horse. In this case, *Vātāyana* means window.

Note 1: *Vātāyanāsana* is the only *āsana* in *Nāḍī-śodhana* sequence, where the *mūla-bandha* is released during the state of the pose.

Note 2 : There are two breathes in the 19th *vinyāsa*.

Samasthitih
Stand straight with feet together and the arms beside the body. Gaze at the tip of the nose.

1 Ekam
Inhale and lift the right foot into half-lotus, as in the 1st *vinyāsa* of the primary series' standing sequence position, *Ardha-baddha-padmottānāsana*. Take the right arm behind the back and firmly grip the right big toe with two fingers and the thumb. Keep the left arm straight beside the body. Gaze at the tip of the nose.

2 Dve
Exhale, release the big toe, bend the upper body down and take both hands to the floor, besides the left foot. Press the chin into the shin. Keep the right leg in half-lotus with the knee about 45 degrees out to the side. Gaze at the tip of the nose.

3 Trīṇi
Inhale, lift the head up and stretch the torso, like in the 3rd *vinyāsa* in *Sūryanamaskāra* A, only the right leg is now in half-lotus. Gaze at the tip of the nose.

4 Catvāri
Exhale, press the palms firmly to the ground, engage *mūla* and *uddīyana-bandha*, lift the left foot from the ground and swing the body back into "one legged" *Catvāri* position. Gaze at the tip of the nose.

5 Pañca
Inhale, put the weight on the arms, straighten the arms slowly and roll the left foot over the toes. The movement is the same as the 5th *vinyāsa* in *Sūryanamaskāra* A, but the right leg is in half-lotus. Keep the left leg straight and the right leg firmly in half-lotus. The right foot, hips and both knees stay up off the ground throughout this *vinyāsa*. Only the left foot and hands touch the floor. Arch the chest, straighten the arms and take the head back. Gaze at the tip of the nose.

Vinyāsa	Prāṇa	Āsana	Dṛṣṭi	Bandha
Samasthitih		Stand straight		
1 Ekam	in	Right foot into lotus-pose take hold of the right big toe		
2 Dve	out	Bend forward, both hands on the floor		
3 Trīṇi	in	Stretch back, head up		
4 Catvāri	out	Catvāri position (with half lotus-pose)		
5 Pañca	in	Upward-facing dog		
6 Ṣaṭ	out	Downward-facing dog		
7 Sapta	in	jump to the right side of the pose, left heel touching the right knee, hands crossed, left arm under the right		
This is the state of the right side āsana, hold for 5 deep breaths				
8 Aṣṭau	in	hands on the floor, lift up		
9 Nava	out	Catvāri position (with half lotus-pose)		
10 Daśa	in	Upward-facing dog		
11 Ekādaśa	out	Downward-facing dog, change the leg		
12 Dvādaśa	in	Jump to the left side of the pose, right heel touching the left knee, hands crossed, right arm under the left		
This is the state of the left side āsana, hold for 5 deep breaths				
13 Trayodaśa	in	hands on the floor, lift up		
14 Caturdaśa	out	Catvāri position (with half lotus-pose)		
15 Pañcadaśa	in	Upward-facing dog		
16 Ṣoḍaśa	out	Downward-facing dog		
17 Saptadaśa	in	Jump forward, grab the left big toe, head up		
18 Aṣṭadaśa	out	Bend forward		
19 Ekonaviṃśatiḥ	in & out	Head up again hold the pose		
20 Viṃśatiḥ	in	Come up, to standing		
Samasthitih	out	Release the leg, arms on the sides		

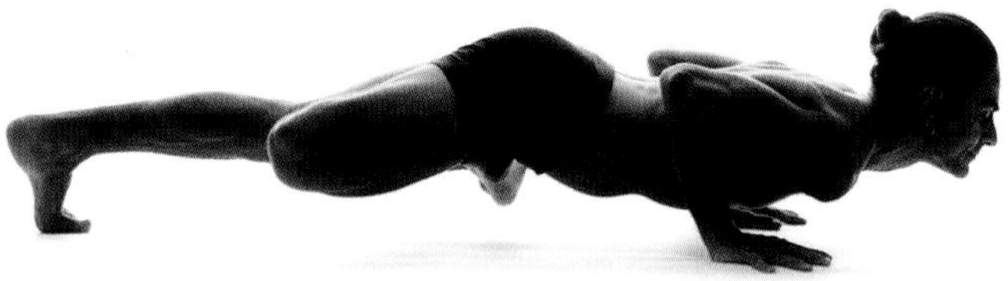

4. *vinyāsa*

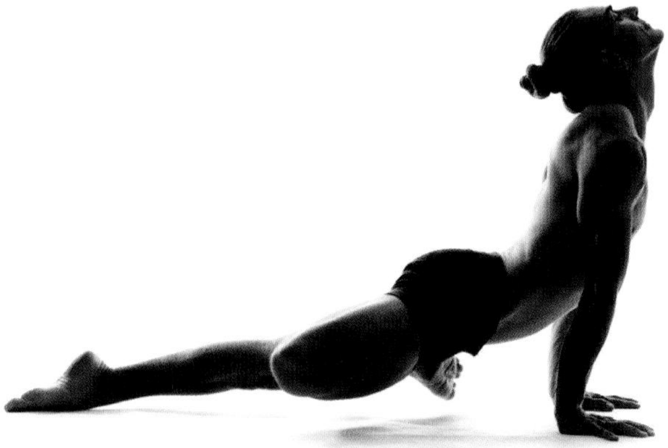

5. *vinyāsa*

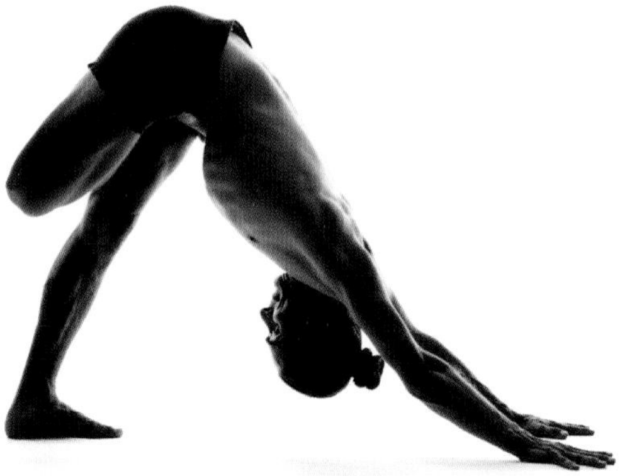

11. *vinyāsa* (right side)

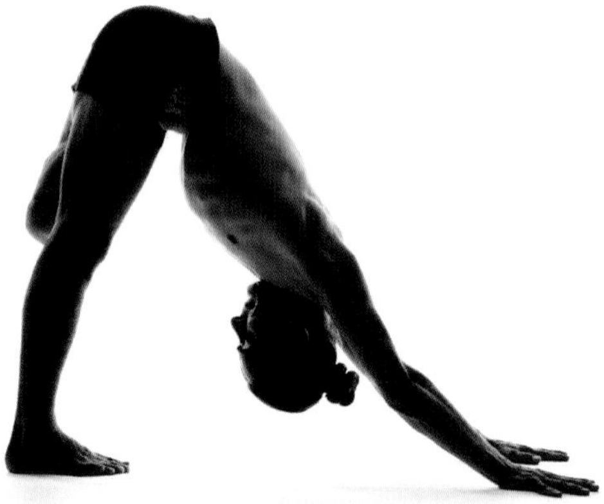

11. *vinyāsa* (left side)

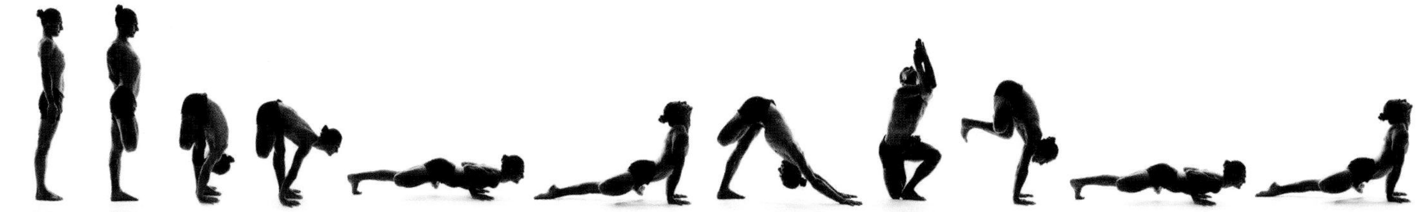
Samasthiti
1. vinyāsa
2. vinyāsa
3. vinyāsa
4. vinyāsa
5. vinyāsa
6. vinyāsa
7. vinyāsa
8. vinyāsa
9. vinyāsa
10. vinyāsa

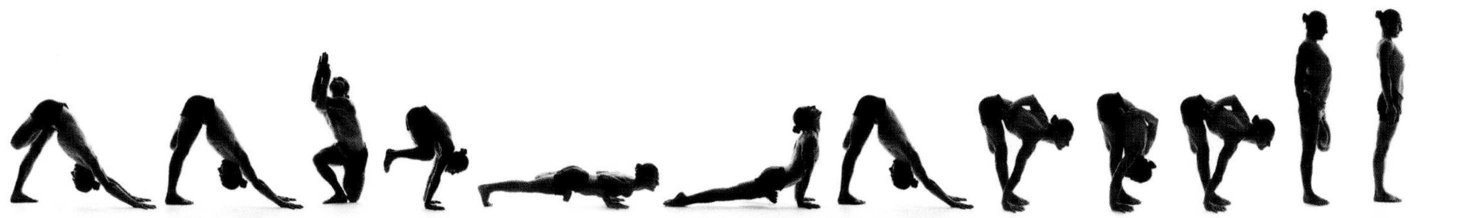
11. vinyāsa
11. continuing
12. vinyāsa
13. vinyāsa
14. vinyāsa
15. vinyāsa
16. vinyāsa
17. vinyāsa
18. vinyāsa
19. vinyāsa
20. vinyāsa
Samasthiti

<u>6 Ṣaṭ</u>
Exhale and lift the hips up like in the 6th *vinyāsa* of *Sūryanamaskāra* A. Make sure that only the hands and the left foot touch the ground during this *vinyāsa*.

<u>7 Sapta</u>
Inhale, jump forward and land the left leg in between the hands. Lower the right knee onto the ground in front of you, place the left heel on the inner edge of the right knee, and turn the left foot about 90 degrees out to the side. Keep the left heel in contact with the inside of the right knee throughout the *vinyāsa*. Press the left foot evenly onto the ground, without lifting the heel up. Take the upper arms across the front of the chest, with the left arm crossing underneath the right. Place the left palm against the right as evenly as possible. Keep the fingers together and avoid modifying the position by crossing the fingers or holding one palm too low, i.e, closer to the wrist. Push the hips forward, extend the spine and open the left knee to the side. Stretch the crossed arms straight up and take the head back. The position of the arms will not allow you to straighten the arms completely; therefore, it is natural that the elbows remain slightly bent.

Relax *mūla-bandha* to facilitate the opening and cleansing of the pelvis, but pull in *uddīyana-bandha* to straighten the back and help with the balance. This is the state of the pose on the right side. Gaze upwards and breathe deeply five times.

<u>8 Aṣṭau</u>
Inhale, release the arms and place the palms on the floor to the sides of the left foot and right knee. Engage with the strength of the arms and both, *mūla* and *uddīyana-bandha*, and lift the body about 1-2 feet into the air, keeping the same position with the feet. There is no need to lift the body all the way up into the handstand. Gaze at the tip of the nose.

<u>9 Nava</u>
Exhale, swing the body behind in the air and straighten the left leg into a "one-legged" *Catvāri* position. Gaze at the tip of the nose.

The 10th and 11th *vinyāsas* are the same as the 5th and 6th *vinyāsas*, but the feet are switched at the end of the exhalation of the 11th *vinyāsa*. Release the right leg from the half lotus and straighten it down. Then prepare the half lotus position on the other side, with the left foot up into the left groin. Use the hand as needed to help set the left foot into the pose. Gaze at the navel.

Vinyāsas 12-16 are the same as *vinyāsas* 7-11, only now the the left leg in half-lotus.

<u>17 Saptadaśa</u>
Inhale, jump forward and land the right foot in between the hands, like the 7th *vinyāsa* of *Sūryanamaskāra* A, with the left leg in half-lotus. After the jump, immediately take the left hand behind the back and grip the left big toe firmly. Lift the head up and stretch the torso. Gaze at the tip of the nose.

<u>18 Aṣṭadaśa</u>
Exhale, bend the upper body down and press the chin into the shin. Gaze at the tip of the nose.

<u>19 Ekonaviṃśatiḥ</u>
Inhale, lift the head up again and stretch the upper body. Exhale and hold the pose. Gaze at the tip of the nose.

<u>20 Viṃśatiḥ</u>
Inhale, come up to standing with the right leg straight and keep holding onto the left big toe, as in the 9th *vinyāsa* of the primary series' standing sequence position, *Ardha-baddha-padmottānāsana*.

<u>Samasthitih</u>
Exhale, release the left leg to the floor next to the right leg and both arms on the sides.

<u>**Benefits:**</u>
Vātāyanāsana is a complex *āsana* with a number of effects. In particular, it stretches the spine and opens the hips. Further, a relaxed *mūla-bandha* releases the hips.
Vātāyanāsana also:
- cleanses the anus and rectum
- cures rectal diseases such as hemorrhoids, constipation and fistula
- straightens and strengthens the spine
- opens the hips, knees and ankles
- stretches the arms
- improves the sense of balance.

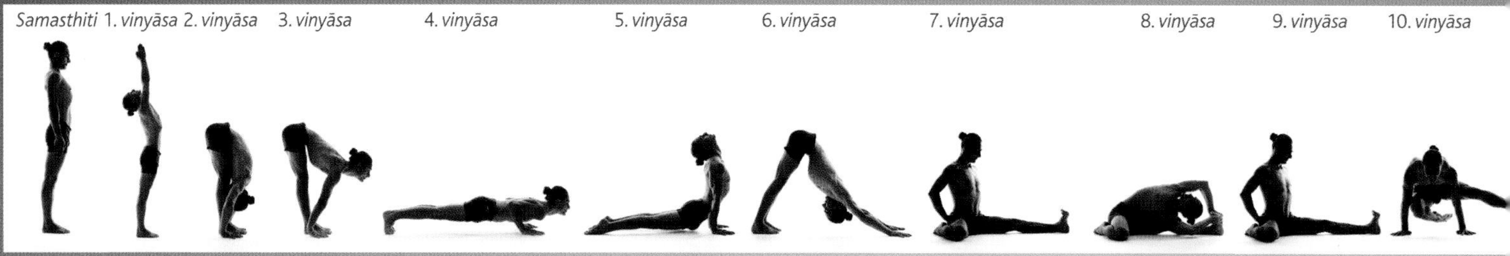
Samasthiti
1. vinyāsa
2. vinyāsa
3. vinyāsa
4. vinyāsa
5. vinyāsa
6. vinyāsa
7. vinyāsa
8. vinyāsa
9. vinyāsa
10. vinyāsa

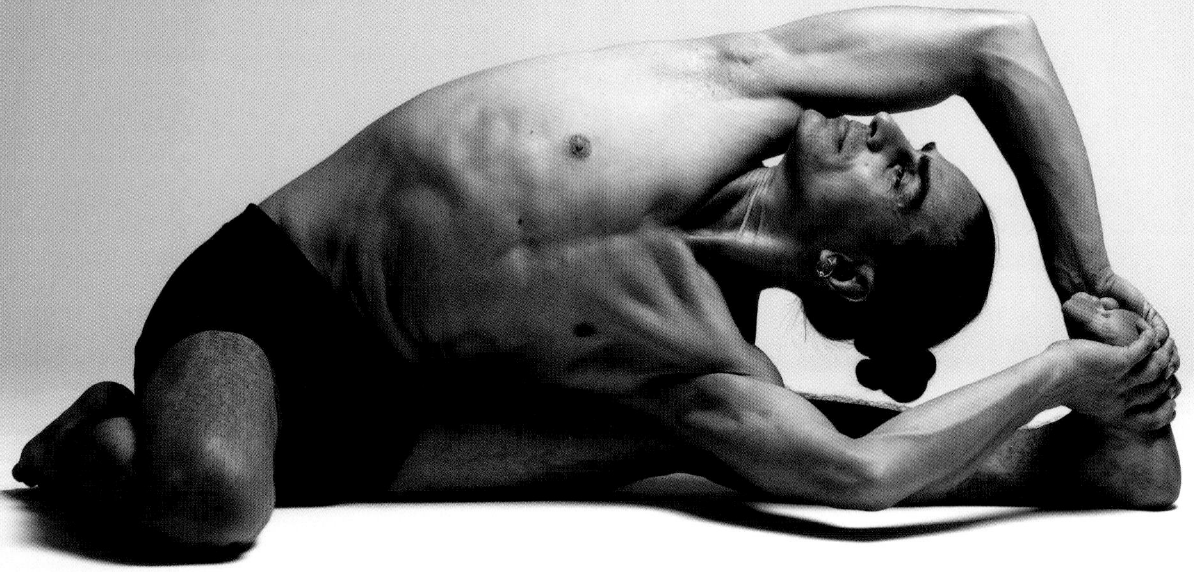

परिघासन

Parighāsana

Gate bar pose | 22 *vinyāsas*

1. vinyāsa 12. vinyāsa 13. vinyāsa 14. vinyāsa 15. vinyāsa 16. vinyāsa 17. vinyāsa 18. vinyāsa 19. vinyāsa 20. vinyāsa

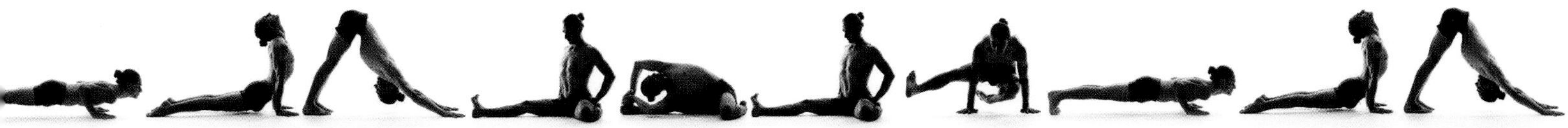

Parighāsana

According to Guruji, parigha refers to a jungle animal, which we couldn't find the exact name for, with tusks or horns and makes a circular movement position. In most sources, parigha is described as an iron or wooden bolt for shutting a gate, hence *Parighāsana* is translated as gate bolt pose or gate bar pose.

Note 1: There are two breathes in the 9th and 16th *vinyāsas*.
Note 2: In the 10th and 17th *vinyāsas*, it is possible to jump back with crossed legs.
Note 3: There are two options for the 7th and 14th *vinyāsas*.

Samasthitih
Stand straight with feet together and arms by the sides. Gaze at the tip of the nose.

Vinyāsas 1–6 are the same as *vinyāsas* 1–6 in *Sūryanamaskāra* A.

7 Sapta
Inhale, jump forward. Bend the right leg back in the air during the jump and keep the left leg straight. Place the bent right leg between the hands and the straight left leg directly behind the left hand 90 degrees out to the left. The right knee faces forward. Place the hands on the hips and align the hips and chest forward. Expand the upper body and lengthen the spine. Gaze at the tip of the nose.

Note: There has been another form from the 7th and 14th *vinyāsas*, where the jump through has been done like in Paścima-tānāsana in the Primary series (inhale jump through, exhale hold the pose and then inhale set the legs as it is described here in the 7th *vinyāsa*). Anyhow, in this book we have the form which I got from Śrī Pattabhi Jois in 2007.

8 Aṣṭau
Exhale, bend the torso straight to the left side on the left leg. Rotate the rib cage upwards, move the hands from the hips and stretch the left upper arm onto the left inner thigh. Take hold with the left hand from the inner edge of the left foot. Stretch the right arm over the head towards the left side of the foot and firmly grip the right hand from the outer edge of left foot. Keep the right foot by the buttock and the knee straight ahead. The legs form a 90 degree angle relative to each other. While taking hold of the left foot, the right hip will usually lift 1-2 inches up from the floor. Do not let the hip move too high; instead, keep pressing it down towards the ground. Stretch the right side, rotate the rib cage and turn the head upwards. Keep the neck straight and the head in the air without pressing it into the shin. This is the state of the pose on the right side. Gaze upwards and breathe deeply five times.

9 Nava
Inhale, release the hands and come back up to the position in the 7th *vinyāsa*, placing the hands on the hips. Exhale and hold the pose. Gaze at the tip of the nose.

10 Daśa
Inhale, place the right hand on the ground outside the right thigh and the left hand in the front of the left thigh. Strengthen the arms and both *mūla* and *uddīyana-bandha* and lift the body off the ground. Gaze at the tip of the nose.

11 Ekādaśa
Exhale, swing the body back and straighten the legs in the air into *Catvāri* position. Gaze at the tip of the nose.

The 12th and 13th *vinyāsas* are the same as the 5th and 6th *vinyāsas* in *Sūryanamaskāra* A.

Vinyāsas 14–18 are the same as *vinyāsas* 7–11, but on the left side, the left knee is bent and the right leg is straight out to the side.

Vinyāsas 19–20 are the same as the 5th and 6th *vinyāsas* in *Sūryanamaskāra* A.

From the Parighāsanas 20th *vinyāsa*, move to the 7th *vinyāsa* in *Gomukhāsana*.

Benefits:
Parighāsana is part of a group of rotation movements, and their most powerful effect is to release the nervous system around the spine. In addition, *Parighāsana*:
- opens the hips
- deeply stretches the hamstrings and sides
- cleanses the internal organs and the lower cakras.

Vinyāsa	Prāṇa	Āsana	Dṛṣṭi	Bandha
Samasthitih		Stand straight		
Vinyāsas 1–6 according to Sūrya-namaskāra A				
7 Sapta	in	Jump through, left leg to the side, hands on the hips		
8 Aṣṭau	out	Bend to the left, twist the arms, take hold of the foot		
This is the state of the right side āsana, hold for 5 deep breaths				
9 Nava	in & out	Up to the sitting, hands on the hips hold the pose		
10 Daśa	in	Hands on the floor, lift up		
11 Ekādaśa	out	Catvāri position		
12 Dvādaśa	in	Upward-facing dog		
13 Trayodaśa	out	Downward-facing dog		
14 Caturdaśa	in	Jump through, right leg to the side, hands on the hips		
15 Pañcadaśa	out	Bend to the right, twist the arms, take hold of the foot		
This is the state of the left side āsana, hold for 5 deep breaths				
16 Ṣoḍaśa	in & out	Up to the sitting, hands on the hips Hold the pose		
17 Saptadaśa	in	Hands on the floor, lift up		
18 Aṣṭadaśa	out	Catvāri position		
19 Ekonaviṃśatiḥ	in	Upward-facing dog		
20 Viṃśatiḥ	out	Downward-facing dog		
21 Ekaviṃśatiḥ	in	Jump forward, head up		
22 Dvāviṃśatiḥ	out	Bend forward		
Samasthitih	in & out	Come up Stand straight		

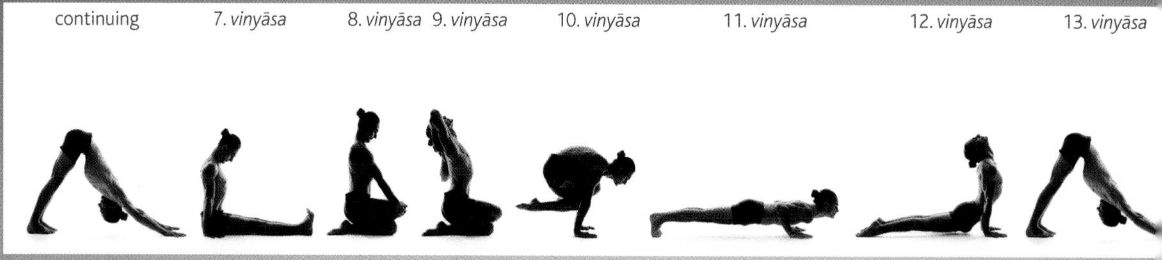

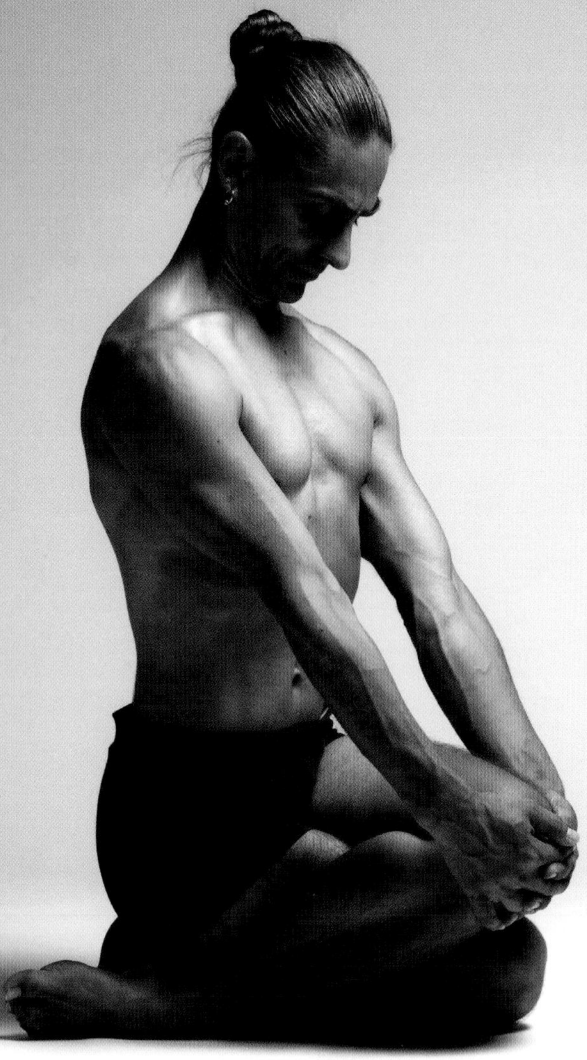

गोमुखासन

Gomukhāsana

Cow face pose | 22 *vinyāsas*

14. *vinyāsa* 15. *vinyāsa* 16. *vinyāsa* 17. *vinyāsa* 18. *vinyāsa* 19. *vinyāsa* 20. *vinyāsa*

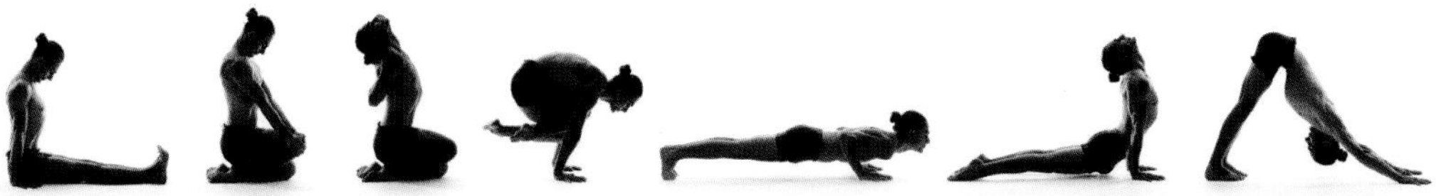

Vinyāsa	Prāṇa	Āsana	Dṛṣṭi	Bandha
Samasthitih		Stand straight		
Vinyāsas 1–6 according to Sūrya-namaskāra A				
7 Sapta	in & out	Jump through to sitting, hold the pose		
8 Aṣṭau	in	Fold left leg under, right crossed on the top, sit on the right heel, take hold of the right knee, chin down		
This is the first state of the āsana, hold for 5 deep breaths				
9 Nava	in	Hands behind the back, left from below, right from above, head back		
This is the second state of the āsana, hold for 5 deep breaths				
10 Daśa	in	Hands on the floor, lift up		
11 Ekādaśa	out	Catvāri position		
12 Dvādaśa	in	Upward-facing dog		
13 Trayodaśa	out	Downward-facing dog		
14 Caturdaśa	in & out	Jump through to sitting, hold the pose		
15 Pañcadaśa	in	Fold right leg under, left crossed on the top, sit on the left heel, take hold of the left knee, chin down		
This is the first state of the āsana, hold for 5 deep breaths				
16 Ṣoḍaśa	in	Hands behind the back, right from below, left from above, head back		
This is the second state of the āsana, hold for 5 deep breaths.				
17 Saptadaśa	in	Hands on the floor, lift up		
18 Aṣṭadaśa	out	Catvāri position		
19 Ekonaviṃśatiḥ	in	Upward-facing dog		
20 Viṃśatiḥ	out	Downward-facing dog		
21 Ekaviṃśatiḥ	in	Jump forward, head up		
22 Dvāviṃśatiḥ	out	Bend forward		
Samasthitih	in & out	Come up Stand straight		

Gomukhāsana

Go – cow; *mukha* – face

Note 1: There are two states in this *āsana*.
Note 2: In the 10th and 17th *vinyāsas*, one can also jump back with the legs crossed.
Note 3 : There are two breaths in the 7th and 14th *vinyāsas*.

Gomukhāsana continues from the 20th *vinyāsa* in *Parighāsana*.

7 Sapta
Inhale, jump through to sitting and straighten the legs in front of you. Gaze at the tip of the nose.

Exhale and hold the pose.

8 Aṣṭau
Inhale, press the palms to the ground and lift the hips up. Bend the left leg and place the sole of the foot under the hips. Lift the right foot across and over the left thigh and take the right sole of the foot onto the left side of the hip. The edges of the feet touch together. Move the hips to the left, place the right heel under *mūla-bandha*. Place the hands under the right knee and cross the fingers. Keep the knee down, gently pull with the hands up from the knee and lower the chin down between the clavicles. Straighten the back and arms and expand the upper body. This is the first state of the pose. Gaze at the tip of the nose and breathe deeply five times.

9 Nava
Inhale, the lower body remains in the same pose as you take the left hand, from below, behind the back and lift it up closer to the neck, in the middle of the spine. Take the right hand, from above, over the right side of the head and pull it closer between the shoulder blades. The left hand takes hold of the right wrist, or as close to the wrist as possible, and the head can tilt back. The right arm stays on the right side of the head (not behind the head, but next to the ear) and the elbow points upwards. Lift the chest, lengthen the upper body and firmly hold *mūla* and *uddīyana-bandha*. This is the second state of the pose. Gaze upwards and breathe deeply five times.

10 Daśa
Inhale and lower the palms onto the ground next to the shins. Engage the *mūla* and *uddīyana-bandha* and arms and lift, rather than jump up, the body off the ground. Keep the feet in the same position and gaze at the tip of the nose.

11 Ekādaśa
Exhale, swing the body back in the air and straighten the legs into *Catvāri* position. Gaze at the tip of the nose.

The 12th and 13th *vinyāsas* are the same as the 5th and 6th *vinyāsas* in *Sūryanamaskāra* A.

Vinyāsas 14–18 are the same as *vinyāsas* 7ç11 but the second side is done with the right leg under and the left arm above.

The 19th and 20th *vinyāsas* are the same as the 5th and 6th *vinyāsas* in *Sūryanamaskāra* A.

From the 20th *vinyāsa* in *Gomukhāsana*, move to the 7th *vinyāsa* in *Supta-ūrdhva-pāda-vajrāsana*.

Benefits:
Gomukhāsanassa combines the effects of the three previous *āsanas*:
• cleanses the rectum and anus
• straightens and strengthens the spine
• stretches the thighs, hips, arms and shoulders.

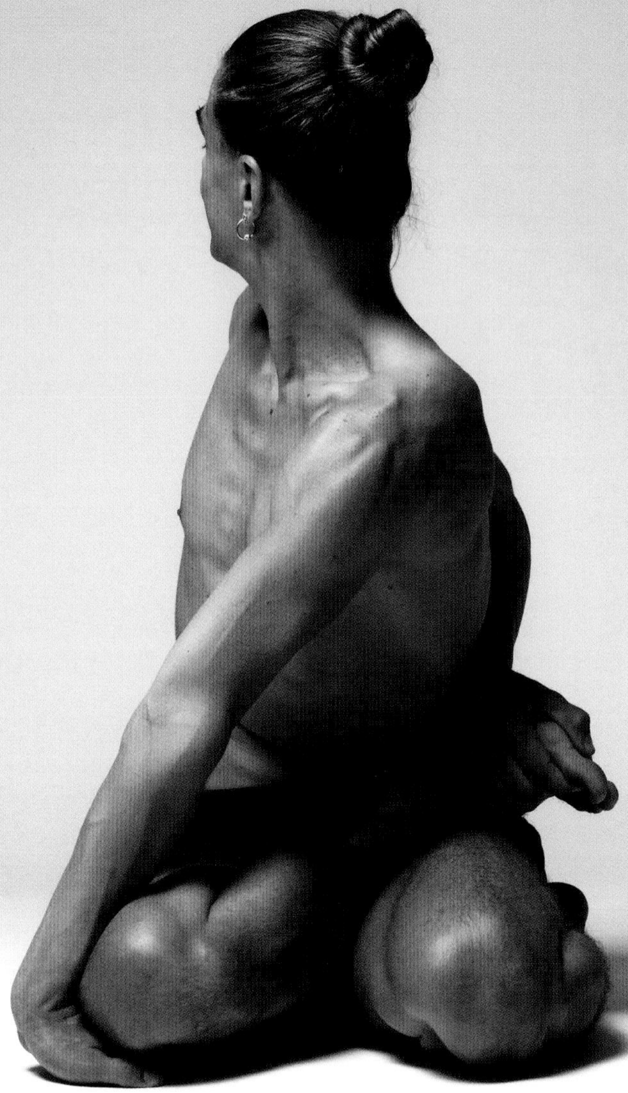

सुप्तोर्ध्वपादवज्रासन

Supta-ūrdhva-pāda-vajrāsana

Sleeping thunderbolt pose with raised foot | 22 *vinyāsas*

Supta-ūrdhva-pāda-vajrāsana

Supta – sleeping, reclining; *ūrdhva* – up; *pāda* – foot; *vajra* – thunderbolt

Note: There are two breaths in the 7th, 8th, 14th and 15th *vinyāsas*.

Supta-ūrdhva-pāda-vajrāsana continues from the 20th *vinyāsa* in *Gomukhāsana*.

7 Sapta

Inhale, jump through to sitting and straighten the legs in front of you. Lie down on your back on the same inhalation. Gaze at the tip of the nose.

Exhale and hold the position, hands on the floor by the hips and the body extended.

8 Aṣṭau

Inhale, press the arms down and lift both legs up and over the head, as in the beginning of the transition from Salamba-sārvangāsana to *Halāsana* (p 131). As you transition the legs back and over you, bend the right knee, bring the right foot into the left groin (half-lotus position), using the hand if necessary, and lower the left leg straight to the ground behind the head. Take the right arm behind the back and firmly grip the right big toe. Then take hold of the left big toe with the left hand (the thumb, forefinger and middle finger). Gaze at the tip of the nose.

Exhale and hold the completed pose.

9 Nava

Inhale, bend the left leg and lift it up from the ground. Change the left-handed grip from the left big toe to the outer edge of the foot. Point the left foot, bend the knee even deeper in, so that the left foot comes close to the left hip. Keep a tight hold on the right big toe. Roll down the spine, over the left arm (with the fingers still holding the left foot), all the way down to sitting. Bring the bent left leg next to the left hip and keep holding the right big toe throughout the roll. Release the grip of the left foot and bring the knees toward each other, as close together as possible.

Place the left palm under the right knee, like in *Bharadvājāsana* (p 83), with the fingers under the thigh and the palm firmly on the ground. Flex the right foot and keep hold of the big toe. Rotate the torso, lengthen the spine to the right side, and press both sitting bones into the ground. This is the state of the right side pose. Gaze towards the right side and breathe deeply five times.

10 Daśa

1. Jump - back technique:
   ...place the hands on the floor next to the hips and hold the legs as they are.
2. Jump - back technique:
   ...release the legs and cross them in the air in the front of the body.
3. Jump - back technique:
   ...bring the bent left leg (in the air) to the front, keeping the right in half-lotus pose.
4. Jump - back technique
   ...bring the left leg to the front and on the top of the right leg into full-lotus pose.

Vinyāsa	Prāṇa	Āsana	Dṛṣṭi	Bandha
Samasthitiḥ		Stand straight		
Vinyāsas 1–6 according to Sūrya-namaskāra A				
7 Sapta	in & out	Jump through to sitting, lie down, hold the pose		
8 Aṣṭau	in	Legs back over head, right leg to half lotus, take hold of the both big toes		
	& out	Hold the pose		
9 Nava	in	Roll up to sitting, left hand under the right knee		
This is the state of the right side āsana, hold for 5 deep breaths				
10 Daśa	in	Hands on the floor, lift up		
11 Ekādaśa	out	Catvāri position		
12 Dvādaśa	in	Upward-facing dog		
13 Trayodaśa	out	Downward-facing dog		
14 Caturdaśa	in & out	Jump through to sitting, lie down, hold the pose		
15 Pañcadaśa	in	Legs back over head, right leg to half lotus, take hold of the both big toes		
	& out	Hold the pose		
16 Ṣoḍaśa	in	Roll up to sitting, right hand under the left knee		
This is the state of the right side āsana, hold for 5 deep breaths				
17 Saptadaśa	in	Hands on the floor, lift up		
18 Aṣṭadaśa	out	Catvāri position		
19 Ekonaviṃśatiḥ	in	Upward-facing dog		
20 Viṃśatiḥ	out	Downward-facing dog		
21 Ekaviṃśatiḥ	in	Jump forward, head up		
22 Dvāviṃśatiḥ	out	Bend forward		
Samasthitiḥ	in & out	Come up Stand straight		

The *vinyāsa* continues:
Strengthen the *mūla* and *uddīyana-bandha* and press the hands firmly on the floor next to the hips. Lift the body up from the ground and take the legs backwards through the arms. Gaze at the tip of the nose.

11 Ekādaśa

Exhale and swing the body in the air back into *Catvāri* position. Gaze at the tip of the nose.

The 12th and 13th *vinyāsas* are the same as the 5th and 6th *vinyāsas* in *Sūryanamaskāra A*.

Vinyāsas 14-18 are the same as *vinyāsas* 7-11, but are done on the left side.

The 19th and 20th *vinyāsas* are the same as the 5th and 6th *vinyāsas* in *Sūryanamaskāra A*.

From the 20th *vinyāsa* in *Supta-ūrdhva-pāda-vajrāsana* move to the 7th *vinyāsa* in *Mukta-hasta-śīrṣāsana*.

Benefits:
Supta-ūrdhva-pāda-vajrāsana combines the effects of the four preceding *āsanas*, as well as from *Bharadvājāsana*:
- stretches the muscles between the ribs, external and internal intercostal muscles
- opens the rib cage
- straightens scoliosis
- cleans and strengthens the heart and *anāhata-cakra*
- improves heart problems, such as arrhythmia
- cleanses the liver and spleen
- stretches the hips, knees and ankles
- releases the nervous system around the spine.

8. *vinyāsa*

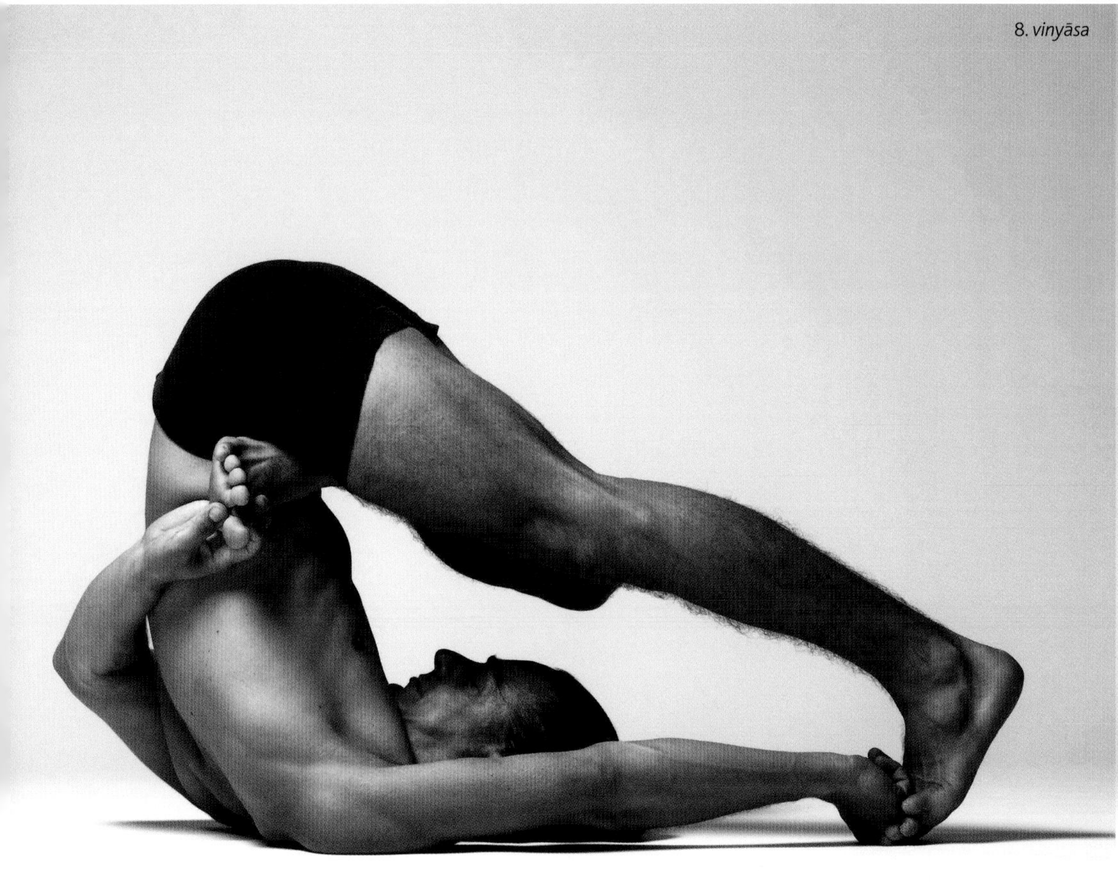

9. *vinyāsa*

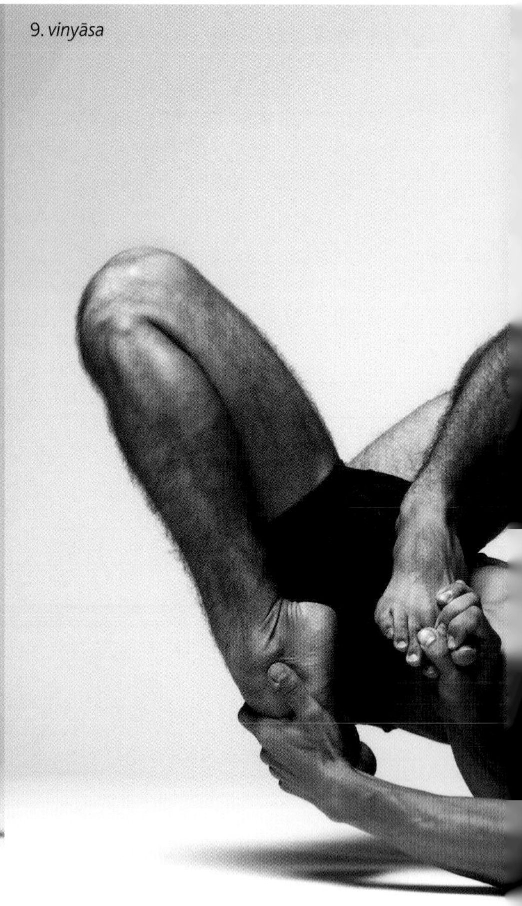

continuing 7. *vinyāsa* 8. *vinyāsa* 9. *vinyāsa* 10. *vinyāsa* 11. *vinyāsa* 12. *vinyāsa*

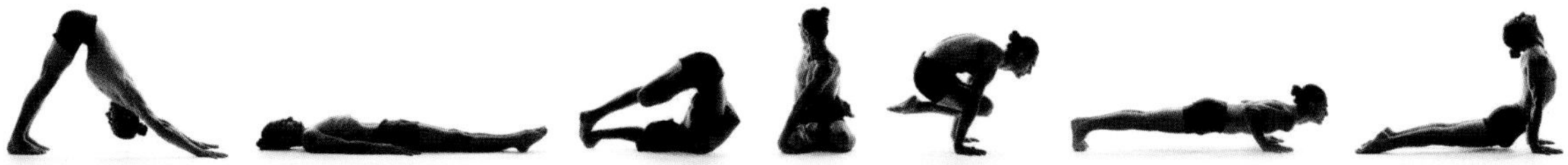

13. *vinyāsa* 14. *vinyāsa* 15. *vinyāsa* 16. *vinyāsa* 17. *vinyāsa* 18. *vinyāsa* 19. *vinyāsa* 20. *vinyāsa*

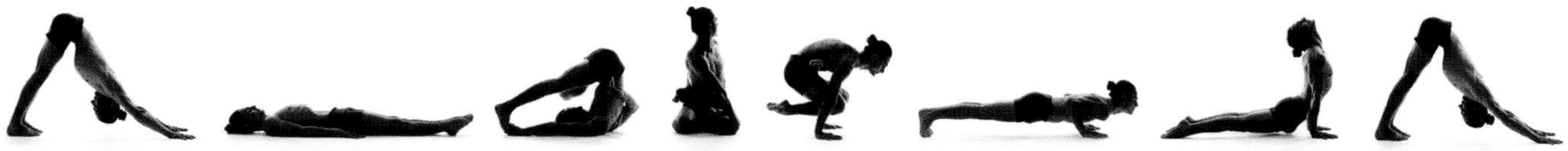

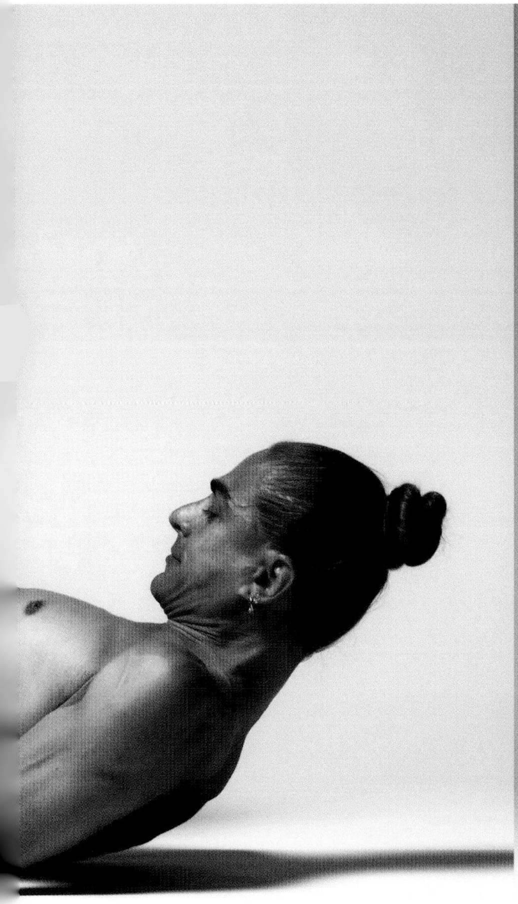

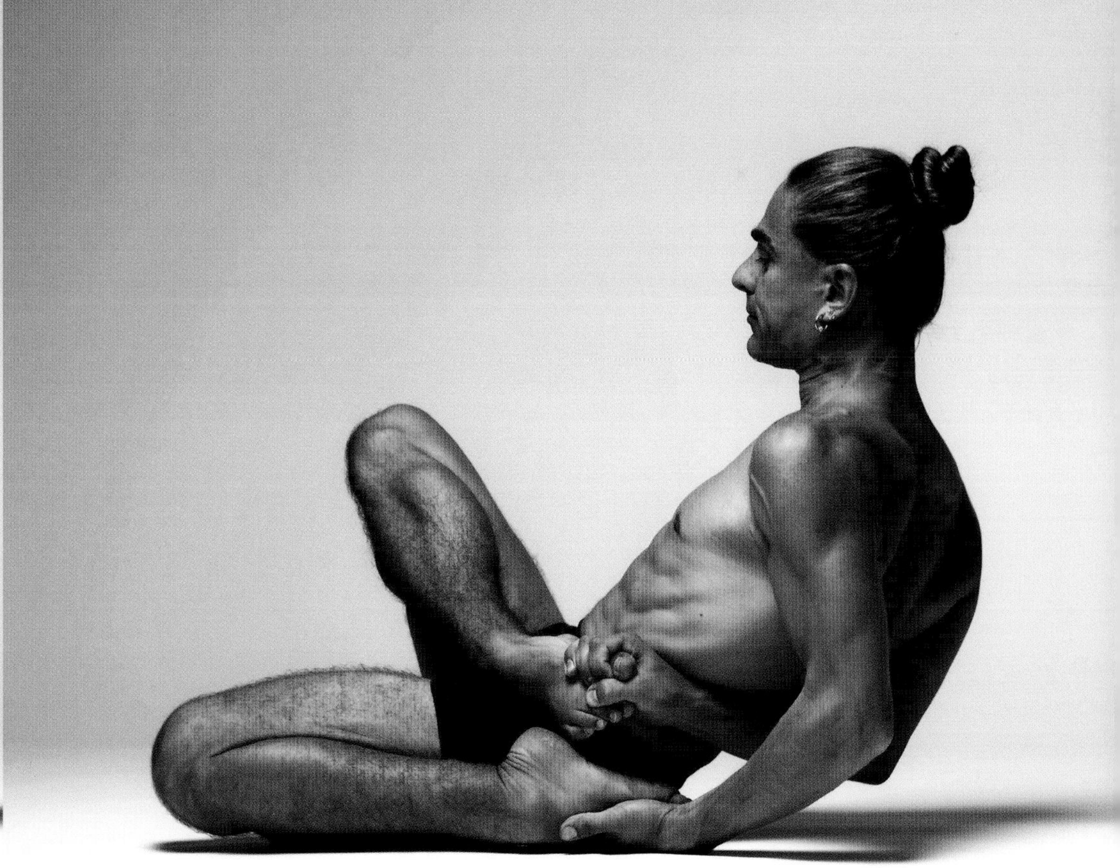

9. *vinyāsa*

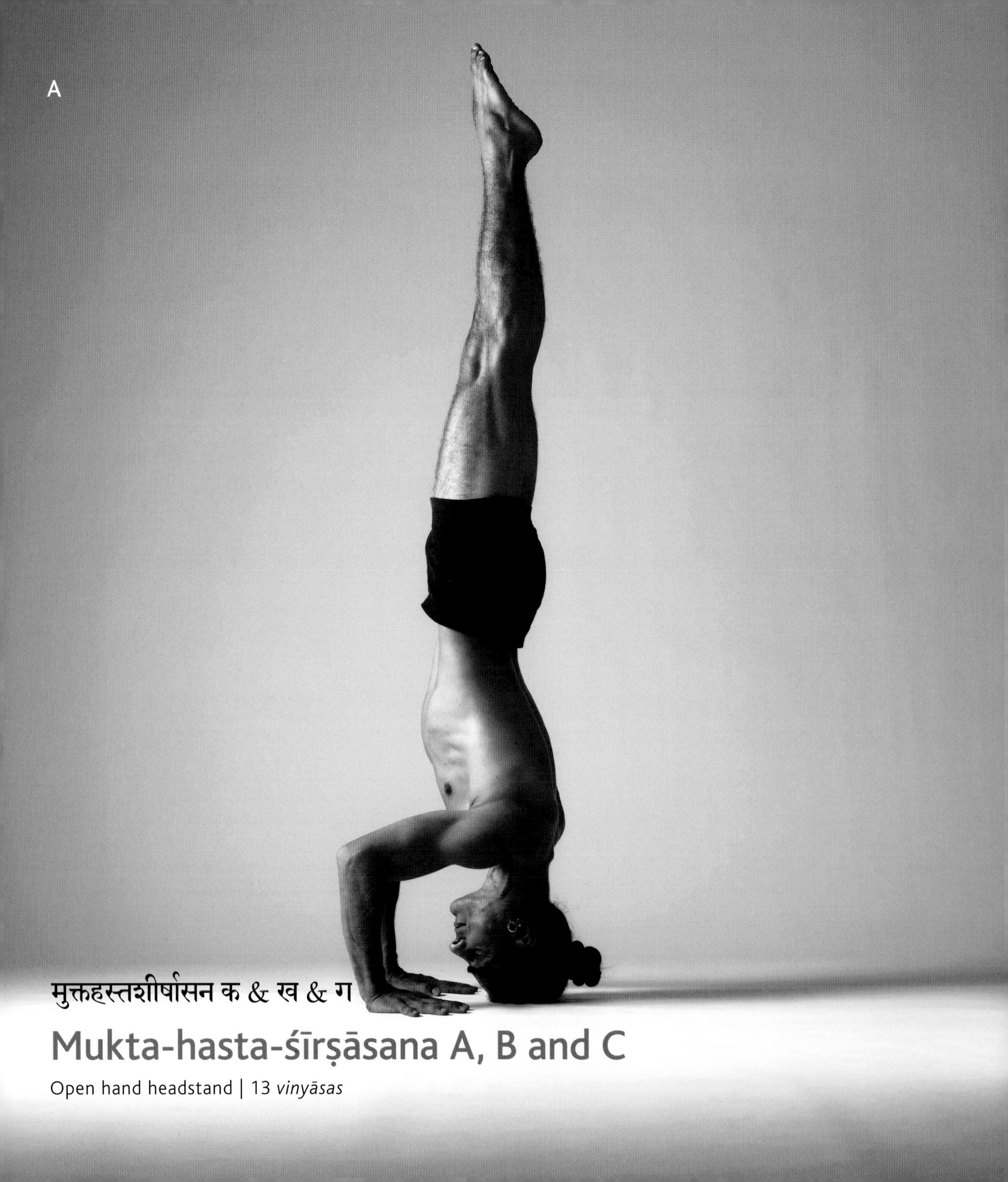

A

मुक्तहस्तशीर्षासन क & ख & ग

Mukta-hasta-śīrṣāsana A, B and C

Open hand headstand | 13 *vinyāsas*

A continuing 7. *vinyāsa* 8. *vinyāsa* 9. *vinyāsa* 10. *vinyāsa* 11. *vinyāsa*

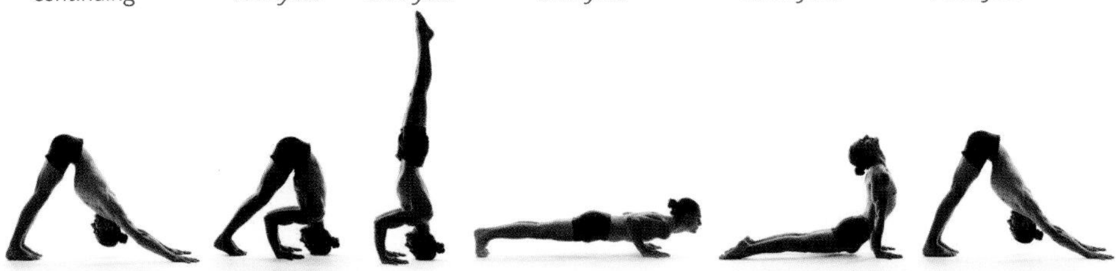

Mukta-hasta-śīrṣāsana A

Mukta – free, open; *hasta* – hand; *sirsa* – head

Note: There are two breaths in the 7th *vinyāsa*.

Mukta-hasta-śīrṣāsana A continues from the 20th *vinyāsa* in *Supta-ūrdhva-pāda-vajrāsana*.

7 Sapta

Inhale, lower the knees to the floor behind the hands and keep the the balls of the feet on the ground. Place the head and arms in the initial state of the A position (listed below).

Exhale and straighten the legs.

A-āsana: (B and C, page 119)

Place the palms, about shoulder-width apart, and the crown of the head, brahma-randhra, on the ground, about 30 centimeters (one foot) in front of the hands. The elbows make a 90 degree angle and the crown point is located approximately five centimeters (two inches) behind the hairline. The head and hands form a triangle. Gaze at the tip of the nose.

8 Aṣṭau

State of the pose

Inhale, engage *mūla* and *uddīyana-bandha*, straighten the back and lift the hips and legs up into headstand. Keep the hands firmly on the ground, feet pointed and the legs straight while moving up. This is the state of the A pose. Gaze at the tip of the nose and breathe deeply five times.

9 Nava

Exhale, with control, fall down with straight legs as you lift the head into the air and land into *Catvāri* position. In the A position, the hands remain in the same place during the fall (in B and C positions, the hands move into the A position). Keep the feet flexed during the fall, so the balls of the feet hit the ground first (not the toes). Gaze at the tip of the nose.

Vinyāsas 10–11 are the same is the 5th and 6th *vinyāsas* in *Sūryanamaskāra* A.

Mukta-hasta-śīrṣāsana continues on the next page.

Vinyāsa	Prāṇa	Āsana	Dṛṣṭi	Bandha
Samasthitih		Stand straight		
Vinyāsas 1–6 according to Sūrya-namaskāra A				
7 Sapta	in & out	Kneel down, set the head and hands on the ground, A: Elbows bent, palms on the floor B: Arms straight out, palms up C: Arms straight out to the sides, palms down Straighten the legs		
8 Aṣṭau	in	Lift the legs up		
This is the state of the āsana, hold for 5 deep breaths				
9 Nava	out	Fall down into cakrāsana		
10 Daśa	in	Upward-facing dog		
11 Ekādaśa	out	Downward-facing dog		
12 Dvādaśa	in	Jump forward, head up		
13 Trayodaśa	out	Bend forward		
Samasthitih	in & out	Come up Stand straight		

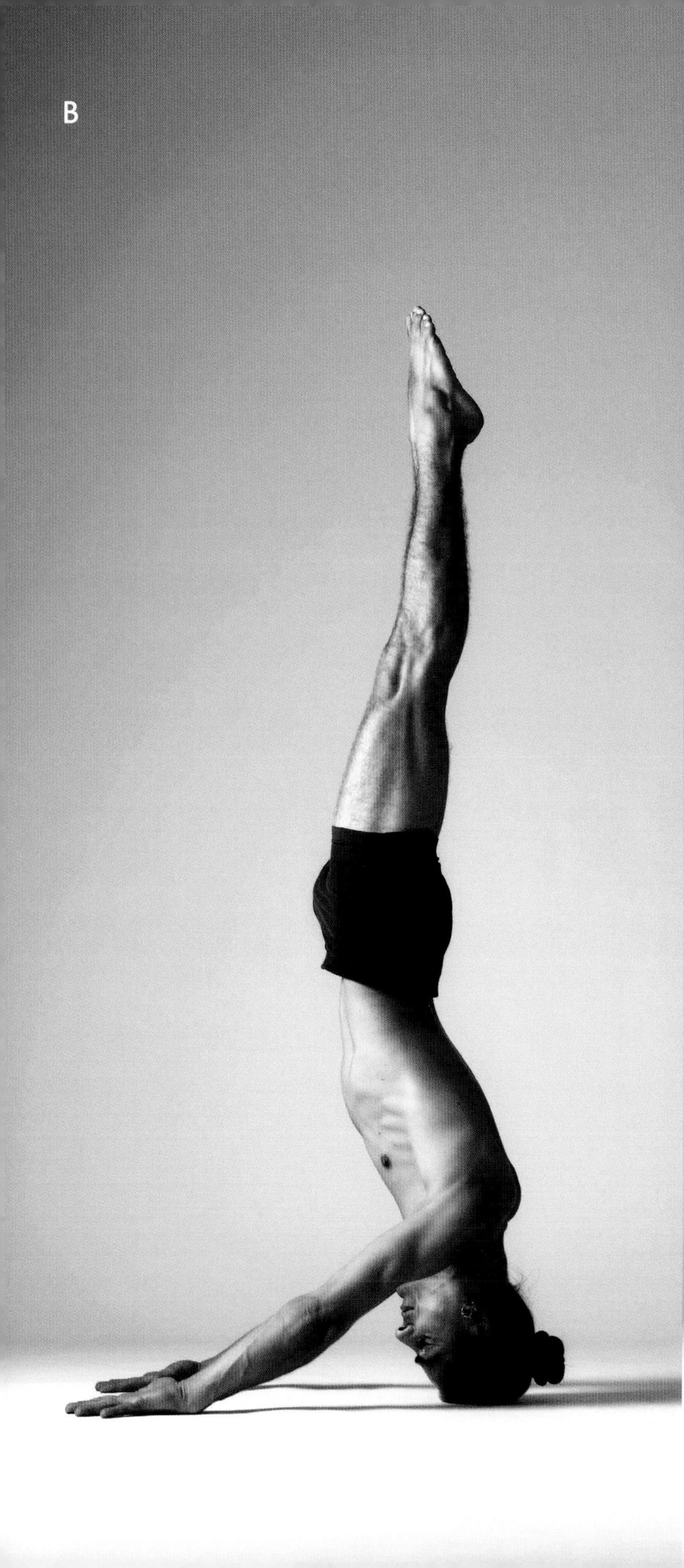
B

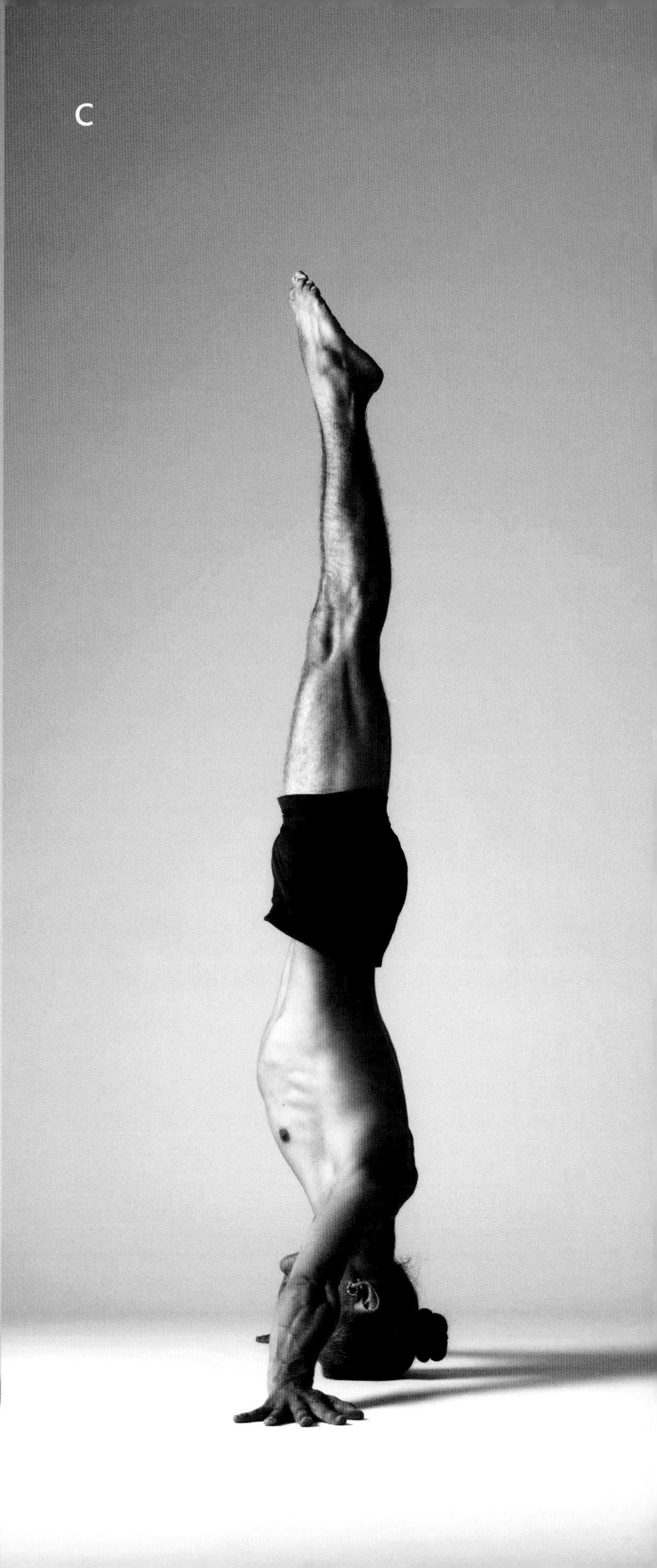
C

B continuing 7. *vinyāsa* 8. *vinyāsa* 9. *vinyāsa* 10. *vinyāsa* 11. *vinyāsa*

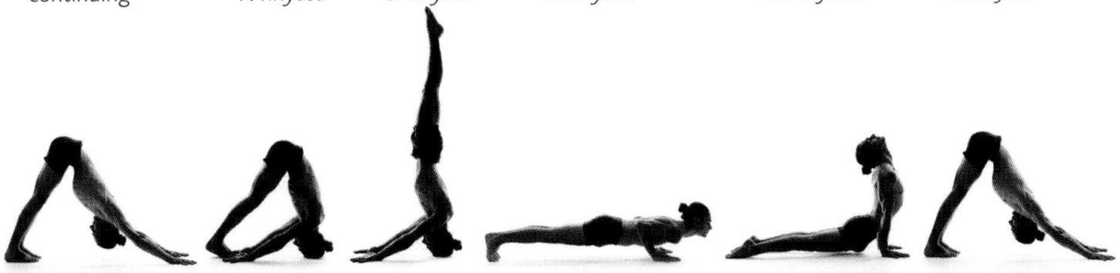

C continuing 7. *vinyāsa* 8. *vinyāsa* 9. *vinyāsa* 10. *vinyāsa* 11. *vinyāsa*

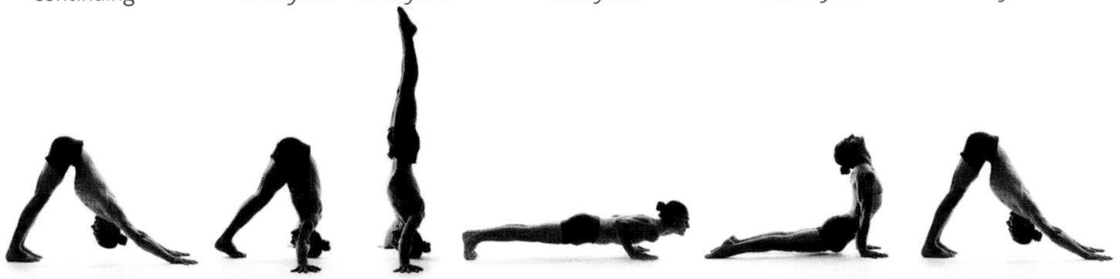

Mukta-hasta-śīrṣāsana B and C

Mukta-hasta-śīrṣāsana B continues from the 11th *vinyāsa in Mukta-hasta-śīrṣāsana A*. Do it all the way to the end, to the *11th vinyāsa,* before continuing with *Mukta-hasta-śīrṣāsana C*.

7 Sapta
Inhale, lower the knees to the floor behind the hands and keep the the balls of the feet on the ground. Place the head and hands in the variation of the B or C position (listed below).

Exhale and straighten the legs.

B-āsana:
Place the crown of the head as in the A position and straighten the arms, shoulder-width apart, in front of the body. Turn the back of the hands down onto the ground and keep the fingers together. Keep the arms straight and maintain a strong position throughout the posture. Press into the back of the hands onto the ground to facilitate balance. Gaze at the tip of the nose.

C-āsana:
(done after the 11th vinyāsa of the B-āsana)
Place the crown of the head on the ground, as in the A posture, and straighten the arms laterally on either side of the head. Keep the arms straight through and position the palms firmly on the ground with the fingers spread wide. Pressing the palms and fingers onto the ground will facilitate with balance. Gaze at the tip of the nose.

8 Aṣṭau
State of the pose
Inhale, engage *mūla* and *uddīyana-bandha*, straighten the back and lift the hips and legs powerfully up to headstand. Keep the hands firmly on the ground, feet pointed and the legs straight while moving up. This is the state of the B and C poses. Gaze at the tip of the nose and breathe deeply five times.

9 Nava
Exhale, move the hands to the A position. Fall down with control, keeping the legs straight, lifting the head into the air and landing in *Catvāri* position. Keep the feet flexed during the fall, so the balls of the feet hit the ground first (not the toes). Gaze at the tip of the nose.

Vinyāsas 10–11 are the same is the 5th and 6th *vinyāsas* in *Sūryanamaskāra* A.

From the 11th *vinyāsa* in *Mukta-hasta-śīrṣāsana* C, move to the 7th *vinyāsa* in *Baddha-hasta-śīrṣāsana*.

Benefits:
Mukta-hasta-śīrṣāsana A, B, and C are part of a group of inverted positions (*viparīta-karaṇi*), and their many effects are similar to the finishing sequence position, *śīrṣāsana*. Different arm positions develop the arms and upper body muscles and improve control of one's balance.

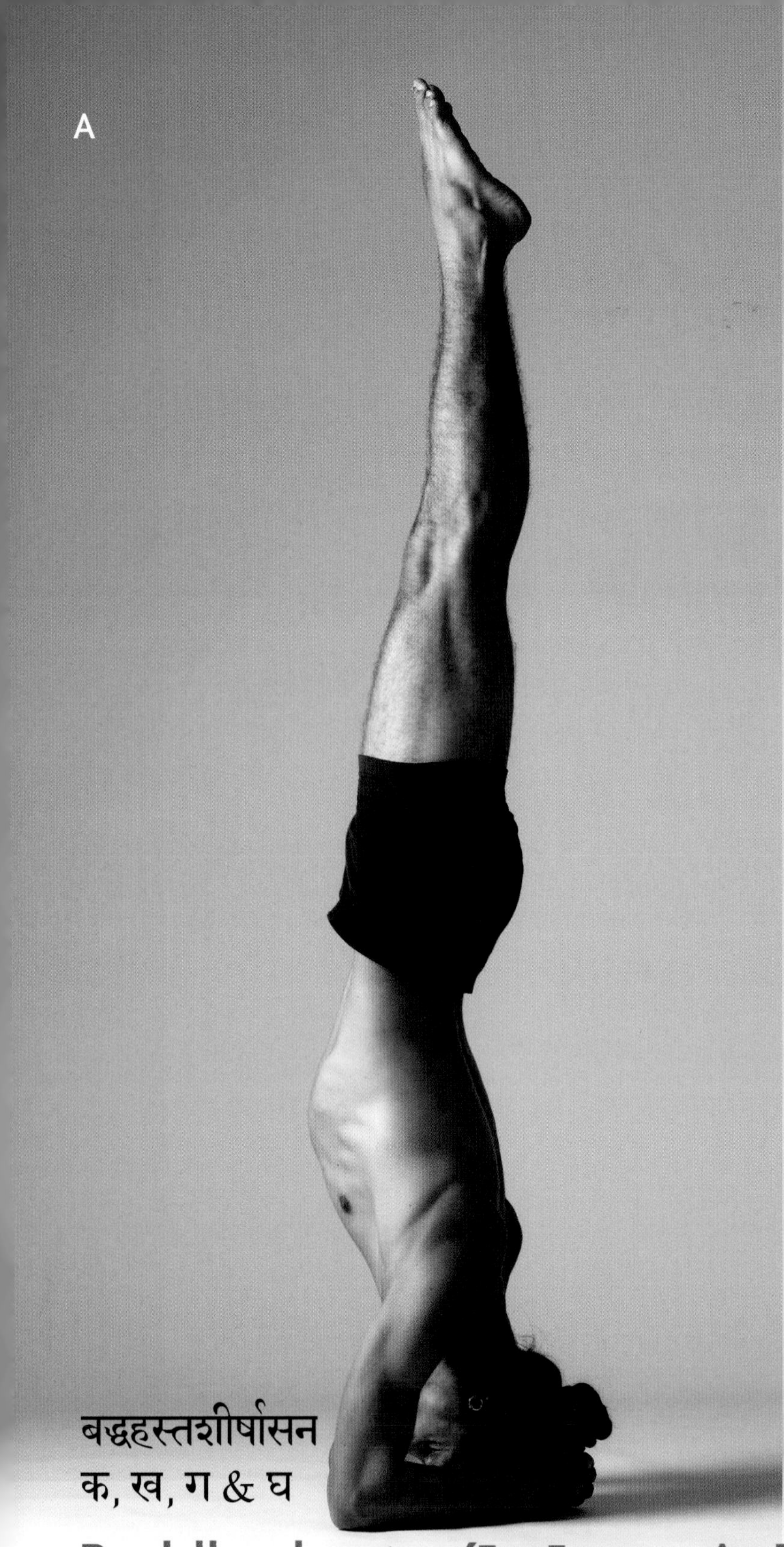

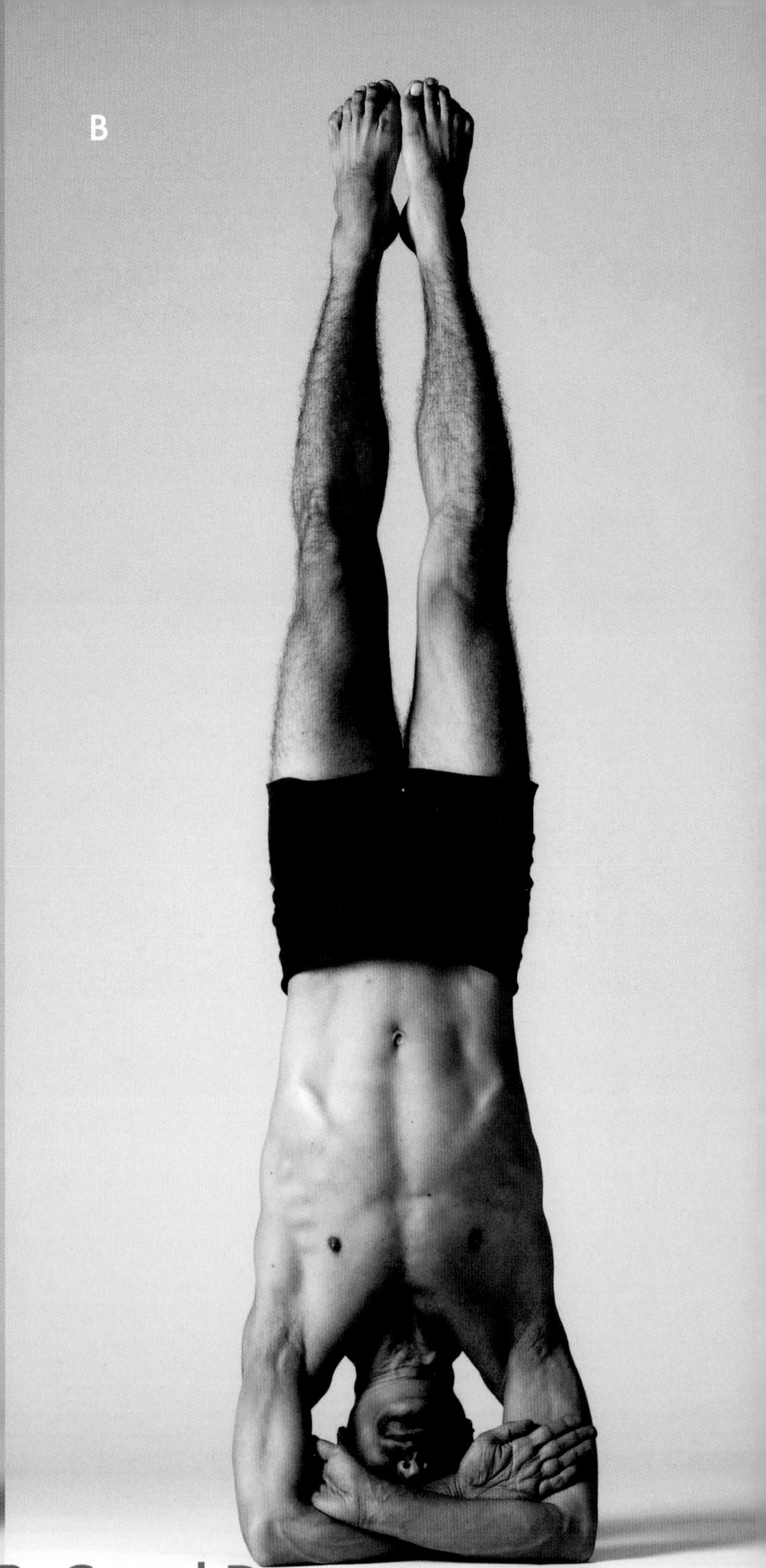

बद्धहस्तशीर्षासन
क, ख, ग & घ

Baddha-hasta-śīrṣāsana A, B, C and D

Bound hand headstand | 13 *vinyāsas*

C

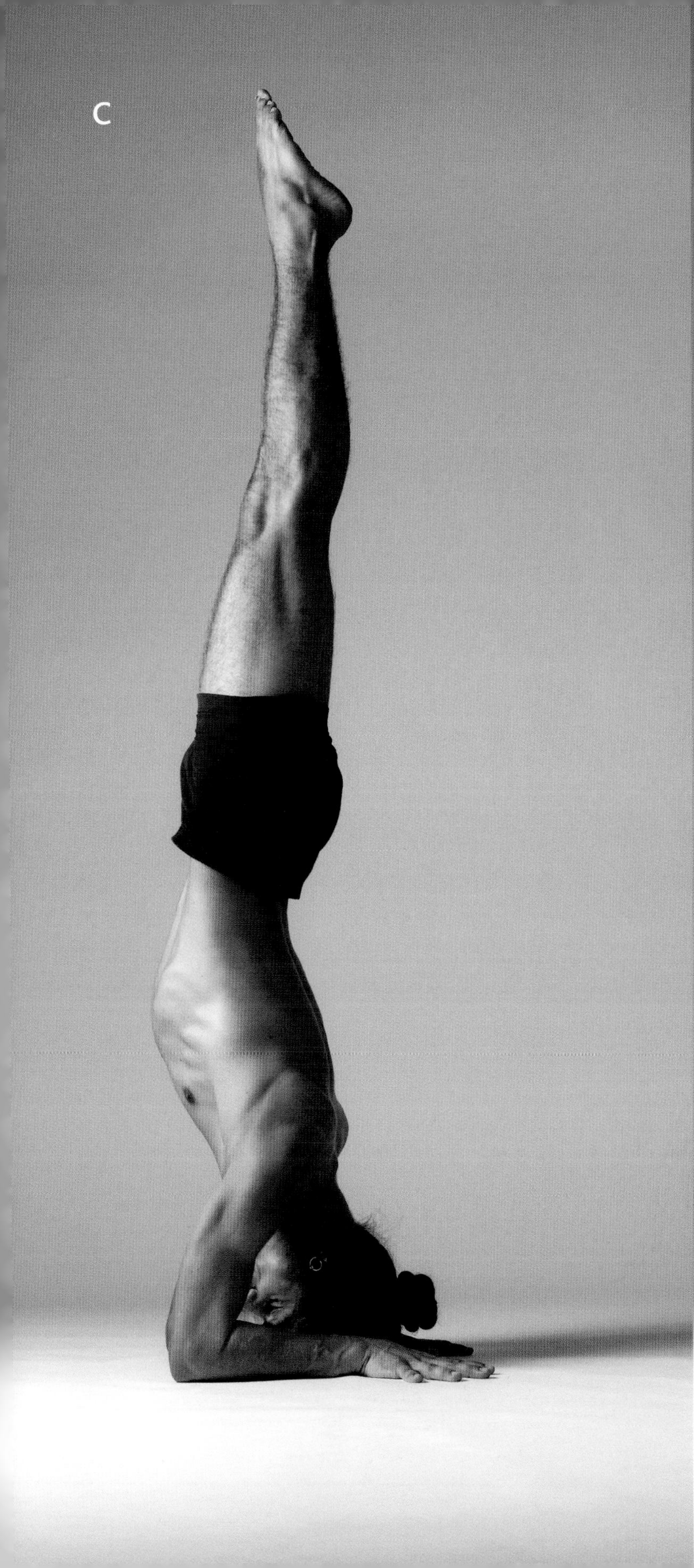

D

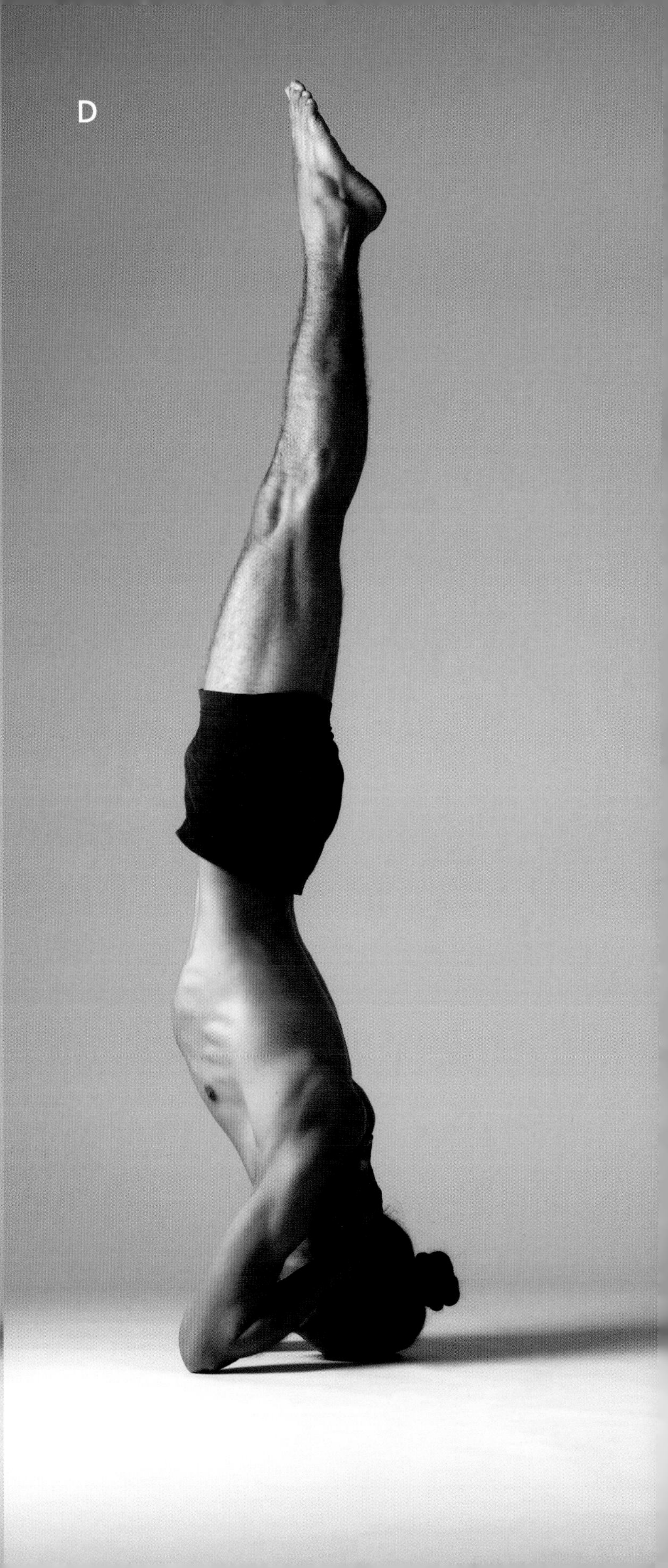

Baddha-hasta-śīrṣāsana A, B, C and D

Baddha – bound; *hasta* – hand; *śīrṣa* – head

Note: There are two breaths in the 7th *vinyāsa*.

Baddha-hasta-śīrṣāsana A continues from the 11th *vinyāsa* in *Mukta-hasta-śīrṣāsana*.

7 Sapta

Inhale, lower the knees to the floor behind the hands and keep the the balls of the feet on the ground. Place the head and arms in the variation of the A, B, C or D positions (listed below).

Exhale and straighten the legs.

A-āsana:

Place the crown of the head onto the ground, with the hands in the same position as in *Śīrṣāsana*, the headstand in the finishing sequence. The fingers are crossed and the back of the head is cradled in the palms. Gaze at the tip of the nose.

B-āsana: (done after the 11th vinyāsa in the A-āsana)

Bring the elbows shoulder width in front of the knees. Place the forearms to the similar setting as in lotus posture. The right hand onto the left upper arm, but the left hand goes behind the right upper arm, crossing the right arm. Both palms are straight and the fingers together (do not hold the arms with the hands). Place the crown of the head on the ground in the middle and in front of the arms. Gaze at the tip of the nose.

C-āsana: (done after the 11th vinyāsa in the B-āsana)

Put the forearms firmly on the floor, facing straight forward and shoulder-width apart. Place the crown of the head right in between the forearms. Gaze at the tip of the nose.

D-āsana: (done after the 11th vinyāsa in the C-āsana)

Place the elbows shoulder-width apart on the ground and the crown of the head about 10 centimeters (4 inches) in front of the elbows. Bend the forearms towards the back sides of the shoulders and place both palms on the shoulders/ upper back. Keep the little fingers on either side of the spine, with all fingers together and straight. Gaze at the tip of the nose.

8 Aṣṭau

State of the pose

Inhale, strengthen *mūla* and *uddīyana-bandha*, straighten the back and lift the hips strongly but softly up. Raise the legs up and point the feet. This is the state of the A,B,C and D pose. Gaze at the tip of the nose and breathe deeply five times.

9 Nava

Exhale, bring the hands in a controlled manner into *Mukta-hasta-śīrṣāsana* A. Fall down with straight legs, and with control, lifting the head in the air and land in *Catvāri* position. Keep the feet flexed during the fall, so the balls of the feet hit the ground first (not the toes). Gaze at the tip of the nose.

Vinyāsas 10–11 are the same is the 5th and 6th *vinyāsas* in *Sūryanamaskāra* A.

From the 11th *vinyāsa* of *Baddha-hasta-śīrṣāsana* D, move to the 7th *vinyāsa* in *Ūrdhva-dhanurāsana* or continue onto Viśvāmitrāsana, which is the first posture found in Sthira-bhāga, the Advanced A sequence of *āsanas*.

Benefits:

Baddha-hasta-śīrṣāsana A, B, C, and D are part of the same group of *āsanas* from the preceding sequence, *Mukta-hasta-śīrṣāsana*. The effects of both *āsanas* are similar to the the finishing sequence position, *Śīrṣāsana*. Different arm positions develop the arms and upper body muscles and improve control of balance.

A continuing — 7. *vinyāsa* — 8. *vinyāsa* — 9. *vinyāsa* — 10. *vinyāsa* — 11. *vinyāsa*

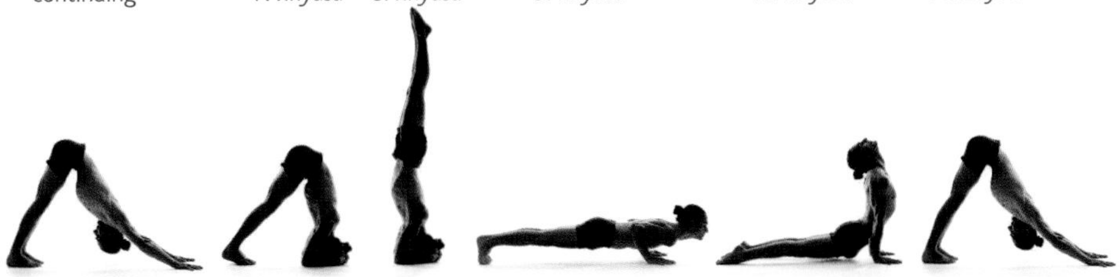

B continuing — 7. *vinyāsa* — 8. *vinyāsa* — 9. *vinyāsa* — 10. *vinyāsa* — 11. *vinyāsa*

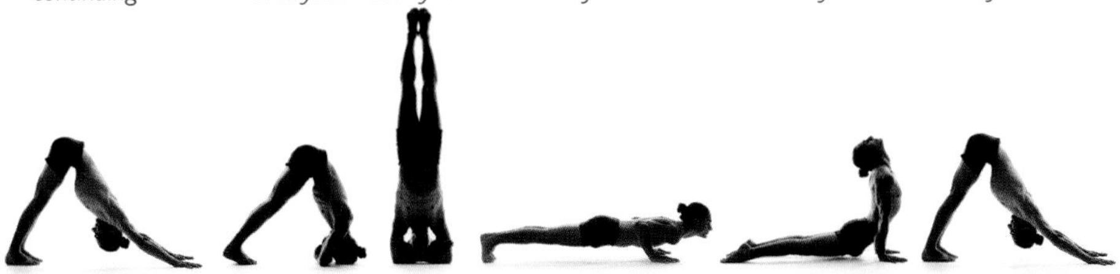

C continuing — 7. *vinyāsa* — 8. *vinyāsa* — 9. *vinyāsa* — 10. *vinyāsa* — 11. *vinyāsa*

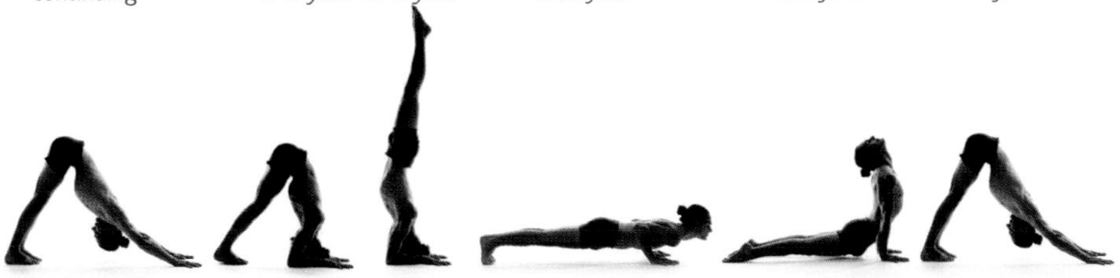

D continuing — 7. *vinyāsa* — 8. *vinyāsa* — 9. *vinyāsa* — 10. *vinyāsa* — 11. *vinyāsa*

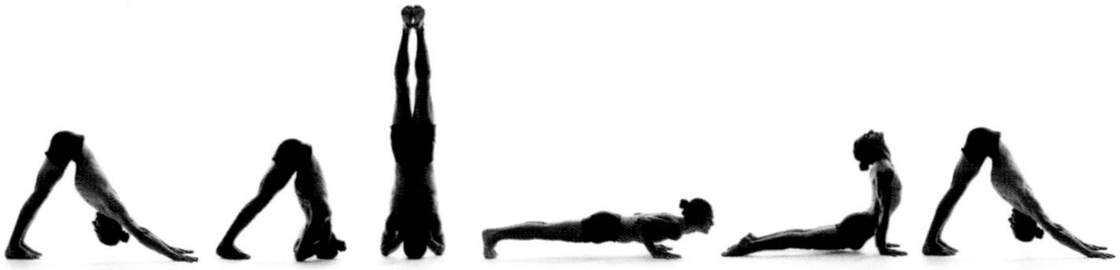

Vinyāsa	Prāṇa	Āsana	Dṛṣṭi	Bandha
Samasthitih		Stand straight		
Vinyāsas 1–6 according to Sūrya-namaskāra A				
7 Sapta	in	Kneel down, set the head and hands on the ground A: Elbows, forearms and head in triangle B: Forearms crossed, straight fingers C: Forearms straight forward D: Palms on the upper back, straight		
	& out	Straighten legs		
8 Aṣṭau	in	Lift the legs up		
This is the state of the āsana, hold for 5 deep breaths				
9 Nava	out	Fall down into cakrāsana		
10 Daśa	in	Upward-facing dog		
11 Ekādaśa	out	Downward-facing dog		
12 Dvādaśa	in	Jump forward, head up		
13 Trayodaśa	out	Bend forward		
Samasthitih	in & out	Come up Stand straight		

Drop back

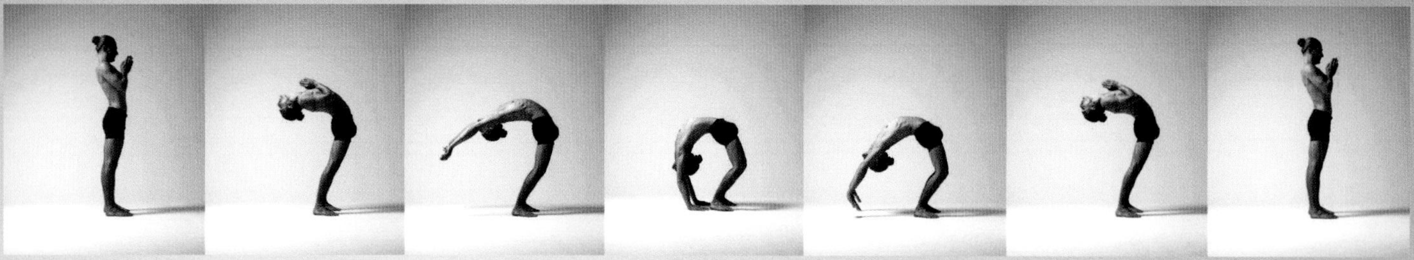

in out out out in in in

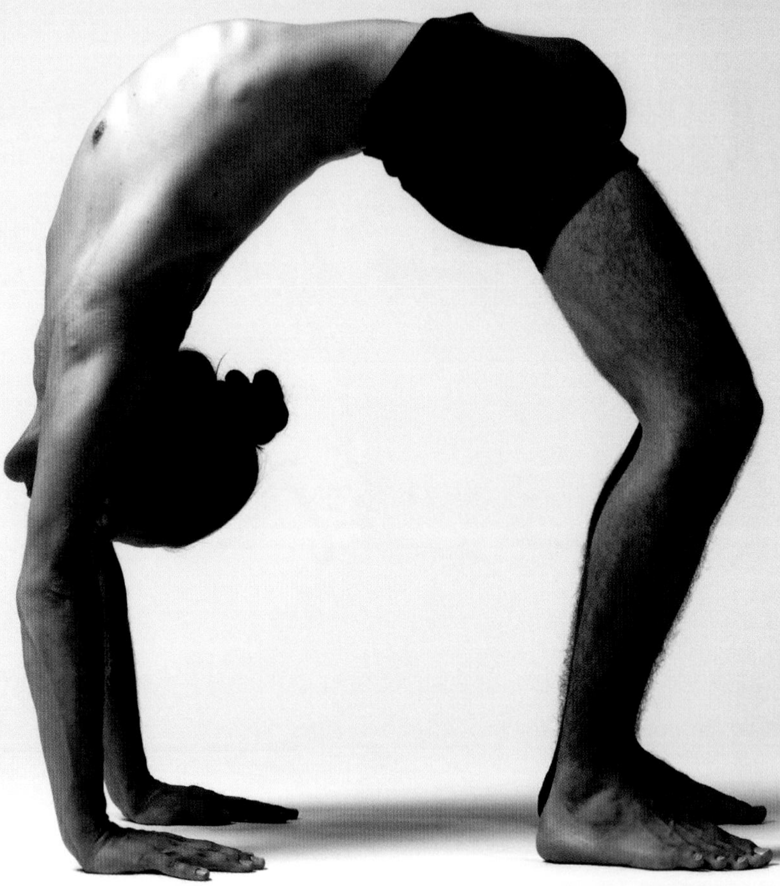

ऊर्ध्वधनुरासन

Ūrdhva-dhanurāsana

Upward bow pose | 15 *vinyāsas*

continuing | 7. *vinyāsa* | 8. in | 8. out | 9. *vinyāsa* | 10. *vinyāsa* | 9. *vinyāsa*

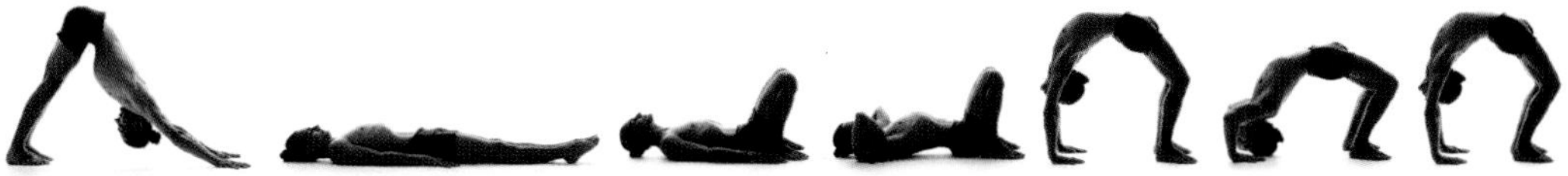

10. *vinyāsa* | 9. *vinyāsa* | 10. *vinyāsa* | 11. in | 11. out | 12. *vinyāsa* | 13. *vinyāsa* | 14. *Paschimatānāsana* (forward bend)

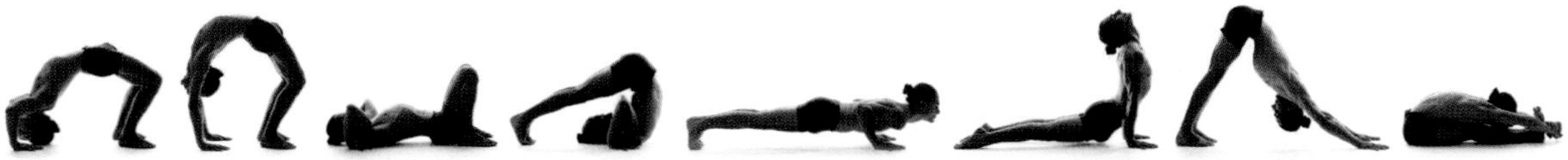

Ūrdhva-dhanurāsana

Ūrdhva – upward; *dhanuḥ* – bow (as in bow and arrow)

Note 1: There are two breaths in the 7th, 8th and 11th *vinyāsas*.
Note 2: Paśchima-tānāsana C follows *Ūrdhva-dhanurāsana*.
Note 3: The state of the pose is repeated three times.
Note 4: The *vinyāsa* chart doesn't include extra backbend techniques or Paśchima-tānāsana C instructions.
Note 5: *Ūrdhva-dhanurāsana* is the last seated posture done in all 6 series (primary, intermediate, the four advanced series) within *Aṣṭāṅga yoga*.

Ūrdhva-dhanurāsana continues from the 13th *vinyāsa* in Setu-bandhāsana.

7 Sapta
Inhale and jump through to sitting. Continue with the inhalation as you lie down onto the floor. Keep the legs together and straight on the floor. Press the palms into the floor by the thighs, expand the chest and lengthen the whole body along the mat. Gaze at the tip of the nose.
Exhale and hold the pose.

8 Aṣṭau
Inhale, bend the knees and pull the heels in, as close to the hips as possible, keeping the feet hip-width apart, with the toes pointing forward.
Exhale and place the hands on the floor by the ears, palms down, fingers spread wide and the fingertips pointing towards the shoulders. Gaze at the tip of the nose.

9 Nava
Inhale, press the hands and feet into the floor. Lift the body up into an arch - "bow" pose, or as it is usually defined as a bridge or backbend. Straighten the arms, and engage the thighs to straighten the knees. Lift up through the chest, shoulders and hips, keeping the back relaxed. Mūla-bandha will keep the hips lifted, lighten the body and help relax the buttocks. Uddīyana-bandha supports the chest and opens the sternum up and into the arch. Lean the head back to release the shoulders and chest. This is the state of the *āsana*. Breathe deeply five times and gaze at the tip of the nose.

10 Daśa
Exhale, bend the elbows and knees and lower the crown of the head, or the whole back, slowly onto the floor. The soles of the feet and the palms should stay firmly in place. On the next inhalation, come back up to the state of the *āsana*, as described in the 9th *vinyāsa*. Repeat this *vinyāsa* three times, taking a minimum of five deep breaths each time. Lifting up to the bridge pose is counted as a 9th *vinyāsa* and lowering down to the floor is the 10th *vinyāsa*. On the second and third attempt up into bridge, try to walk the hands closer to the feet, bending the elbows to help bring the hands in, and straightening the arms again into the state of the *āsana*.

Option 1: Check the drop-back sequence on the left page
After the third repetition of *Ūrdhva-dhanurāsana*, come to stand up on an inhalation, and continue on with further back-bending techniques, drop backs etc., according the teacher's advice. After the last backbend variation, sit down and do the counter pose, the 9th *vinyāsa* in Paschimatānāsana C (primary series forward bend with the wrist grip, if possible). Breathe deeply ten times and gaze at the tip of the nose or to the toes.

Option 2: Check the backbend sequence above
After the third lift-up into the 9th *vinyāsa*, lie back down on the exhalation on the 10th *vinyāsa*. Do not straighten the legs here but move straight into the 11th *vinyāsa* (cakrāsana). Gaze at the tip of the nose.
From *Catvāri* pose, do *Ūrdhva-mukha-śvanāsana* (12th *vinyāsa*, upward-facing dog) and *Adho-mukha-śvanāsana* (13th *vinyāsa*, downward-facing dog) and follow *vinyāsas* 7-14 in *Paschimatānāsana* C (primary series forward bend with a wrist grip; more detailed *vinyāsas* for this are explained in my primary series book). Breathe deeply ten times and gaze at the tip of the nose or to the toes.
The 14th *vinyāsa* in Paschimatānāsana C is the same pose as the 13th *vinyāsa* in *Ūrdhva-dhanurāsana* (both poses are Adho-mukha-śvanāsana). You can continue on from here to the *next āsana, the 7th vinyāsa in Salamba-sarvāṅgāsana.*

Benefits:
- releases muscle and nerve tension
- realigns the spine
- extends the front of the thighs, chest and shoulders
- stretches and strengthens the wrists
- engages and releases the arms and shoulders simultaneously
- strengthens the inner organs
- releases and purifies the stomach
- improves digestion
- expands the chest
- purifies the lungs, throat and esophagus.

Vinyāsa	Prāṇa	Āsana	Dṛṣṭi	Bandha
Samasthitih		Stand straight		
Vinyāsas 1–6 according to Sūrya-namaskāra A				
7 Sapta	In & out	Jump to sitting, lie down hold the pose		
8 Aṣṭau	In & out	Place the feet and hands		
9 Nava	In	Lift up to bow		
This is the state of the āsana, hold for 5 deep breaths				
10 Daśa	out	Head or back to floor		
Back up to vinyāsa 9 on an inhale; repeat 3 times, for 5 breaths Follow your teacher's instruction for further backbend techniques				
11 Ekādaśa	In & out	Cakrāsana, back-roll, into Catvāri pose		
12 Dvādaśa	In	Upward-facing dog		
13 Trayodaśa	out	Downward-facing dog		
Continue here with the 7th vinyāsa in Paschimatānāsana C (forward bend)				
14 Caturdaśa	In	Jump forward, head up		
15 Pañcadaśa	out	Bend forward		
Samasthitih	In & out	Come up Stand straight		

The benefits of the finishing sequence

It is recommended to conclude your practice with a series of primarily-inverted postures known as *viparīta karaṇi* which guide the energy in the body upwards, after the seated *āsana* sequence. The poses are held longer than in the standing or seated *āsanas* and are done at a slower pace with long, extended breathing. The finishing sequence can be divided into five parts, each with its own specific focus.

1. The first five *āsanas* are made up of the shoulderstand and its four variations. Shoulder stand strengthens and purifies the muscles and joints in the body.

This *āsana* and its variations benefit the heart by slowing down the heart rate. Blood circulation and the quality of blood (and other bodily fluids) improves. The effect of gravity on the body is reversed when doing inversions, thus relieving pressure from the organs and tension in the muscles and nervous system. Furthermore, reversed blood flow relieves the build-up of fluid in the legs and aids in proper circulation, while delivering restorative life-energy to the head. Illnesses such as dry cough, digestive problems, constipation, high-blood pressure and chronic hiccups can be cured.

Shoulder standing works on the energy channels (*nāḍīs*), the energy centers (*cakras*), the blood vessels and nervous system (*dhamani*), the three *dosas* (*vāta, pitta, kapha*), the metabolism and the digestive fire (*jaṭharāgni*).

The body's lower regions are purified, including but not limited to, the stomach, lower back, intestines, anus and sexual organs. The digestive and elimination systems also benefit from shoulderstand.

As these *āsanas* stimulate the throat and neck, the energy center located here, *viśuddha-cakra*, is purified and strengthened. The two lowest energy centers (mūladhara and svādhiṣṭhāna cakra) are also stimulated, which release the three energy knots (*granthi-traya – Brahmā, Viṣṇu* and *Rudra*), so that *prāṇa* can flow without restriction through the *suṣumnā-nāḍī*.

In the shoulderstand, warm blood which pathways has been heated during the standing and seated sequences, can flow easily throughout the upper body, nourishing, among others, the following systems in the body: the digestive organs; skin, lungs, heart, brain; cell reproduction. Moreover, the shoulder-standing sequence creates equilibrium in the body's inner energetic system.

Shoulder standing and head standing generate *amṛta-bindu*, (drop of the nectar of immortality; there is detailed description in my Primary series book) which has been created in part through digestion, so that it can move up from the stomach to the *Brahmarandra*, or *Brahmas* opening, located on the crown of the head. In this way, practicing inversions, along with getting plenty of fresh air, leading a sattvic lifestyle and following the principles of *brahmachārya*, increases the amount of *amṛta-bindu* in *Brahmarandra*.

2. Matsy*āsana* and *Uttāna-pādāsana* are counter-poses to the shoulderstand *āsanas*.

3. Headstand is a continuation of the inverted positions and has similar effects as the shoulderstand. When performed correctly, the head shouldn't press down too strongly, if at all, on the floor. This activates the *sahasrāra cakra*, or crown *cakra*. In order to get the full effects of headstand, it should be done consistently and held for a considerable amount of time. *Yoga Mala* recommends holding the headstand anywhere from a minimum of five minutes to as long as three hours.

4. *Padmāsana* and its variations: *Baddha-padmāsana* and *Yoga-mudrā* are strengthening and cleansing positions. They prepare the body for *Padmāsana*, which is the ideal position for stabilizing the mind and breath. *Padmāsana* is the most beneficial for meditation, chanting, *prānāyāma* and other spiritual practices. According to ancient texts, through the purification process in the *Padmāsana* sequence, the body will be cleansed of impurities and the mind freed from latent karmic impressions known as saṃsāra or the "big sins" (*pāpa*). *Utplutiḥ* strengthens the bandhas and arms, and prepares the practitioner for the relaxation pose that completes the practice.

5. The *āsana* series culminates with the final relaxation pose, giving the practitioner enough time to recover while restoring energy to the body and mind. In addition, the relaxation pose allows the nervous system to process the effects of the deep purification that has taken place throughout the *āsana* sequence.

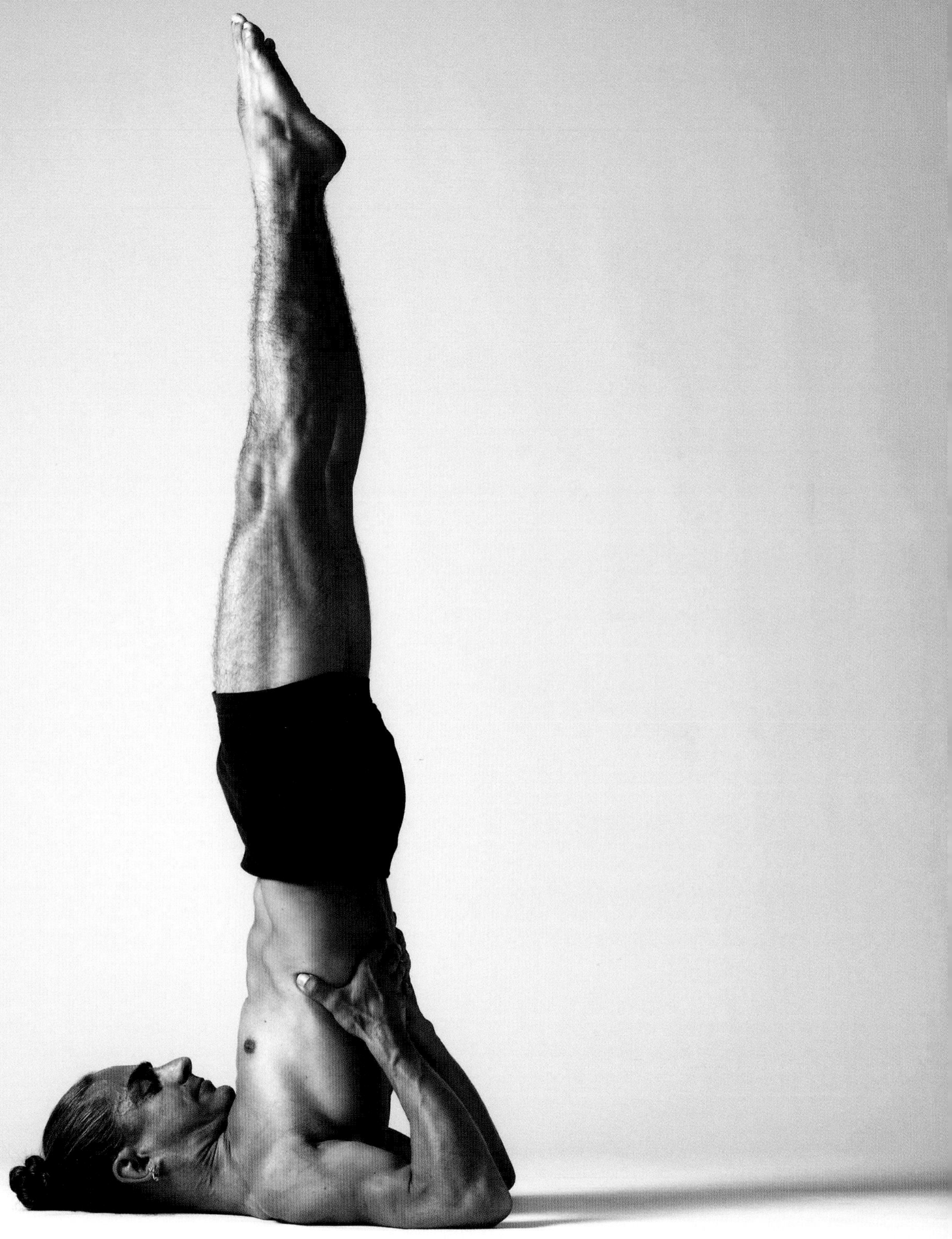

सलम्बसर्वाङ्गासन

Salamba-sarvāṅgāsana

Shoulderstand | 13 *vinyāsas*

continuing 7. *vinyāsa* 8. *vinyāsa*

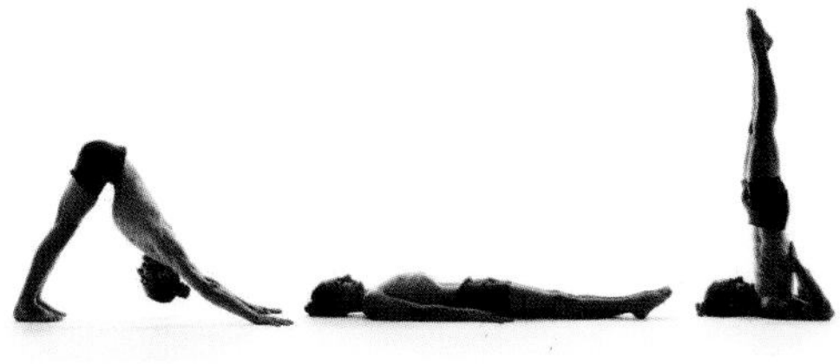

Salamba-sarvāṅgāsana

Salamba – supported; *sarva* – all, full; *aṅga* – limbs

Note 1: There are one to five breaths in the 7th *vinyāsa*.

Note 2 : The breathing in the finishing sequence is slower than in the standing and sitting poses.

Salamba-sarvāṅgāsana follows directly after the 14th *vinyāsa* in *Paścima-tānāsana*.

7 Sapta

Inhale, jump through to sitting. Continue the inhalation, slowly roll down on your back keeping the legs on the floor straight and together. Press the palms into the floor and expand the chest, lengthening the body along the mat. Let the mind calm down and start to breathe slower and longer. Gaze at the tip of the nose.

Exhale only once or stay for five deep breaths. These five breaths are added here often to slow down the pace for the finishing sequence.

8 Aṣṭau

The state of the pose

Inhale, press the palms into the floor, next to the thighs. Draw in the *mūla* and *uddīyana-bandha* and lift the legs, hips, and spine straight up, keeping the legs straight and together. Point the feet towards the ceiling. Bend the elbows and support the torso by placing the hands on either side of the spine. The fingers face up towards the hips and the thumbs are out to the sides. Draw the elbows in, shoulder-width apart, and move the shoulders closer together to support the body's straight alignment. Most of the weight is supported by the shoulders, so the neck should not be pressing uncomfortably into the floor. Only the shoulders, upper arms, elbows, and back of the head touch the floor. Tuck the chin in between the collarbones and sternum. According to Śrī Pattabhi Jois, this is not *Jalandhara-bandha*, even though the positions look similar. *Jalandhara-bandha* is done in *prāṇāyāma* while performing *kuṃbhaka*. This is the state of the *āsana*. Breathe deeply for 10–25 breaths and gaze at the tip of the nose.

After the last inhalation in the 8th *vinyāsa*, go directly to the next *āsana*, the 8th *vinyāsa* in *Halāsana*.

Benefits:

It is said that this *āsana* cures all ailments. The benefits of the *āsana* will increase the longer you hold the pose. In addition to the following list, refer to the benefits of the finishing sequence (p 127):

- improves posture and opens the chest and shoulders
- releases tension in the back and corrects the alignment of the spine
- purifies the throat and stimulates viśuddha-cakra
- clarifies the voice and makes it melodious
- cures ailments of the throat, asthma, and heart-related illnesses
- revives the lungs, heart, and limbs
- balances the thyroid gland hormones
- helps cure insomnia and mental illnesses (through long-term, sustained practice).

Vinyāsa	Prāṇa	Āsana	Dṛṣṭi	Bandha
Samasthitih		Stand straight		
Vinyāsas 1–6 according to *Sūrya-namaskāra* A				
7 Sapta	in & out	jump to sitting lie back hold the pose, breathe 1 to 5 calm breaths		
8 Aṣṭau	in	lift legs to shoulderstand, hands support the back		
This is the state of the āsana, hold for 10-25 deep breaths				
9 Nava	in & out	Cakrāsana, back-roll into Catvāri position		
10 Daśa	in	Upward-facing dog		
11 Ekādaśa	out	Downward-facing dog		
12 Dvādaśa	in	Jump forward, head up		
13 Trayodaśa	out	Bend forward		
Samasthitih	in & out	Come up Stand straight		

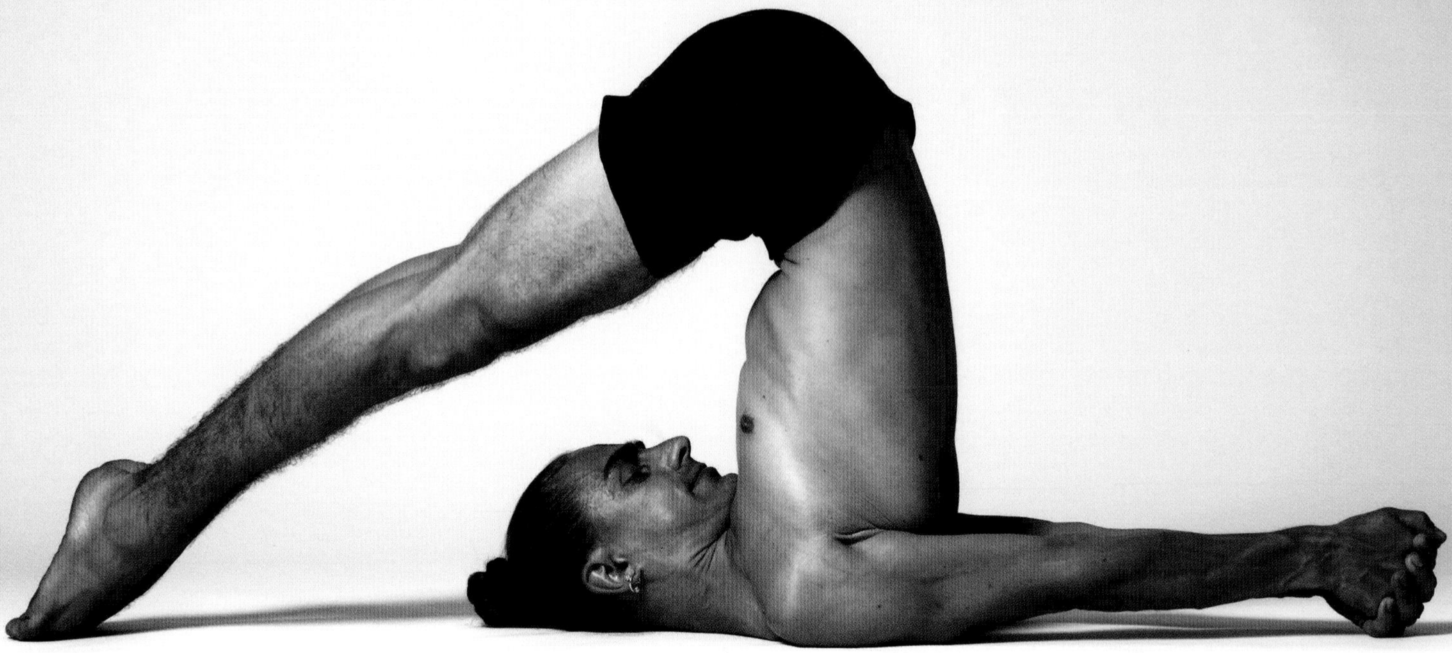

हलासन

Halāsana

Plough pose | 13 *vinyāsas*

continuing 8. *vinyāsa*

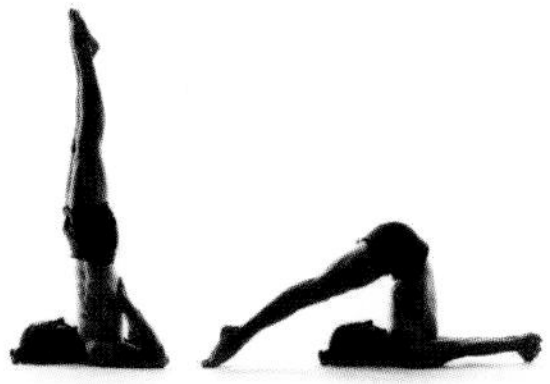

Halāsana

Hala – aura

Halāsana follows directly after the 8th *vinyāsa* in *Salamba-sarvāṅgāsana*.

8 Aṣṭau
The state of the pose
Exhale, bring the legs down behind the head. Keep the legs straight, point the feet and stretch through the toes. Lower the hands from the back, and interlace the fingers, squeezing the palms together and pressing the arms, straight out onto the floor. The shoulders and back of the head are on the floor. However, keep the back of the neck lifted up off the floor. Engage *mūla-bandha* to support and lift the hips, and to relax the buttocks. Engage *uddīyana-bandha* to open the back, and to straighten and lift the spine. This is the state of the *āsana*. Breathe deeply eight to ten times. Gaze at the tip of the nose.

After the last inhalation, go directly to the 8th *vinyāsa* in *Karṇa-pīḍāsana*.

Benefits:
In addition to the list, refer to the benefits of the finishing sequence (p 127):
- aligns the hips
- purifies and strengthens the hips, intestines and stomach
- cures all ailments of the throat and chest, including respiratory problems such as asthma and chronic bronchitis; heart problems, sore throat, unclear speech and loss of speech.

Vinyāsa	Prāṇa	Āsana	Dṛṣṭi	Bandha
Samasthitih		Stand straight		
Vinyāsas 1–6 according to *Sūrya-namaskāra* A				
7 Sapta	in & out	Jump to sitting, lie back hold the pose		
8 Aṣṭau	in & out	Lift legs lower legs behind the head		
This is the state of the āsana, hold for 8-10 deep breaths				
9 Nava	in & out	Cakrāsana, back-roll, into Catvāri position		
10 Daśa	in	Upward-facing dog		
11 Ekādaśa	out	Downward-facing dog		
12 Dvādaśa	in	Jump forward, head up		
13 Trayodaśa	out	Bend forward		
Samasthitih	in & out	Come up Stand straight		

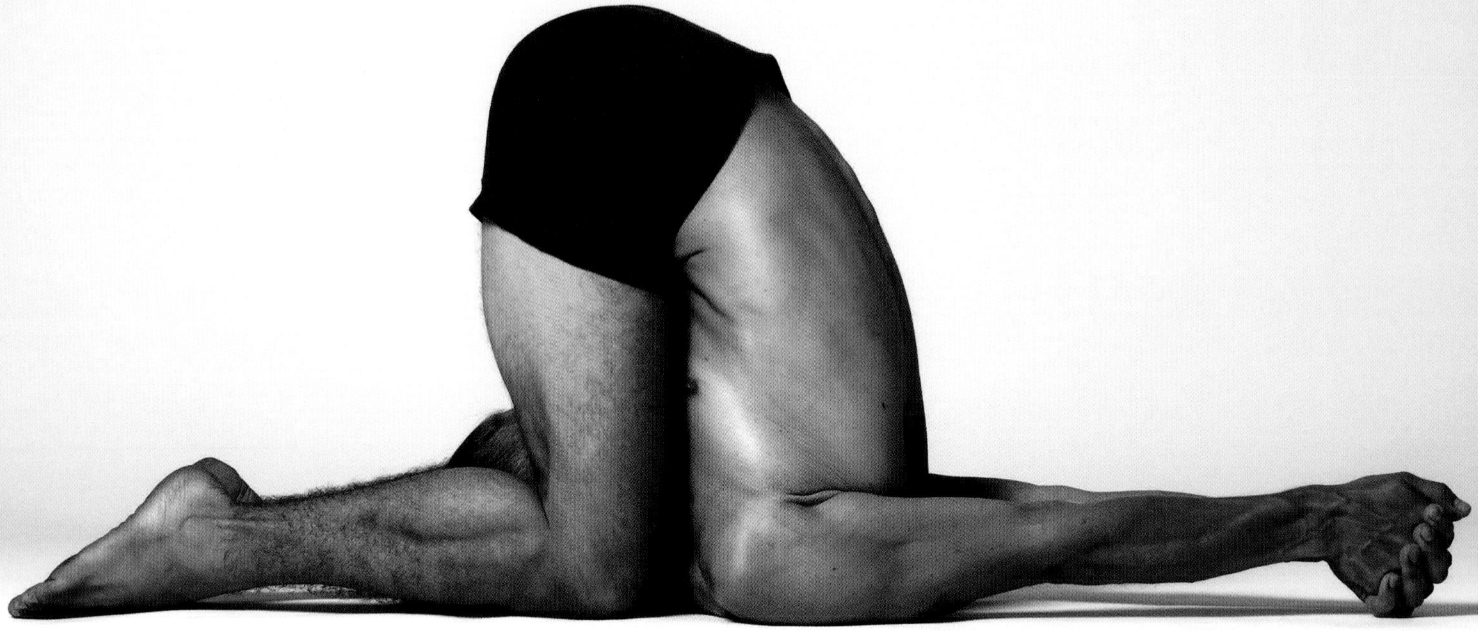

कर्णपीडासन

Karṇa-pīḍāsana

Ear pressure pose | 13 *vinyāsas*

continuing 8. *vinyāsa*

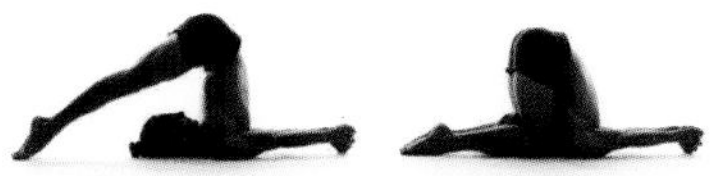

Karṇa-pīḍāsana

Karṇa – ear; *pīḍa* – pressure, pain

Karṇa-pīḍāsana follows directly after the 8th *vinyāsa* in *Halāsana*.

8 Aṣṭau

The state of the pose

Exhale, lower the knees to the floor right behind the shoulders, and squeeze the inner knees into the ears. Keep the feet and toes together with the feet pointed. The hands and arms stay behind the back, as they were in *Halāsana*. This is the state of the *āsana*. Breathe here eight to ten times and gaze at the tip of the nose.

After the last exhalation, go directly to the 8th *vinyāsa* in *Ūrdhva-padmāsana*.

Benefits:

In addition to the list, refer to the benefits of the finishing sequence (p 127):

- alleviates ear infections, tinnitus and other ear-related problems
- purifies the ears and improves the sense of hearing.

Vinyāsa	Prāṇa	Āsana	Dṛṣṭi	Bandha
Samasthitih		Stand straight		
Vinyāsas 1–6 according to *Sūrya-namaskāra* A				
7 Sapta	in & out	Jump to sitting lie back hold the pose		
8 Aṣṭau	in & out	lift legs, bend knees to ears		
This is the state of the āsana, hold for 8-10 deep breaths				
9 Nava	in & out	Cakrāsana, back-roll, into Catvāri position		
10 Daśa	in	Upward-facing dog		
11 Ekādaśa	out	Downward-facing dog		
12 Dvādaśa	in	Jump forward, head up		
13 Trayodaśa	out	Bend forward		
Samasthitih	in & out	Come up Stand straight		

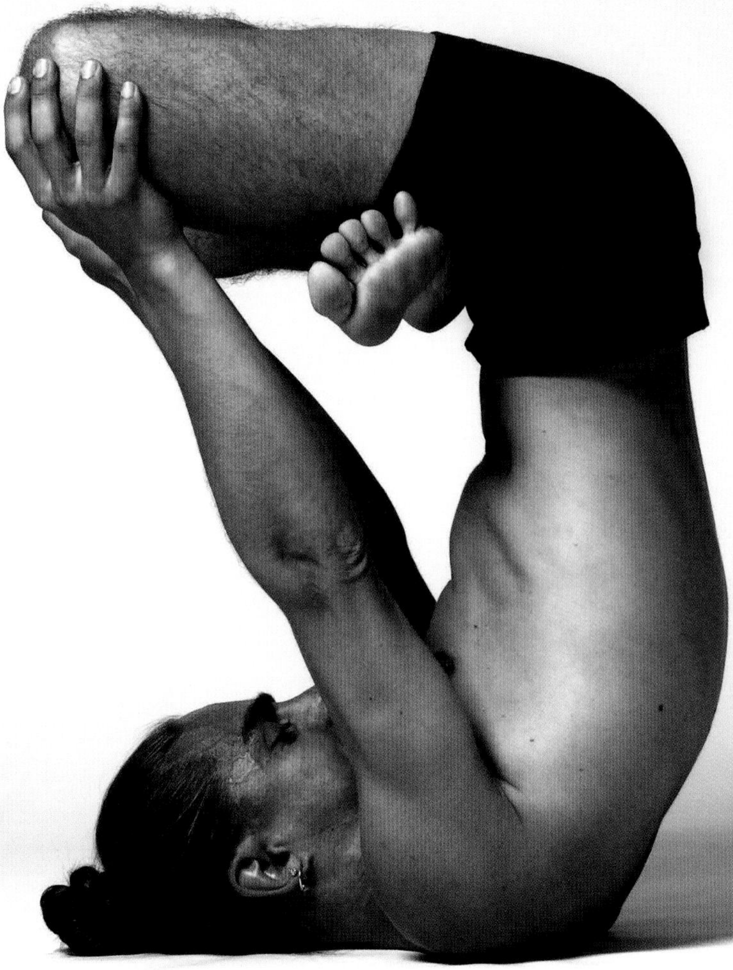

ऊर्ध्वपद्मासन

Ūrdhva-padmāsana

Upward lotus pose | 14 *vinyāsaa*

continuing 8. *vinyāsa* 9. *vinyāsa*

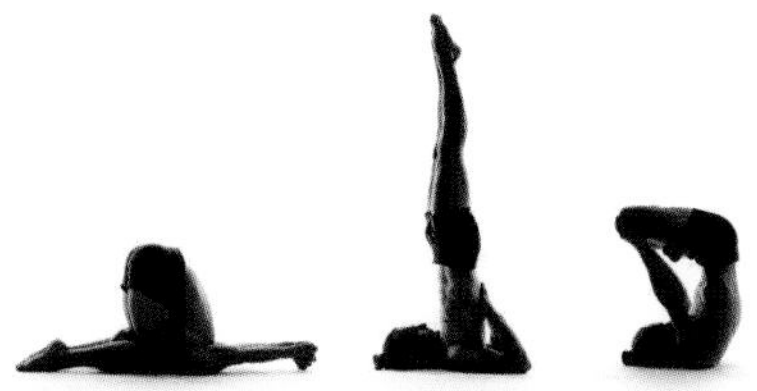

Ūrdhva-padmāsana

Ūrdhva – upward, raising; *padma* – lotus

Ūrdhva-padmāsana follows directly after the 8th *vinyāsa* in *Karṇa-pīḍāsana*.

8 Aṣṭau
Inhale, raise the legs and move the hands back to support the spine, as in *Salamba-sarvāṅgāsana*. Gaze at the tip of the nose.

9 Nava
The state of the pose
Exhale, lower the right foot into the left groin. The heel is pointing towards the left side of the navel. Then draw the left foot in, likewise, to the right groin, with the heel towards the right of the navel. This is an upside-down lotus, *Padmāsana*, position.

Note: Advanced students can work to bring the legs into lotus without using the hands to help. In this case, the hands would stay on the back, and one would move into lotus using the strength of the muscles, the breath, and the rhythm of the movement.
Continue the *āsana* by straightening the spine, opening the chest and engaging the *mūla* and *uddīyana-bandha*. Place the palms to the knees with the fingers on the kneecaps and straighten the arms. This is the state of the *āsana*. Breathe deeply eight to ten times. Gaze at the tip of the nose.

After the last inhalation in the 9th *vinyāsa*, go directly to the 9th *vinyāsa* in *Pindāsana*.

Benefits:
In addition to the list, refer to the benefits of the finishing sequence (p 127)
- purifies the rectum and urinary tract when the lotus position is set correctly and the heels are pressing the stomach
- strengthens the stomach and back.

Vinyāsa	Prāṇa	Āsana	Dṛṣṭi	Bandha
Samasthitih		Stand straight		
Vinyāsas 1–6 according to Sūrya-namaskāra A				
7 Sapta	in & out	Jump to sitting, lie back hold the pose		
8 Aṣṭau	in	Lift legs to shoulderstand		
9 Nava	out	Legs to lotus pose, hands to knees		
This is the state of the āsana, hold for 8–10 deep breaths				
10 Daśa	in & out	Cakrāsana, back-roll, into Catvāri position		
11 Ekādaśa	in	Upward-facing dog		
12 Dvādaśa	out	Downward-facing dog		
13 Trayodaśa	in	Jump forward, head up		
14 Caturdaśa	out	Bend forward		
Samasthitih	in & out	Come up Stand straight		

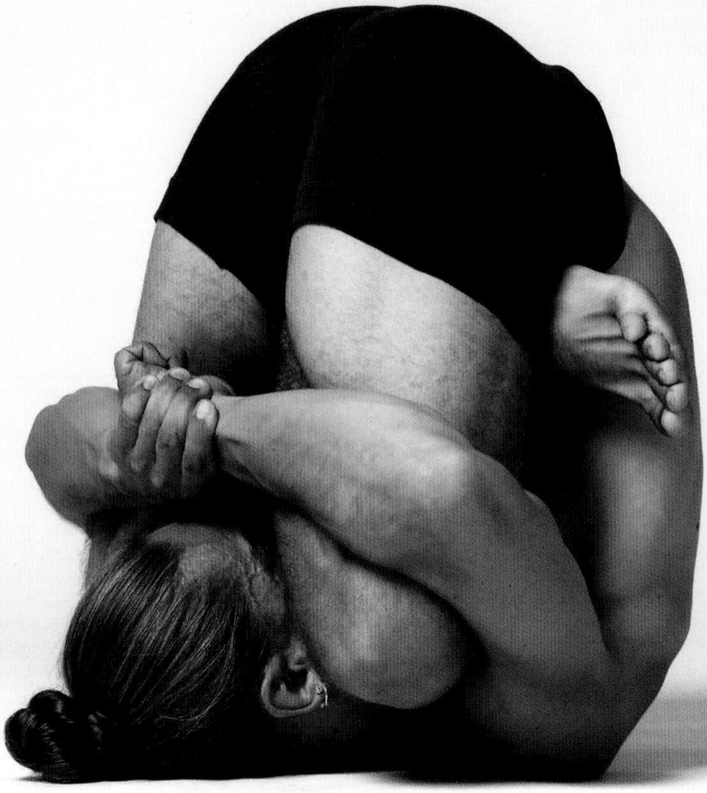

पिण्डासन

Piṇḍāsana

Embryo pose | 14 *vinyāsas*

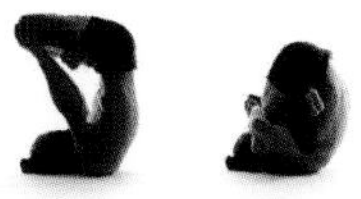

Piṇḍāsana

Piṇḍa – embryo

Pindāsana follows directly after the 9th *vinyāsa* in *Ūrdhva-padmāsana*.

9 Nava

The state of the pose

Exhale and lower the legs (still in lotus) towards the chest, rounding the spine. The shins will come to either side of the face and the knees on either side of the head. Wrap the arms around the outsides of the thighs, bind one wrist and make a soft fist with the free hand. You can also take hold of the fingers instead of the wrist. Draw the lotus into the chest with the arms, but do not force the knees towards the floor. Balance on the shoulders. This is the state of the *āsana*. Breathe deeply eight to ten times and gaze at the tip of the nose.

After the 9th *vinyāsa*, move into the next *āsana*, the 8th *vinyāsa* in *Matsyāsana*.

Benefits:

In addition to the list, refer to the benefits of the finishing sequence (p 127)

- the lotus pose and the fold upper body stimulates purification of the stomach, intestines, liver, spleen and spine.

Vinyāsa	Prāṇa	Āsana	Dṛṣṭi	Bandha
Samasthitih		Stand straight		
Vinyāsas 1–6 according to *Sūrya-namaskāra* A				
7 Sapta	in & out	Jump to sitting, lie back hold the pose		
8 Aṣṭau	in	Lift legs to shoulderstand		
9 Nava	out	Legs to lotus pose, legs into chest, bind hands		
This is the state of the āsana, hold for 8–10 deep breaths				
10 Daśa	in & out	Cakrāsana, back-roll, into Catvāri position		
11 Ekādaśa	in	Upward-facing dog		
12 Dvādaśa	out	Downward-facing dog		
13 Trayodaśa	in	Jump forward, head up		
14 Caturdaśa	out	Bend forward		
Samasthitih	in & out	Come up Stand straight		

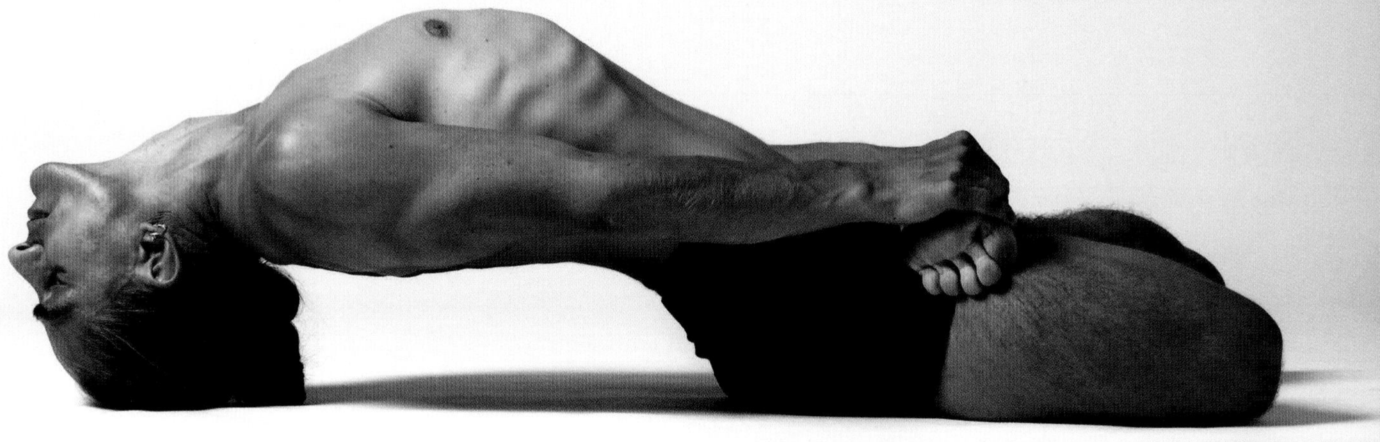

मत्स्यासन

Matsyāsana

Fish pose | 13 *vinyāsas*

continuing 9. *vinyāsa*

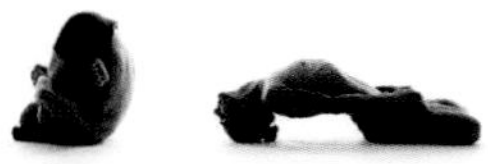

Matsyāsana

Matsya – fish

Matsyāsana follows directly after the 9th *vinyāsa* in *Pindāsana*.

8 Aṣṭau

The state of the pose

Exhale and straighten the arms back onto the mat with the palms down. Round the back, and slowly lower the legs, keeping them in lotus, down to the floor. The back of the head stays on the floor as you roll down. Continue exhaling and lift the upper back off the floor into an arch and place the crown of the head on the floor. Take hold of the middle parts of the feet and pull back, creating an opposing action to the upward arch. Press the knees down into the floor and straighten the arms. This is the state of the *āsana*. Breathe deeply eight to ten times. Gaze at the tip of the nose.

After the last inhalation in the 8th *vinyāsa*, go directly to the 8th *vinyāsa* in *Uttāna-pādāsana*.

Benefits:

This *āsana* works as a counter-pose to the shoulderstand *āsanas*. In addition to the list, refer to the benefits of the finishing sequence (p 127):

- releases tension in the back of the neck
- increases mobility through the neck
- purifies the esophagus and lungs and strengthens the heart
- opens the throat and clarifies the voice
- purifies the anus, rectum, liver and spleen
- strengthens the perineum muscles and *mūla-bandha*
- stimulates the *mūlādhāra cakra*, root cakra.

Vinyāsa	Prāṇa	Āsana	Dṛṣṭi	Bandha
Samasthitih		Stand straight		
Vinyāsas 1–6 according to Sūrya-namaskāra A				
7 Sapta	in	Jump to sitting, lie down		
8 Aṣṭau	out & in	Legs in lotus pose, (come down) chest up, crown of head to floor		
This is the state of the āsana, hold for 8–10 deep breaths				
9 Nava	in & out	Cakrāsana, back-roll, into Catvāri position		
10 Daśa	in	Upward-facing dog		
11 Ekādaśa	out	Downward-facing dog		
12 Dvādaśa	in	Jump forward, head up		
13 Trayodaśa	out	Bend forward		
Samasthitih	in & out	Come up Stand straight		

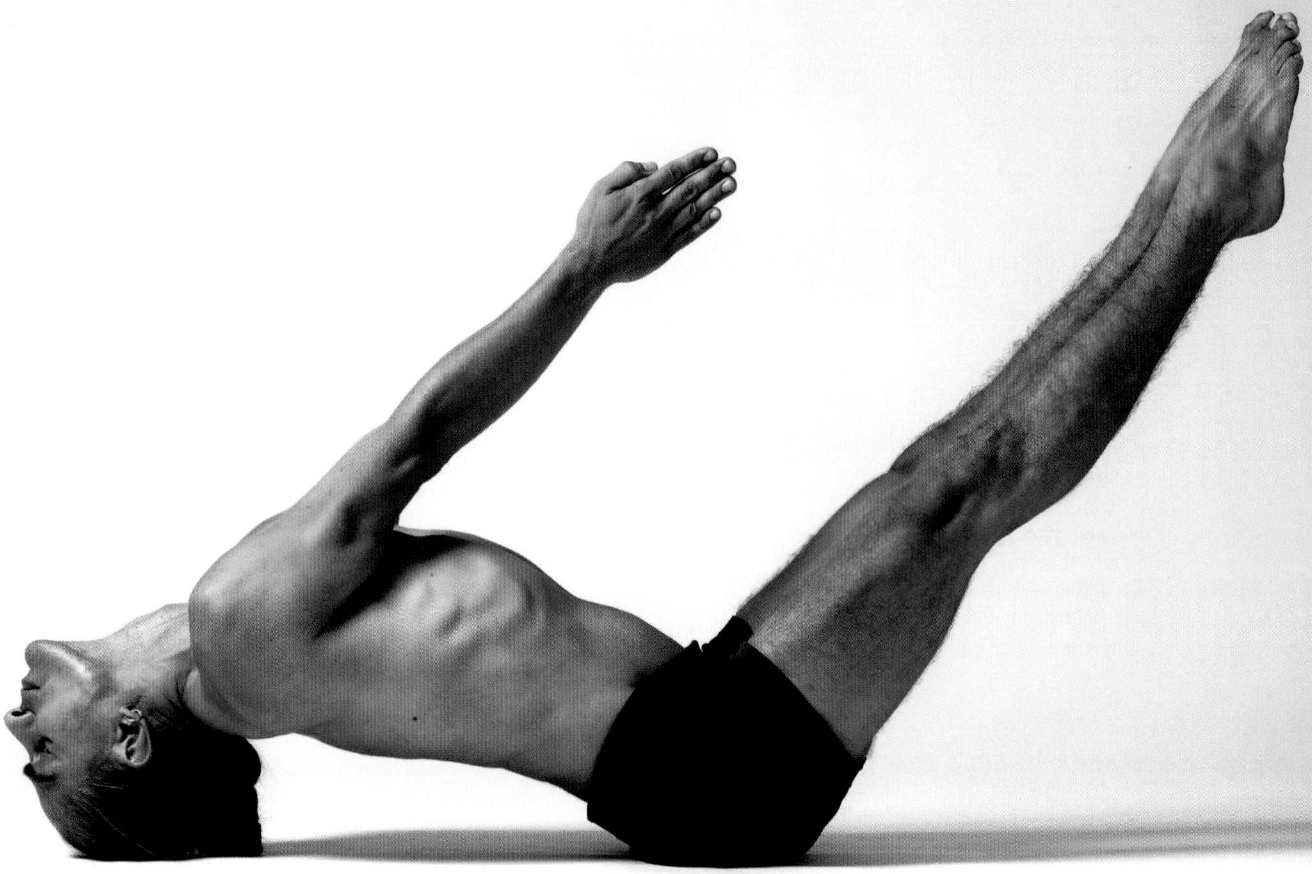

उत्तानपादासन

Uttāna-pādāsana

Extended foot pose | 13 *vinyāsaa*

continuing | 8. *vinyāsa* | 9. in | 9. out | 10. *vinyāsa* | 11. *vinyāsa*

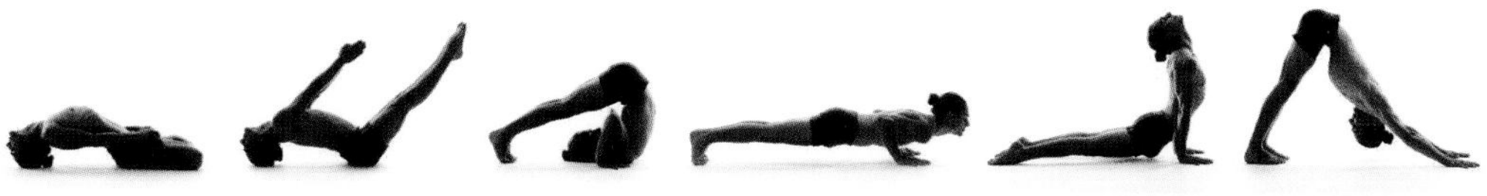

Uttāna-pādāsana

Uttāna – strong, deep stretch; *pāda* – leg

Note: There are two breaths in the 9th *vinyāsa*.

Uttāna-pādāsana follows directly after the 8th *vinyāsa* in *Matsyāsana*.

8 Aṣṭau
The state of the pose

Exhale, leave the chest and head where they are and release the lotus pose by straightening out the legs and lifting them into the same angle as in the boat pose, *Navāsana* (in the primary series). Lift the arms up, align them parallel to the legs and press the palms together. Point the feet and keep an extension in the arms by lengthening through the shoulders. *Mūla-bandha* will support the hips as *uddīyana-bandha* opens and expands the chest and spine. This is the state of the *āsana*. Breathe deeply eight to ten times. Gaze at the tip of the nose.

9 Nava

Inhale, relax the head and back to the floor while the legs stay in the same position. Place the hands on the floor by the ears, fingers towards the shoulders. Engage the bandhas to support the body and raise the hips and back up off the floor. Keep the legs together and lift them straight overhead. Lower them onto the floor behind the head, about a foot apart from each other. Round the spine and the back of the neck and, using the strength of the arms, lift the body off the floor, roll in a straight line over the head, through cakrāsana and into *Catvāri*.

Exhale, straighten the body and land in *Catvāri* position. Gaze at the tip of the nose.

Vinyāsas 10 and 11 are the same as the 5th and 6th *vinyāsas* in *Sūrya-namaskāra* A.

After *vinyāsa* 11, go directly to the next *āsana*, the 7th *vinyāsa* in *Śīrṣāsana*.

Benefits:

This is the counter pose for a long shoulderstand sequence. The benefits of this *āsana* are similar to *Matsyāsana*. In addition to the list, refer to the benefits of the finishing sequence (p 127):

- strengthens the legs, hips, neck and stomach muscles
- releases the tension on the shoulders and hips.

Vinyāsa	Prāṇa	Āsana	Dṛṣṭi	Bandha
Samasthitih		Stand straight		
Vinyāsas 1–6 according to Sūrya-namaskāra A				
7 Sapta	in & out	Jump to sitting, lie back hold the pose		
8 Aṣṭau	in & out	Chest up, crown of head to floor lift arms and legs to angle		
This is the state of the āsana, hold for 8-10 deep breaths				
9 Nava	in & out	Cakrāsana, back-roll, into Catvāri position		
10 Daśa	in	Upward-facing dog		
11 Ekādaśa	out	Downward-facing dog		
12 Dvādaśa	in	Jump forward, head up		
13 Trayodaśa	out	Bend forward		
Samasthitih	in & out	Come up Stand straight		

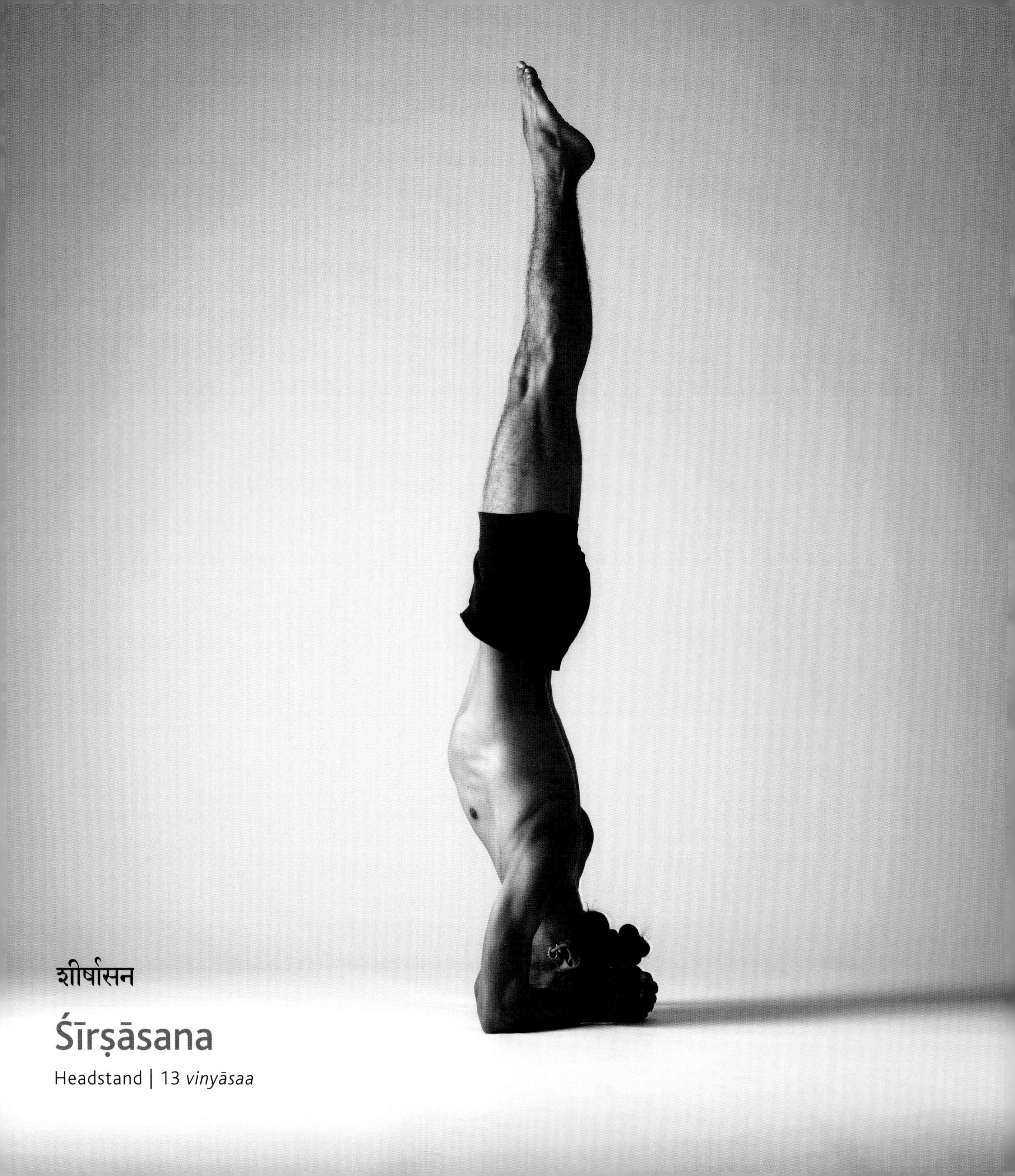

शीर्षासन

Śīrṣāsana

Headstand | 13 *vinyāsaa*

continuing | 8. *vinyāsa* | 8. continuing | 9. *vinyāsa* | 9. continuing | 10. *vinyāsa* | 11. *vinyāsa*

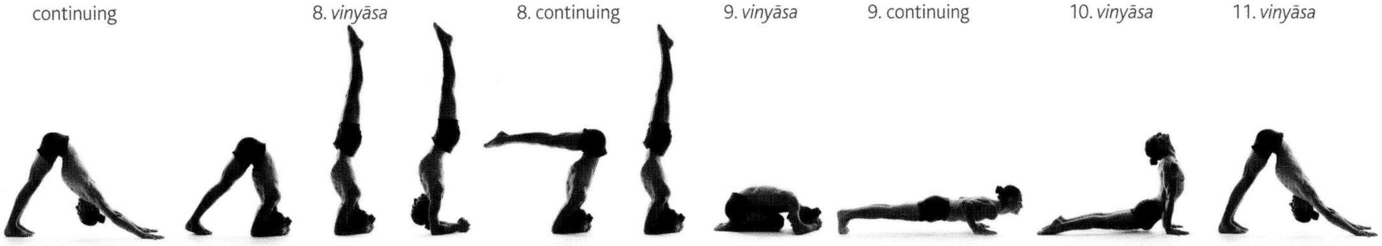

Śīrṣāsana

Śīrṣa – head, spot on the head which is on the floor in headstand

Note 1: There are two breaths in the 7th *vinyāsa* and three breaths in the 9th *vinyāsa*.
Note 2: Lifted up headstand in the 8th *vinyāsa* is an extra pose.
Note 3: Relaxation is part of the 9th *vinyāsa*.
Note 4: *Vinyāsa* 8 includes an extra variation: the 90 - degree bend.
Śīrṣāsana is done after Uttana Padāsanas *vinyāsa* 11.
Śīrṣāsana follows directly after the 11th *vinyāsa* in *Uttāna-pādāsana*

7 Sapta

Inhale, lower the knees to the floor behind the hands and curl the toes under so that the balls of the feet are on the ground. Place the elbows on the floor, in front of the knees, a forearm's length apart. You can measure this distance by placing both hands over the forearms, fingertips touching each elbow. Open the hands out and interlace the fingers. Place the outside edge of the hands into the mat, keeping the palms open, forming a rounded base as a 'cup'. The hands and the elbows should make a triangle, which serves as the foundation for the headstand. Place the front part of your head (the area between the forehead and the crown of the head called *Brahma-randhra* or *śīrṣa*) on the floor. Press the crown of the head onto the 'cup' you have made with your interlaced fingers and palms.

Exhale, straighten the legs, and walk the feet in until the spine is straight and approximately in line with the shoulders. The hips should point up towards the ceiling. Keeping the toes on the floor with the heels up and legs together, press the forearms and outer edges of the hands into the floor. Try to distribute the weight of the body more on the hands than on the head.

8 Aṣṭau

The state of the pose

Inhale, straighten the legs and lift them up with control, keeping the legs together and the feet pointed. This is the state of the *āsana*. Take 10–50 deep breaths here. Gaze at the tip of the nose.

The head can be slightly lifted up off the floor, or at least not bearing too much weight and is supported by the forearms and shoulders. This relaxed position of the head is beneficial for blood circulation and for the necks health. It enables the release of energy from the more delicate *sira-nāḍīs*, the nervous system in the crown of the head.

Note: *Yoga Mala* states that one can practice *Śīrṣāsana* for a minimum of five minutes up to a maximum of three hours, and anywhere in between, in order to receive the full benefits of this *āsana*.

Raised headstand:

Stretch through the shoulders and strengthen the arms by pressing the forearms even more into the floor. Lift the head up in between the shoulders and draw the chin in towards the chest. Point the feet and gaze up at the toes. Balance and breathe deeply. This is an additional position for the strength.

90-degree angle:

After holding *Śīrṣāsana* for minimum 10 breaths, exhale and lower the legs to a 90-degree angle, keeping the legs straight and the feet pointed. Gaze at the tip of the nose and stay here for ten deep breaths.

On an inhalation, lift the legs back up once more to *Śīrṣāsana*.

Note: As soon as you can remain steady in *Śīrṣāsana* for an extended amount of time, you can begin to practice this variation as well. Since it is part of the 8th *vinyāsa* (or additional pose), it does not have its own *vinyāsa* number.

9 Nava

Exhale and slowly lower straight legs down, gently touching the toes first, to the mat. Without lifting the head, bend the knees and place the shins on the floor. Sit back on your heels and place your forehead on the floor in *Balāsana* (child's pose). The hands and arms are in front of you and remain in the same position as they were in headstand, but the elbows are released out to the sides. Breathe deeply here for a minute or two, balancing out the blood pressure and circulation. Gaze at the tip of the nose.

Note: After a longer headstand (more than five minutes), it is essential to rest in child's pose for a sufficient amount of time. Take rest for at least two minutes.

Continue by inhaling and lifting the head up. Place the hands on the floor, next to the shoulders and curl the toes under so that the balls of the feet are on the ground. Jump back on the exhalation, straightening the legs as you go, and land in *Catvāri* (this is still part of the 9th *vinyāsa*). Gaze at the tip of the nose.

Vinyāsas 10 and 11 are the same as the 5th and 6th *vinyāsas* in *Sūrya-namaskāra* A.

After *vinyāsa* 11, move into the next *āsana*, the 7th *vinyāsa* in *Baddha-padmāsana*.

Benefits:

Headstand belongs to the group of inverted finishing poses (*viparīta-karaṇī*) and many of its benefits are listed on p 127. Because of its many benefits, it is considered to be the "king of the *yoga āsanas*" and is said to:

- improve balance and increase confidence
- engage the muscles needed for balance, and familiarize one with being upside-down
- rejuvenate the *nāḍīs* and carries blood to the head
- improve and increase sensitivity in the senses of sight, smell and hearing
- improve memory and clear and brighten the eyes
- release tension in the muscles and nerves throughout the whole body
- encourage feelings of lightness, relaxation and peace of mind
- purify the *sahasrāra-cakra*, the crown *cakra*, and help gather and contain *amṛita-bindu* within the head.

Vinyāsa	Prāṇa	Āsana	Dṛṣṭi	Bandha
Samasthitih		Stand straight		
Vinyāsas 1–6 according to Sūrya-namaskāra A				
7 Sapta	in & out	Hands and head to floor, straighten the legs		
8 Aṣṭau	in	Lift the legs to headstand		
This is the state of the āsana, hold for 10–50 deep breaths Exhale legs down to 90 degrees, inhale back up				
9 Nava	out in & out	Legs down, rest for 1-2 mins, hands on the floor jump to Catvāri position		
10 Daśa	in	Upward-facing dog		
11 Ekādaśa	out	Downward-facing dog		
12 Dvādaśa	in	Jump forward, head up		
13 Trayodaśa	out	Bend forward		
Samasthitih	in & out	Come up Stand straight		

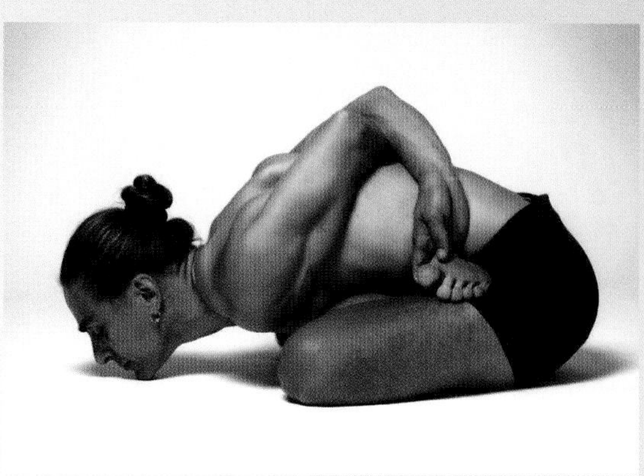

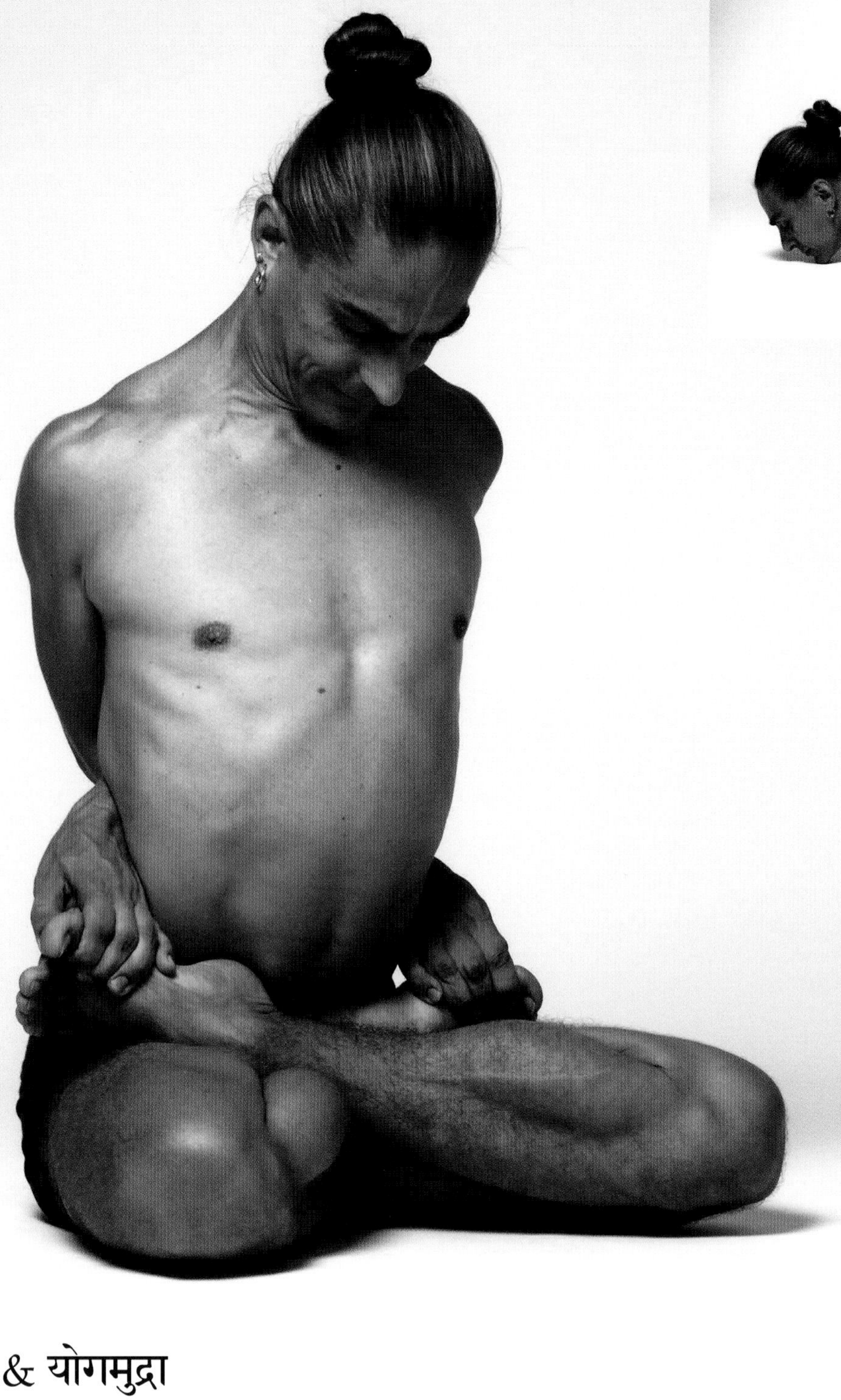

बद्धपद्मासन & योगमुद्रा

Baddha-padmāsana & Yoga-mudrā

Bound lotus & sealed pose | 16 *vinyāsas*

continuing 7. *vinyāsa* 8. *vinyāsa* 9. *vinyāsa* 10. *vinyāsa*

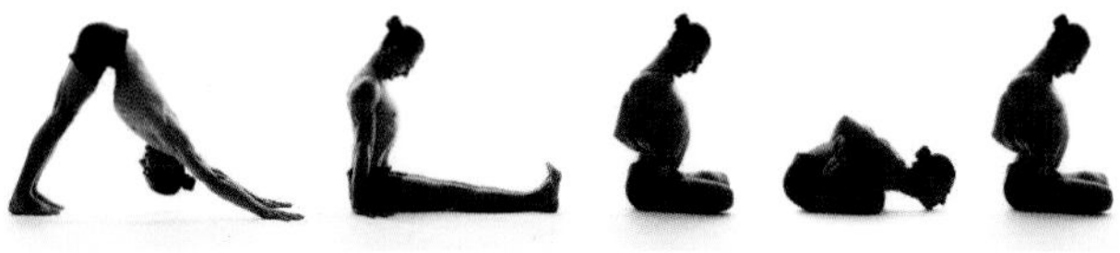

Baddha-padmāsana & Yoga-mudrā

Baddha – bound; *padma* – lotus; *yoga* – path to *samādhi*, liberation; *mudra* – close, set a seal on

Note 1: In the 9th *vinyāsa* (*Yoga-mudrā*), you can also keep the gaze at the tip of the nose.
Note 2: There are two breaths in the 8th and 10th *vinyāsas*.

Baddha-padmāsana follows directly after the 11th *vinyāsa* in *Śīrṣāsana*.

7 Sapta

Inhale, jump through to sitting. Gaze at the tip of the nose.

8 Aṣṭau

Exhale, bring the right foot up into the left groin. Turn the foot so the sole of the foot faces up; the back of the foot presses into the crease of the inner left thigh and groin, and the heel points towards the left side of the navel. Relax in the right hip joint to lower the right knee towards the floor, at a 45-degree angle away. Lift the left foot over the right calf, and place it likewise into the right groin. This is lotus pose, *Padmāsana*.

Note 1: Advanced students can try to bring the legs into lotus without the help of the hands, using the bandhas, breath and momentum. Leave the palms on the floor by the hips as you fold the legs into lotus.

Note 2: There is another common way to enter to *Padmāsana* position. It is 7 Sapta, jump through while inhaling and exhale hold the pose. Then 8 Aṣṭau, inhale and lift the legs to Lotus pose. In my last interview with Guruji in February 2007, he told me to do all the Padm*āsanas* in any sequences with an exhalation (not only the inverted positions, but also the seated poses). So I've been following his advice and all the Padm*āsanas* here are done with an exhalation.

Continuing with the exhalation, extend the left shoulder and wrap the left arm around the back to bind the left big toe with the first two fingers and thumb. The palm is turned down. Do the same with the right hand, binding the right big toe. Pull lightly on the toes, press the knees down towards the floor and flex the feet so the heels press in to the sides of the navel. Bow the head and lower the chin down. This is *Baddha-padmāsana*. Take a slow inhalation here, open the chest and lengthen the upper body. Gaze at the tip of the nose.

9 Nava

Exhale, straighten the head and keep the chest open while bending the body forward and down onto the heels and shins, reaching the chin out towards the floor. Grip the big toes firmly while still pressing the heels into the navel area, massaging the intestines and stimulating the inner organs and energy channels. Draw in *uddīyana-bandha* to lengthen the body out and to create space for the heels and calves. *Mūla-bandha* presses the hips down, counter-balancing the forward bending. This is the state of *Yoga-mudrā*. Take ten deep breaths here. Gaze in between the eyebrows.

10 Daśa

Inhale, keep hold of the big toes and come back up to *Baddha-padmāsana* with a strong back and bandhas. Gaze at the tip of the nose.

After *vinyāsa* 10, move into the next *āsana*, the 7th *vinyāsa* in *Padmāsana*.

Benefits:

In addition to the list below, refer to the benefits of the finishing sequence (p 127):

- simultaneously strengthen and increase flexibility in the ankles, knees, hips and lower back
- open the chest, shoulders and upper back
- *Yoga-mudrā* purifies the intestines, liver, lower back, spleen, when the heels are pressing the abdomen
- purify the anus and rectum
- remove excess fat from the waist and hips.

Vinyāsa	Prāṇa	Āsana	Dṛṣṭi	Bandha
Samasthitih		Stand straight		
Vinyāsas 1–6 according to Sūrya-namaskāra A				
7 Sapta	in	Jump to sitting		
8 Aṣṭau	out & in	Legs in lotus pose, bind toes open chest		
This is the state of Baddha-padmāsana, hold for 1 deep inhalation				
9 Nava	out	Bend forward, chin to floor		
This is Yogā-mudrā, hold for 10 deep breaths				
10 Daśa	in & out	Back to Baddha padmāsana hold the pose		
11 Ekādaśa	in	Hands on the floor, lift up		
12 Dvādaśa	out	Catvāri position		
13 Trayodaśa	in	Upward-facing dog		
14 Caturdaśa	out	Downward-facing dog		
15 Pañcadaśa	in	Jump forward, head up		
16 Sodasa	out	Bend forward		
Samasthitih	in & out	Come up Stand straight		

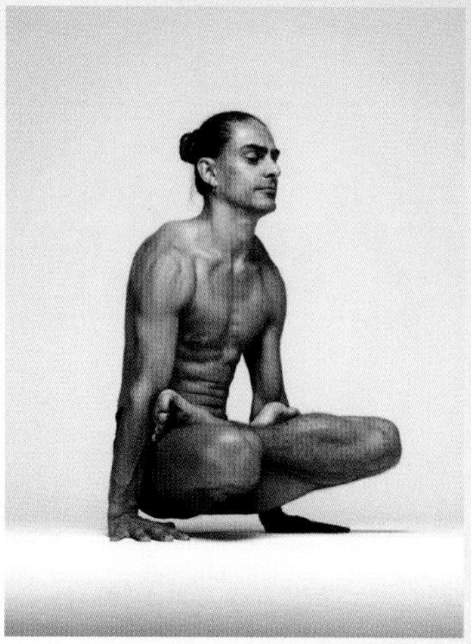

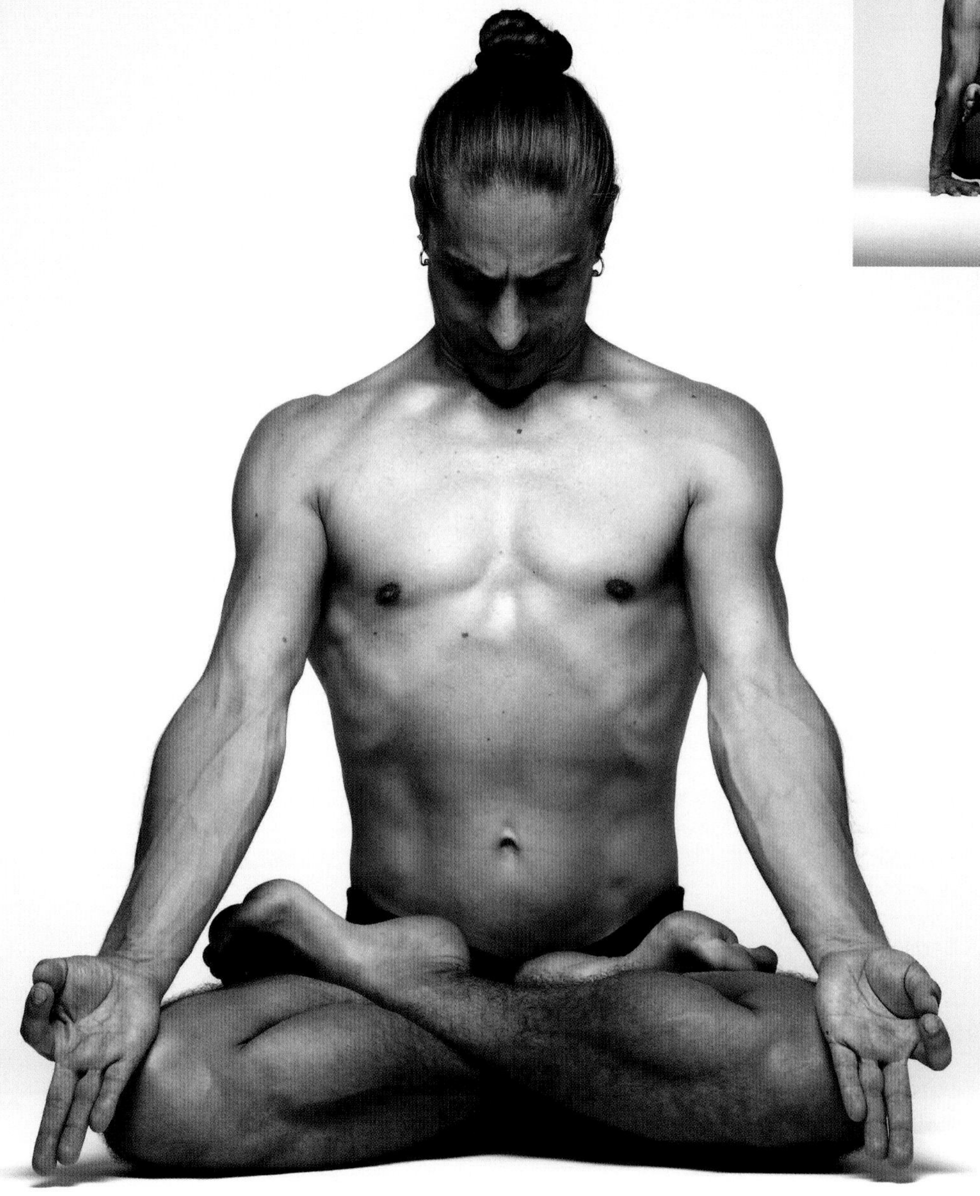

पद्मासन & उत्प्लुति

Padmāsana & Utplutiḥ

Lotus pose & strong lift | 14 *vinyāsas*

continuing 8. *vinyāsa* 9. *vinyāsa* 10. *vinyāsa* 10. continuing 11. *vinyāsa* 12. *vinyāsa* 13. *vinyāsa* 14. *vinyāsa* *Samasthitih*

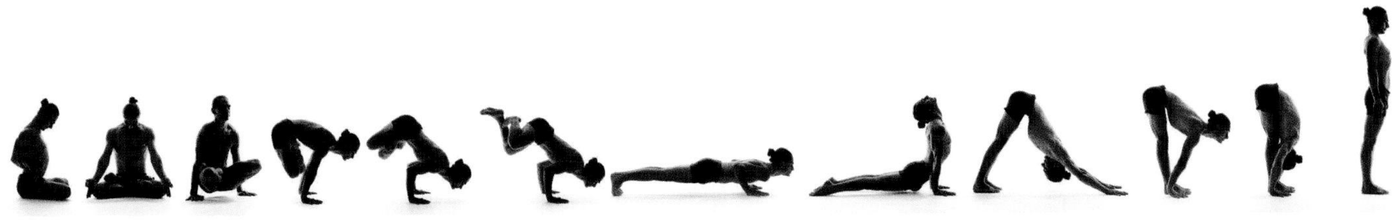

Padmāsana & Utplutiḥ

Padma – lotus, lotus blossom; *ut* – deep, strong; *pluti* – lift, take off, rise

Note 1: The breath is even longer and deeper now than in the earlier finishing poses.
Note 2: After *Padmāsana*, take the *vinyāsa* up to *Samasthitiḥ* to chant the closing invocation (p 26).
Note 3: From the 10th *vinyāsa*, try to jump back without touching the floor.

Padmāsana follows directly after the 10th *vinyāsa* in *Baddha-padmāsana*.

8 Aṣṭau
Exhale, straighten the arms and place the hands (palms up) on the tops of the knees. Touch the tips of the index finger and thumb and straighten the middle, ring and little fingers together. Keep them together and pointed towards the floor. This position of the hands is *jñāna-mudrā*. Lift *mūla-bandha* to ground the body; engage *uddīyana-bandha* to elongate the spine, and to expand and broaden the chest. Widen the shoulders and draw the chin down towards the collarbones. Lower the knees to the floor and flex the feet. Push the lower abdomen slightly forward, so that the heels press in on either side of the navel. Separate the knees wider than in other lotus-based positions to open the hips, support the energy flow into the *nāḍīs* and to increase the lengthening of the spine. This is the state of the *āsana*. Hold for 10–25 deep breaths. Gaze at the tip of the nose.

Note: According to *Yoga Mala*, advanced students can sit in this *āsana* and meditate for over three hours. This opens the *āsana* up on a profound level; the mind can reach new states of clarity while the body becomes light and free.

9 Nava
Inhale, press the palms into the floor by the hips. Stretch through the shoulders, engage the arms and lift the body up off the floor, still keeping the legs in lotus. The upper body and legs should create, more or less, a 90-degree angle at the hip crease. Using *mūla* and *uddīyana-bandha* will increase the sense of lightness in this *āsana*, while building strength in both bandhas. Straighten the spine, keep the head up and open the chest. This is the state of *Utplutiḥ*. Hold for 10–25 deep breaths. Gaze at the tip of the nose.

With the last inhalation, lift the hips up higher and move the legs through the arms without touching the feet to the floor.

10 Daśa
Exhale, release the lotus pose and straighten the legs (in the air). When the feet touch the ground, bend the elbows and land in *Catvāri* position. If the legs do not stay in the air during the entire jump-back, keep them lifted as long as you can. Then release the lotus, touch the feet to the floor, and jump back into *Catvāri* position. Gaze at the tip of the nose.

Vinyāsas 11–14 are the same as the 5–8 *vinyāsas* in *Sūrya-namaskāra A*.

Samasthitih
Inhale, come up to standing with a straight body, arms to the sides, and gaze at the tip of the nose. Traditionally, one chants the closing invocation (p. 26) here, with the head bowed and hands together in front of the heart (*kara-mudrā* or *añjali-mudrā*).

Benefits:
It is an ideal position for meditation, *prāṇāyāma* and other spiritual practices. In addition to the list below, refer to the benefits of the finishing sequence (p 127):

- bring flexibility to the ankles, knees, hip joints and lower back
- facilitate the flow of energy through the *nāḍīs*
- calm the mind and focus the concentration
- unlock the three energy knots, *granthi-traya*, allowing pranic energy to flow to the *suṣhumnā-nāḍī*
- burn off old *karma* and heal all ailments (according to ancient texts)
- *Utplutiḥ* develop the strength and awareness of the *mūla* and *uddīyana-bandha*.

Vinyāsa	Prāṇa	Āsana	Dṛṣṭi	Bandha
Samasthitih		Stand straight		
Vinyāsas 1–6 according to Sūrya-namaskāra A				
7 Sapta	in	Jump to sitting		
8 Aṣṭau	out	Legs in lotus pose, hands in jñāna-mudrā		
This is Padmāsana, hold for 10–25 deep breaths				
9 Nava	in	Lift up		
This is Utplutiḥ, hold for 10–25 deep breaths				
10 Daśa	out	Jump-back to Catvāri position		
11 Ekādaśa	in	Upward-facing dog		
12 Dvādaśa	out	Downward-facing dog		
13 Trayodaśa	in	Jump forward, head up		
14 Caturdaśa	out	Bend forward		
Samasthitih	in & out	Come up Stand straight		

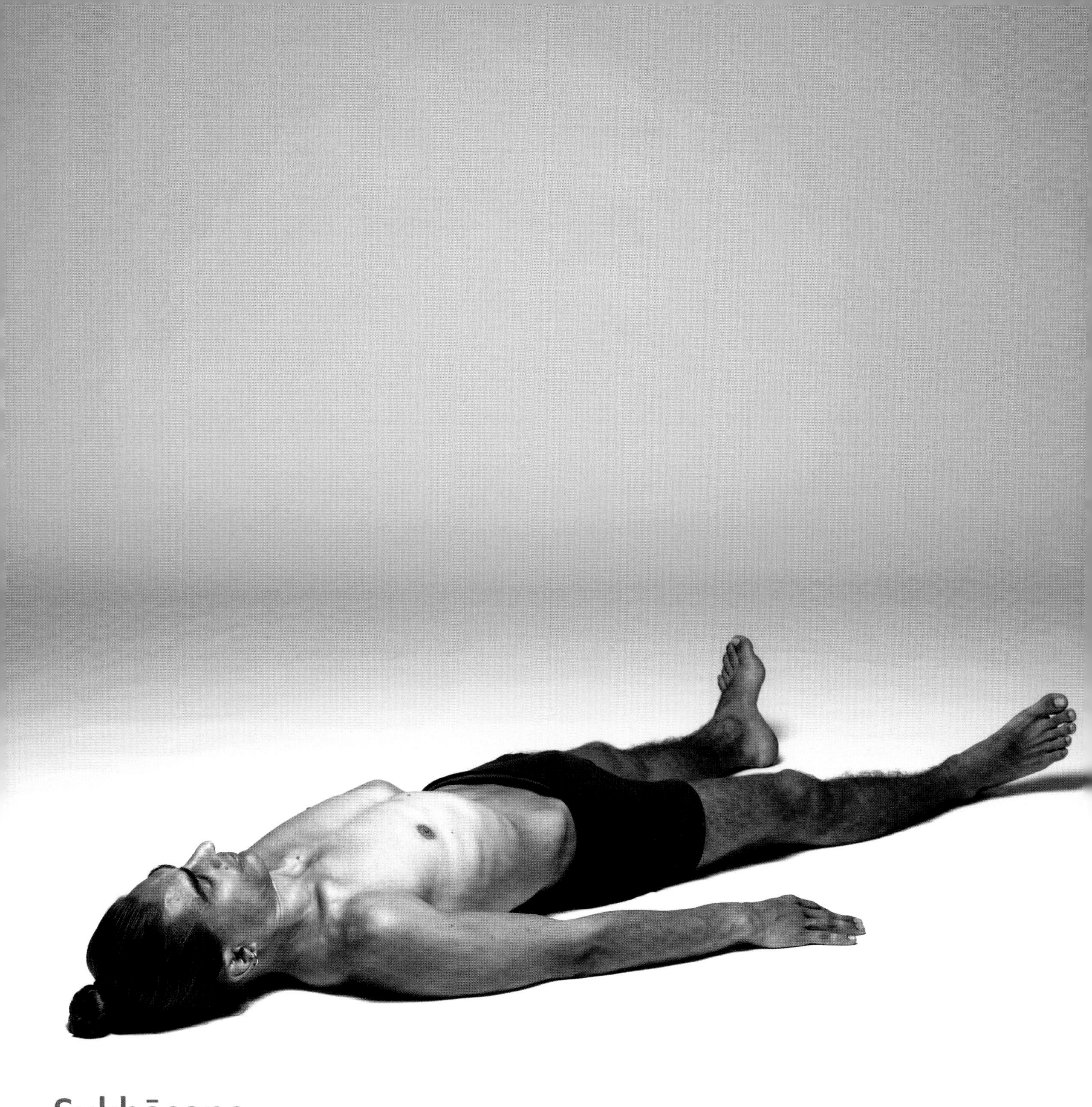

Sukhāsana

Relaxation pose

Samasthitih 1. *vinyāsa* 2. *vinyāsa* 3. *vinyāsa* 4 *vinyāsa* 5. *vinyāsa* 6. *vinyāsa* 7. *vinyāsa*

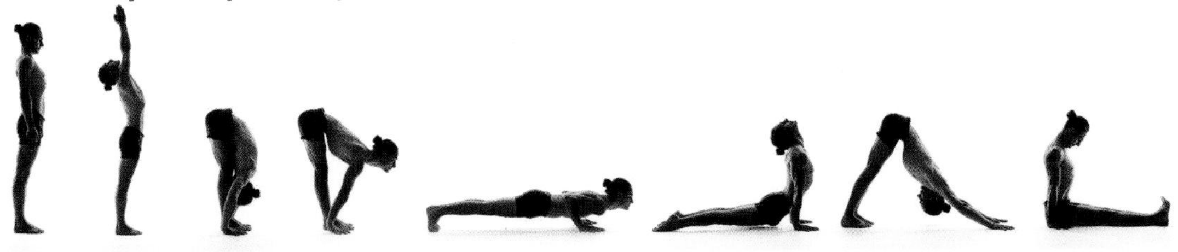

Sukhāsana/Sāvāsana

Note: Śrī Pattabhi Jois called this pose resting pose; Sharath Jois calls it *Sukhāsana*, easy pose. It is also commonly known as *Sāvāsana*, corpse pose or relaxation pose.

Sukhāsana, relaxation pose, is done after *āsana* and *prāṇāyama* practice. Prepare yourself for comfortable relaxation by keeping the body warm and making sure you will not be disturbed. Put on warm, dry clothes or use a blanket that will protect you from any draft or chill. The final resting pose is of utmost importance as the body and mind need some time to recover after the practice. Muscles receive the chance to soften and the nervous system can settle down, bringing a peaceful state to your mind and deserved release for your body.

Do *vinyāsas* 1–6 of *Sūrya-namaskāra* A after chanting the closing invocation.

7 Sapta

Inhale, jump through to sitting and come to lie down. Open the legs and arms so that the feet are about mat-width apart, with the hands by the sides. The palms can either face up towards the ceiling or face down and touch the floor. Lengthen the back of the neck by drawing the chin down slightly. Close the eyes and relax the eyelids. Lengthen the hips by stretching the legs out. Relax and widen the shoulders and let the spine settle comfortably along the floor. Slow the breathing down even more, releasing all tension from the body and mind. Open the mouth slightly and release the body further, including more subtle areas, such as your facial muscles, scalp, tongue, corners of the mouth, fingers and toes. Relax the body effortlessly and breathe calmly. If other thoughts arise, simply return the focus peacefully to your breathing. Allow the feelings of light, freedom and happiness to be fully absorbed within. If you continue to feel tension arising in a specific area of the body, direct the breath to that place, release the tension using your breath and return to relaxing the entire body.

Stay here for 5 to 15 minutes.

In this resting pose, the mind can become conscious of the different phases and levels of relaxation. Avoid drifting off into sleep, as that will lessen the body's ability to create restorative energy, increasing the level of tamo-guṇa (tamas = ignorance, darkness) instead.

When you have finished resting, take a deep, energizing inhalation and exhalation. Wake the body up again with small movements and stretches (e.g. move the fingers and toes, circle the ankles and wrists, stretch the arms over the head, bring the knees into the chest, and roll slowly onto the back). Open your eyes and slowly come up to sitting. You should feel peaceful, clear-minded, renewed and fully energized.

We should never forget
to carry the torch of divine light
of yogic knowledge,
which has been passed down to us
with our Vedic culture,
and to keep its flame alight for all eternity.

– Yoga Mala

Saraswathi Jois interview

I was born on the 11th of September 1941 in Mysore (mother "Ammaji" Savitri and father Śrī Pattabhi Jois; more about them in my first book's chapter on Śrī Pattabhi Jois's history) and started practicing *Aṣṭāṅga yoga* in 1947 with my father, Guruji. The first four years we were playing with the postures. My grandmother (from my mother's side) was very scared of our playing and was scolded Guruji. We did a few warm up positions and then quickly went into deep backbends. For us it was fun, but it had to look dangerous for my grandmother. From the age of 10 to 22, I regularly and systematically practiced the *Aṣṭāṅga yoga* method and I also started to take my first steps in teaching *Aṣṭāṅga* in public.

I got married in 1967 in Mysore and we moved to Chamchatpur, a small village near Calcutta. My husband worked in a Tata Company and I was teaching *Aṣṭāṅga yoga* to young boys. My husband was not interested in *yoga* but I never left my *yoga* practice, even if I wasn't practicing all the time with Guruji.

Education and teaching experience

When I first got pregnant in 1969 I came back to Mysore to my parent's house and stayed there for 1 1/2 years. Then I went back to my husband in Calcutta. I got pregnant again and my parents asked me to move back home, as my husband was moving around with his work and we couldn't follow him with the children. Sharath was born on the 29th of September 1971 in Mysore. It was better for the children and the family to have a stable life in Mysore. We stayed there for 14 years and I continued to practice and assist in the shala.

In 1974 I got an opportunity to teach classes of my own. I taught *Aṣṭāṅga* at the beautiful Venkateshwamy palace temple for 11 years. My classes became very successful and some people didn't like it, they were envious of me. My mother didn't like me to teach there anymore either, and so when we moved to my recently built house in Gokulam, I started to teach in Gokulam.

My mother died in December 1997. Four months later Guruji also moved to Gokulam, opposite of where the new *yoga* shala is now located.

I never practiced at the shala. I always went to the Sanskrit College with my brother Manju, where Guruji was teaching *Aṣṭāṅga*. For 13 years I practiced there in the afternoon at 4.30. Before Guruji retired (in 1973), I only practiced there.

For 3 years I went to the Sanskrit College in the morning at 7.30 to study Sanskrit. At 10.30am, I started regular school where I studied up to the 11th standard. My mind was so interested in *yoga* that I wanted to stop school and study only *yoga* with Guruji.

Childhood memories

There are some fun memories from my childhood and about the *yoga āsanas* with Guruji, but mainly it wasn't funny at all. The teaching method was hard at that time, Guruji used a stick and beating us up every time we did something wrong. It was painful, serious study.

One time Manju wanted to take a tabla lesson at the same time as there was a *yoga* class, at 4.30pm. Guruji didn't like it and made holes in the tablas.

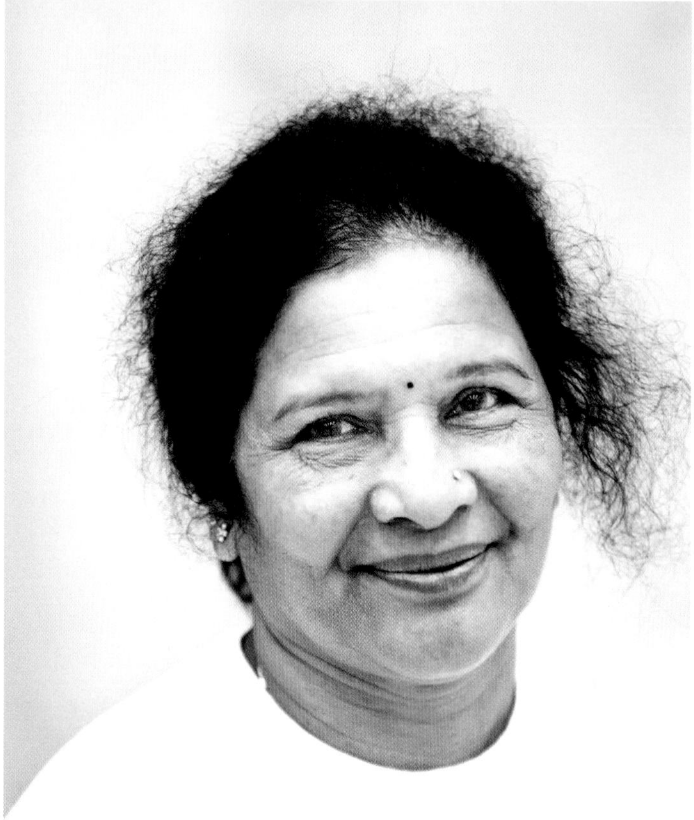

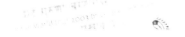

When the tabla teacher came and they started to play there was no sound on the tablas. They inspected the tablas and found the holes. Manju said, "One day, he's beating and the other day, there are no tablas." The teacher became very angry with Guruji, took hold of Manju, threw him into Guruji's lap, left and never came back. But Guruji was happy to get his son back to the *yoga* shala.

I saw the first Westerners at the Lakshmipuram *yoga* shala in the mid 60s. Belgian yogi Andre van Lysbeth (considered as the first western *Aṣṭāṅga* practitioner) wrote a book *Prāṇāyāma*, in French and was written mainly from his experience in 1964 in Mysore shala with Guruji. That brought many French-speaking people to Mysore. They stayed upstairs at the house and we used to cook for them with my mom. After that, I started to see more and more Westerners coming to practice with Guruji. Now I've gotten used to them, even though they have such a different culture. They practice very honestly every morning around the same time and are disciplined. Many Indians were also like that before, but lately, they became lazy and don't want to practice regularly. Like many of the Western students, they also follow after too many teachers, which only makes their minds confused. It is important to practice every day at the same time and with one teacher only.

Students should have the patience to practice for years before they start to teach. Some students want to teach after only two months of practicing, which is impossible. If you don't know anything about *yoga*, how can you teach it to the people?

I saw Krishnamacharya many times. I actually did my Intermediate series exam with him. I still have a certification from that. It was in the late 50s. The last time I saw him was in 1984–85, when we went to visit him in Chennai. I couldn't get the visa with my two children to see my husband in Saudi-Arabia, so I travelled instead to Chennai to see Krishnamacharya.

Advice for yoga practitioners

I used to cook for my family for many years, but for the last three years now, I have been busy with teaching and haven't been able to cook that regularly. A sattvic vegetarian diet is important for Aṣṭāṅgis. We can't use too oily, heavy or spicy food. Once a week we can eat more spices but not too often. We also use lots of fresh cow milk which we boil, filter and then drink. Boiling is important for getting rid of unnecessary bacteria. We can also add some figs or butter to the boiling milk to make it tasty. Buttermilk, curd (yoghurt) with rice, cow ghee (purified butter), dahl (lentils) and fruits are all good ingredients. As a Brahmin (in the old caste system, Brahmin is the highest caste) family, we never eat garlic and onion. Garlic is good only for the moms with newborn babies as it helps with milk production and keeps the body strong. Anyhow, I never ate garlic and I'm still very strong (laughing).

For body purification, besides the practice, a castor oil bath is the most beneficial once or twice in a week. Traditionally, married women take a bath on Tuesday and Friday mornings. A warm body (heated from a hot bath) can hold oil for a longer time, but the cold body can hold it only for half an hour. After a bath, take a hot shower and wash the oil off with soap. For men, the best days for an oil bath are Monday and Saturday, but for married women, the days are more important. Tuesday and Friday are special pūjā days and castor oil day for married woman. For the unmarried or widow woman (like me), the days are not that important. Tuesday's pūjā is traditionally made for Gaṇeśa and Friday's for Lakṣmī.

I also used to do pūjās but now Lakshmish, does all the pūjās in the house. I take my bath in the morning and make namaskāras (salutations) to Gaṇeśa. Now the God is inside (not soap outside... laughing). Lakshmish blesses the rice every day in the pūjā and afterwards, people can eat it.

Before, when we used to have brick ovens with an open fire, the woman used to do more pūjās in the kitchen, they put down cow dung – the powder and polished the kitchen. Afterwards, they made rangoli designs (drawings) around the oven and then started to cook. Now, with a gas oven and modern time things has changed a lot, not many people do the old rituals.

I love Gaṇeśa. Every morning after waking up and before seeing anybody else, I make prayers to Gaṇeśa. Then I go to work. He's the first who I see in the morning and the last at night.

For *āyurvedic* treatments, castor oil is best. Āyurvedic treatments are good. There are no side effects, but it is slow, not like allopathic medicine. There are also some good pain oils and treatments, but massage is not good for Aṣṭāṅgis. Practice is the best body and mind therapy.

Aṣṭāṅga yoga is good for everybody, for healthy and sick people... in any case, it's important to take the practice slow, there's no reason to try to do all the *āsanas* in the same day. In India, married women need only do Primary series. They work so much at home, therefore the primary series is enough. In any case go slow and you will be happy!

Saraswathi Jois (Saraswathi Rangaswamy)
Mysore, India, February 2007

Sharath Jois interview

I was born in Mysore on 29th of September 1971. In 1977 I started to do some Primary series *āsanas* with my grandfather, Śrī K. Pattabhi Jois, at the Lakshmipuram *yoga* shala. At that time, it was not a systematic practice, more like children's *yoga*, just for fun. In 1985 my family moved from Lakshmipuram to Gokulam and I stopped going to Guruji. Then, in 1990, I started to practice again, now more seriously. Gradually Guruji also started to show me how to give adjustments (hands on) in the *yoga āsanas* and how to teach *Aṣṭāṅga yoga*. So I became his assistant in the shala.

Many local people from our neighborhood used to come to practice with Guruji, businessmen and workers. First there were lots of Indian people and only few foreigners, but then in the 90s, it turned the other way around.

Since I was born in a yogic family, I understood the *yoga* tradition and why all the Westerners came to practice with my grandfather. Anyhow, it was only when I started to practice seriously, I realized the real value of my grandfather and *Aṣṭāṅga yoga* method.

When I started practicing in 1990, I already knew the Primary and part of the Intermediate series from my childhood. For the first six or seven months, I practiced in the afternoon, at around 4pm, but after Guruji came back from his teaching tour in France in 1991, I switched to the morning, starting between 4.30-5.00am. At that time we had only five or six foreign students at the shala and we used to adjust them in almost every posture. Most of them were beginners, so we had to show them all the *āsana* techniques. Now most students know the positions before they come here. They've been studying with other teachers at home or they've been coming here for many years and they doesn't need so much help anymore. There are more dedicated students nowadays, even though there is still lots of ignorance. And there are also more advanced students who need only one or two adjustments per practice; any more adjustments would just make harm for their bodies and also minds. We are able to watch their practice and help only when they have difficulties in certain postures. The teaching has matured... it's been developing since 1990.

A good Aṣṭāṅga yoga teacher

Teachers have to understand Guruji's traditional *Aṣṭāṅga yoga* method. This is possible only with long experience of the practice and by being together with their Guru, who comes from the *yoga* master's lineage – the paraṃparā. In paraṃparā, the knowledge has been passed straight from the Guru to the students.

If somebody teaches and develops his or her own method, this person will be alone and the source of the knowledge will be cut off. After three or four years of practicing, they cannot have enough understanding about the *Aṣṭāṅga yoga* system. Marketing *yoga* with nice, fancy postures doesn't mean anything. The real teacher should have a deep knowledge and understanding; only then they are ready to teach to others.

The real essence of the *yoga* practice is tapas – involve yourself totally to the practice, dedicate yourself to the Guru. After two or three years of constant studies we are ready to think about the philosophy and read texts like *Bhagavad-gīta, Yoga-sūtras, Haṭha-yoga-pradīpikā*, the *Upaniṣads*... the list is never ending. There is always more to learn.

A good yoga student

Good *yoga* students listen to the teacher, who wants to keep the yogic lineage alive. They respect their teacher by always mentioning their teacher's name. I'm (Sharath), the student of Śrī Pattabhi Jois and a grandson, but first I am the student. The fact that he's my teacher is more important than the fact that he's my grandfather. People recognize the student from his or her Guru and there is a deep respect for Guru. Śrī Pattabhi Jois always talked about Krishnamacharya, his Guru, also in the West on his tours. He brought up Krishnamacharya's name and respected him as his teacher, a big yogi and philosopher.

Daily rhythm

I get up at 1.30am, shower, clean myself and drink half a glass of water. Then I go to practice the *āsanas* from 2 to 4 am. At 4 am I make coffee for the family and then we go downstairs to teach at the big shala at around 4.30am. At 8am I switch shalas, just a couple of blocks away, and teach my students at my house until 12.30 pm (this was in 2007). After that, I come home to eat and take a long nap between 1–3pm. Then I get up, clean myself again, take a cup of cafe and go downstairs to teach the afternoon classes for Indians and work in the office with Guruji. After 7pm we all have dinner: chapati, dosa, sambar. Then I have a little time for rest with my family and then go to bed at 8.30pm.

Other yogic studies

I do prāṇāyāma early in morning when I have time for it, usually a few times in a week, and I read *yoga* philosophy and perform *pūja* (Hindu ritual). I used to study Sanskrit when I was younger, but now I've been too busy for it.

On religion

We are Hindu Brahmins. Our family has one Guru: Ādi Śaṅkarācarya (lived around 700 AD) and we follow his Advaita Vedānta philosophy. I do the *pūjā* at our house for Gaṇeśa on Saturdays when it's my day off from the practice and there is good time for that. Otherwise Lakshmish, the Sanskrit and chanting teacher at the shala, does it every day.

How important are the *āsanas* and is it necessary to do the most advanced postures?

When you develop in your *āsana* practice, you also develop in your spiritual process. You become more concentrated, strong minded, tolerant, clear. The *āsanas* deepen the whole yogic practice, *Aṣṭāṅga yoga*. For the *āsana* practice, the *vinyāsa* system – breathing, gazing and bandhas are very important. What Guruji teaches has been the same for a long time, but people want to change the system. They misunderstand the method and don't have enough determination to keep it pure.

What is the main difference between *yoga* in India and in the West?

Not all *yoga* practitioners are yogis in India. That's a misconception that Westerners have. Just because somebody is Indian doesn't meant that they are big yogis, or that they know anything about *yoga*. Yoga is a universal practice, as Guruji mentioned many times.

Is it possible for the westerners to reach the goal of *yoga*?

Challenging question. Yoga means liberation or in another perspective the union between the soul and the divine. Yoga is not only the *āsana* practice; *āsana* is only one part of it. For many people, *yoga* is physical exercise. They don't feel the spirit, they just do the *āsanas* and whatever they want after the practice. They continue with their life as if nothing happened in their practice.

In my opinion, that is not real *yoga*.

After Krishnamacharya and Guruji, there haven't been many students who have been practicing like them, waking up at 1.30am, practicing, teaching, studying, living a fully yogic life. Some Westerners are very good students, but there is still a long way to go.

Can Westerners attain the Brahma-vidyā? (Some people think that only Indian Brahmins can attain the highest truth)

Anybody, not only Indian Brahmins, can attain the yogic knowledge, the union. Yogis need to be strict, disciplined and have a strong will for the spiritual *yoga* - *Yoga-sādhana*. To live a yogic life is not easy, especially if you are not ready to change your attitude, habits and behaviors. To born in a Brahmin family doesn't mean that the person has yogic knowledge as a gift. They can have also many other duties in their life. Even in my family not everybody is dedicated for *yoga* even though it would be easy for them. The understanding has to come from you, it depends on how much you have interest for *yoga*.

What types of food do you eat?

Rice, *sambar* (clear spicy sauce with vegetables), *chapati* (thin wheat bread) and *dahl* (lentils), only twice a day, lunch and dinner. Besides that I have one big glass of boiled warm milk at lunch time and two to three cups of coffee.

What's your opinion on Ayurvedic treatments?

Every Saturday I take a purifying and refreshing castor oil bath. We don't need other kinds of treatments (like *āyurvedic* massage), only if we feel sick, but we shouldn't take them all the time. If we are healthy, practice is our therapy, it is enough. I have never taken any kind of massage in my life without a real need for it.

What's the key for a good *yoga* practice?

Dedication and discipline towards the practice. Your mind should always think about your *yoga* practice.

How does the inner process of God realization come about?

Realization of God rises slowly from inside of us. God is the supreme power, Param Brahma; it doesn't have any form. The sculptures, pictures and statues of deities are all man made, they represent God, the creator, but are not the same God. Gradually we will notice that everything is actually God.

To feel God we have to think about God, to live the way that the realization is possible. The practice, breathing, *dṛṣṭis* and *bandhas* will be a big help in that progress.

How is the photography is connected to yoga?

We should appreciate nature, it is part of mankind. To keep focus on the animals, recognize and take pictures of them is very exciting. Some of those species may not even exist in 50–60 years' time. I started photography three years ago and I'm totally into it.

There are also many *yoga āsanas* which the animals perform. I shot a picture of the bird which did *Kāraṇḍavāsana* and another did *Mayūrāsana*. It is a full meditation to follow one bird for a long time, observing their movements and behavior with your mind focused only on that.

It is also balancing for my very hectic life of teaching and adjusting hundreds of people at the shala every day. Sometimes I just have to take off, go to nature and recharge myself; breathe the clean air and just be.

What do you think about the future of *Aṣṭāṅga yoga*?

It is very scary... (joking)

It depends on Guruji's students who teach and practice *Aṣṭāṅga*. If they respect the tradition and keep it pure, *Aṣṭāṅga* will have a very good future. The students have to practice with patience and get the real experience of *yoga*.

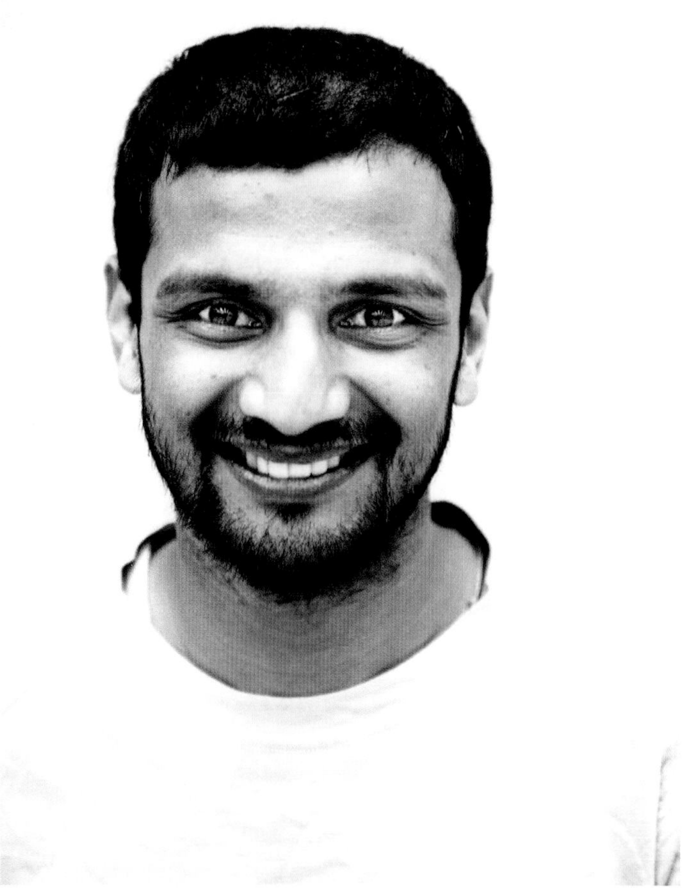

Guruji founded the *Aṣṭāṅga* Yoga Nilayam in 1948 and started to call the method *Aṣṭāṅga yoga*, as it is in Patanjali's *Yoga-sūtras*. His Guru, T. Krishnamacharya, didn't call it *Aṣṭāṅga yoga*. Then 50 or 60 years later, many other *yoga* lineages started to call their methods *Aṣṭāṅga yoga* as well, which created some confusion for the people. We've been thinking to add Śrī K. Pattabhi Jois's name there (Śrī K. Pattabhi Jois's *Aṣṭāṅga yoga*) to make clear that this is the method taught by Śrī K. Pattabhi Jois and his Guru, T. Krishnamacharya.

When *Aṣṭāṅga yoga* became popular everywhere, many people started to use Śrī Pattabhi Jois's name, even if they teach something else. Then their students will get the wrong information and misunderstand the *Aṣṭāṅga* method. This authentic *vinyāsa-krama* comes from Śrī Pattabhi Jois. Even though some other people were practicing in Mysore with Krishnamacharya (between 1932-1953), none of them have been teaching the *vinyāsa* in the same way as Krishnamacharya taught it in Mysore. *Vinyāsa-krama* is important. It is our responsibility to keep it pure and living.

Sharath Jois (Sharath Rangaswamy)

Mysore, India, February 2007

An interview from 2013

How has the 2013 American and European tour been so far?

Everything has been working out very well. There are a lot of enthusiastic *yoga* practitioners coming up now in the *yoga* world. I'm happy to see that more and more people are practicing *Aṣṭāṅga yoga* in the proper way. Many students will come to know and experience the real *Aṣṭāṅga yoga*. This has been my mission: to educate my students and give them the experience and knowledge that I got from Śrī Pattabhi Jois and through my own 23 years of practice.

Reflecting back on the recent history of *Aṣṭāṅga yoga*, there seems to be quite a noticeable difference between how Guruji and you taught in the 70s, 80s and 90s, compared with today. How has the teaching attitude and method changed over the years?

Yes, there are many reasons for this change. It is true that the general attitude was tougher before and that we gave students plenty of strong adjustments. The problem with this approach is that students might get too dependent on teachers so that it becomes very important to receive lots of adjustments in every class. Students could then potentially put less effort in learning *yoga* by themselves and therefore make less progress in their own self-practice. Teachers can teach the techniques for the students, but the students themselves have to then make their own research and get the experience of what the teacher has been teaching. They have to go deep into the practice and understand the meaning of *yoga*, and investigate what is behind the teachings and why something has been taught specifically to them. In this way, we can begin to understand *yoga* as a spiritual practice.

You have been running the main shala in Mysore now since Guruji's passing in 2009. How has this been for your teaching and personal life?

When Guruji was still alive, we had many ideas on how to improve the teaching and how to help people understand this practice. Guruji's English was limited, but his yogic knowledge was impressively vast. Some students might not understand how much he had to share. He couldn't express himself in English the way he could in Kannada (the language in Karnataka state). The physical practice doesn't need much language, so many people thought that this was what Guruji was mainly teaching. I'm now trying to correct this misunderstanding and to share his yogic knowledge. This is only thing on my mind, how to make the students understand more about *yoga* and not just the physical side of the practice. *Āsana* is not everything, even though it provides important benefits for the body and mind. Through the eight limbs of *yoga*, we are able to experience spiritual transformation.

Do you feel Guruji's presence in the shala and while you are teaching?

Definitely I feel his presence. I spent so much time with him and practiced in his presence daily for 18 years. He is always with me in my teaching. I don't want to imitate him, but many of the things he said are fresh in my mind. He put the *yoga* philosophy into the practice. He really knew how this *yoga* should been practiced.

How is it to run the main shala in Mysore?

Someone has to lead the institute and I'm doing my best to make it happen successfully. Nothing should disturb one's personal *sādhanā*. I don't want any big position in life. It is not an easy task. I don't think about these things too much. It all happened very naturally and I will teach *Aṣṭāṅga yoga* while I still have strength in my limbs. This is my *karma*, to teach *yoga*, and I love doing it.

Your primary series book was released earlier this year (March 2013). At the end of the book, you show some therapeutic *āsanas* and a light *prāṇāyāma* sequence. Are these something new to the *Aṣṭāṅga* tradition?

Nothing is new in *yoga*. It has been around for several thousands of years. The primary series is *Yoga-cikitsā* and shows a way to cure various diseases and ailments. I've been teaching these breathing techniques to many ill people and the results have been encouraging. Some light *prāṇāyāma* is useful if you have certain respiratory issues like allergies or asthma. People breathe in polluted air in big cities and this causes a lot of stress. I thought that this *prāṇāyāma* technique would be helpful to share with everyone. This is not *Kumbhaka-prāṇāyāma*, just simple breathing. For *Kumbhaka-prāṇāyāma*, the student must reach a certain level of proficiency, and the teacher who has proper knowledge of *yoga* can determine who is ready to start it. This is how it has been over the ages. Nowadays many teachers show all kinds of *prāṇāyāma* sequences to anyone who is interested. They sympathize with the students, but perhaps aren't aware of the potential danger in teaching these sequences. Since *prāṇāyāma* purifies the more subtle energy and mental kośas, more so than *āsana* even, the fourth limb requires a gradual and safe progression, using the right method.

Many people suffer from back pain and that is why I added a few therapeutic *āsanas* at the end of the book. These can be done as extra poses at the end of the *āsana* practice.

Aṣṭāṅga yoga has received the reputation of being a physical or acrobatic, 'jumping' form of *yoga*. What do you think about this?

This is how it has been projected in the Western world. People bend their bodies and jump around without knowing why they are doing so. Only through grounded *yoga sādhanā* (spiritual path or practice) can we reach higher stages of *yoga*. It's pretty simple, really. There is no trick to it.

You started doing *yoga āsanas* when you were very young. At what age do you think children are ready to start practicing this systematic approach to *yoga*?

They are developmentally ready at around ten or twelve. If they wish to imitate their parents and play with the *āsanas* earlier, that is no problem. Anything goes. This is how I also started and *āsana* was fun and interesting.

However, the *vinyāsa krama* is not easy to understand for a children who are too young. The child has to have a certain level of maturity before he or she can understand how the system works.

The word *vinyāsa* has a very wide definition and is used in many different contexts. How would you describe it?

Vinyāsa cannot be considered as one *āsana*. The main *āsana* has to be supported by the surrounding *āsanas*, as well as the breathing technique. This is *vinyāsa*. *Aṣṭāṅga yoga* is not circus. Correct use of the *vinyāsa* method helps the blood circulate throughout the body, nourishing each and every organ and providing benefit for the nervous system. We must approach *vinyāsa* in a systematic and scientific way, by being precise with how we link the breath with the movement.

What do you think about the idea that many Western yogis have lost the original meaning of *yoga*?

The understanding of *yoga* is limited in the West and also in India. For a proper *yoga* practice we need a healthy foundation. We need stability in our minds. Without stability, we create a lot of frustration, which will then come out through our speech and actions. People blame and criticize each other, and create fights and instability in the community. The change has to start from within. Through the continual practice of *yoga* with an experienced teacher, we can purify our bodies and minds.

Many people direct their attention, and get stuck on, external values such as money, fame, a fit body, you name it. How to attract many people to have a successful *yoga* business? They produce books, DVDs and CDs, but most of these are just nonsense, part of the *yoga* industry. The internal experience is left aside. We don't talk so much about the spirit in *yoga* philosophy. Everyone experiences the life force within him or herself, which is God. We should try to think how to make progress in the practice, how to look within, how to purify our ego and work through our unique and individual accumulation of karma. That is real stability. It is humble and simple process.

Patanjali's *Yoga-sutras* dedicates the third chapter to describing siddhis, the yogic powers that come as a result of continuous and uninterrupted *yoga sādhanā*. These siddhis, however, are not usually discussed in the *yoga* field. What is your experience with them?

How can one talk about *siddhis*? They are always experienced, not expressed. When you have a strong foundation from practicing the first four limbs (aṅgas) of *Aṣṭāṅga yoga*, the last four will automatically happen. If you want to plant a rose, how will you start? We cannot pull the plant out to try and make it grow faster. First, we need to nourish the roots of the plant, which is the base for growth. It needs soil, the earth, a foundation. Then, the nutrients provided with fertilizer, water, sunlight and air can be seen as the *yama, niyama*, *āsana* and *prāṇāyāma*. After these have been supplied to the plant, then the rose will naturally, spontaneously blossom within you.

You talked about *Brahmacharya* in the conference and mentioned that it means celibacy. I imagine celibacy has a wider definition in India than how we understand it in the West?

When you have a strong focus in your *yoga* practice, things of a sexual nature don't disturb your mind. There is no distraction. Celibacy for married couples means honesty and remaining faithful. When you are honest with your partner, you are also honest with yourself. In this case, a sexual life is not prohibited. The *gṛhasta* stage (*gṛha*=household, house, home) means that there is a bond between yourself and your partner. If you follow this, you are practicing *Brahmacharya*. Changing partners consistently and habitually is a false attraction. Love is for life. In Indian mythology, *Śiva* and *Pārvatī* represent that lifelong bond, connection. *Īśvara* (*Śiva*) is the lengthened breath of the universe and *Pārvatī* is the energy. When the breath joins with the energy, they become one living, breathing entity and the universe comes into existence.

You said that it is important to find your *Iṣṭa-devatā*, personal god. Is it not enough to feel directly connected with *Brahman*, the ultimate soul?

Iṣṭa-devatā (cherished divinity) represents different forms of God: *Śiva, Kṛṣṇa*, Allah, Jesus, among many others. The ultimate soul is always *Brahman*. It doesn't have any form. When you pray to your personal God, it always goes to *Brahman*. It is one and the same. The ultimate God is one, whereas the *Iṣṭa-devatā* reflects the preferences in people's hearts. If you have a connection with Jesus, then you pray to Jesus, if you have connection with *Kṛṣṇa*, then you pray to *Kṛṣṇa*. Through your personal God, you will get closer to Brahman. This is not religion. This is reflection. My personal God is *Kṛṣṇa*. I get connected through *Kṛṣṇa*.

In the Hindu tradition, every family has their own *Iṣṭa-devatā*, family God. Together, the family makes offerings at least once a year to their *Iṣṭa-devatā*. They pray for good fortune, that every member be protected, and ask for blessings for the family.

Iṣṭa-devatā is whichever form of God you like, but everything is run by the ultimate soul, *Para-Brahmaṇ* (*para*=beyond).

Sharath Jois
Helsinki, Finland, August 2013

Bibliography

Websites

www.kpjayi.org
www.saraswathiashtanga.com
www.petriraisanen.com
www.petriandwambui.com
www.astanga.fi
www.alexberg.com
www.namarupa.org
www.ayny.org
www.ashtangawambui.com
www.pinterandmartin.com
www.otava.fi

References and literature

Jois, Śrī K. Pattabhi. *Yoga Mala*. Translated into English by Eddie Stern. New York: North Point Press, 1999. Print.

Miele, Lino. *Astanga Yoga: Śrī K. Pattabhi Jois*. Rome: Self-Published by Lino Miele, 1994. Print

Shankaracharya, Adi. *Yoga Taravali* (800th century). Trans and Commentary. T.K.V & Kaustab Desikachar. Chennai: Krishnamacharya Yoga Mandiram, 2003. Print.

Swatmarama, Yogi. *Haṭha-yoga-pradīpikā*. Trans. Swami Vishnu-Devananda. Karnataka: Motilal Banarsidass Publishers & Om Lotus Publications, 1987. Print.

Prasad, Ramananda. *The Bhagavad Gita*. 2nd. ed. Delhi: Motilal Banarsidass Publishers, 1996. Print.

Siva Samhita. 1914 ed. Trans. Rai Bahadur Śrīsa Chandra Vasu. Delhi: Munshiram Manoharlal Publishers, 1999. Print.

Gheranda Samhita. 1914 ed. Trans. Rai Bahadur Śrīsa Chandra Vasu. Delhi: Munshiram Manoharlal Publishers, 2001. Print.

Viveka Cudamani of Śrī Sankaracharya. Trans. Svami Turiyananda. Chennai: Śrī Ramakrishna Math, 2003. Print.

Svetasvatara Upanisad. Trans. Swami Lokeswarananda from the Adi Shankaracharya's notes. Calcutta: The Ramakrishna Mission Institute of Culture,1994. Print.

Iyengar, B.K.S. *Light on the Yoga Sutras of Patanjali*. New Delhi: Harper Collins, 1993. Print.

Yogacarya T. Krishnamacharya. *Yoga Makaranda: The Nectar of Yoga*. Media Garuda, 2011. Print.

A.G. Mohan and Dr. Ganesh Mohan. *Haṭha-Yoga-Pradīpikā*. Svastha Yoga, 2017. Print.

T.K. Sribhashyam. *Emergence of Yoga*. Les Editions Yogakshemam, 2014. Print.

Several editions of *Namarupa* and *Ananda* magazines.

Acknowledgements

Thank you to my students, as well as anyone who reads this book and contributes to its dissemination.

To the following people: I am grateful to all of you from the depths of my heart.

My Guru:

Sri K. Pattabhi Jois

My teachers within the *Aṣṭāṅga* lineage:

Sharath Jois, Saraswathi Jois,
Derek Ireland, Radha Warell, Tove Palmgren, Lino Miele and Eddie Stern

My teachers, dear friends and supporters:

Manju Jois, Savitri "Ammaji" Jois, Ior Bock, Raimo Holtti, Måns Broo, Juha Javanainen, Vijaya Kumar Manja, Dr. M.A.Jayashree, M.A.Narasimhan, A.G.Mohan, Shankaranarayana Jois, Jocelyne Stern, Noah Williams, Guy Donahaye, Rolf and Marci Naujokat, Alexander Takis, Vyaas Houston, Alexander Berg, Erica Fae, Alexander Medin, Richard Freeman, Tina Pizzimenti, A.S. Hari, Hamish Hendry, Anna Wise, Chuck Miller, Betty Lai, Ulrica and Fredrik Salevik, Fredrik Gabrielsson, Timo Kiiskinen, Ilona Silenti, Njuguna "Guka" Mwangi, Celia "Cucu" Nyamweru, Wanjiru Njuguna, Roger Washbourn, Kati Rosendahl, Heikki Rosendahl, Kaija Rosendahl, Alexander, Sveta & Varya Smirkin, Leonid Lanin, Dimitry Barnishnikov, Tom Rosenthal, Nina Grubin, Jeff Lewis, Everett Berger, Raquelle and Rochelle (from Circus Yoga Brooklyn NY), Bess Hochstein, Jarmo Mösö, Niko Tanska, Eija Tervonen, Heidi Parviainen, Tero Valtonen, Hanna Kjellberg, Otava Publishers' Noora Sällström and Emma Alftan, YogaWords and Pinter & Martin Publishers' Paul Walker, Martin Wagner, Zoë Blanc and Zoë Hutton.

My loving parents, sister and her husband:

Matti and Ritva Räisänen, Karola Räisänen, Ilkka Salomaa

My lovely wife and our family:

Wambui Njuguna-Räisänen, Julian, Sesam and Sumu Räisänen

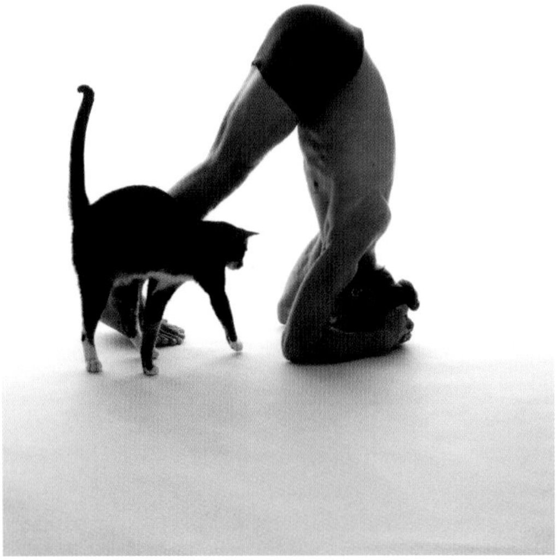